ALCOHOL
AND THE LIVER

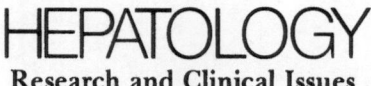

HEPATOLOGY
Research and Clinical Issues

Volume 1 ● Viral Hepatitis

Edited by M. M. Fisher and J. W. Steiner
Canadian Medical Association Journal
(Vol. 106, Special Issue, pp. 417–528, 1972)

Volume 2 ● Jaundice

Edited by C. A. Goresky and M. M. Fisher

Volume 3 ● Alcohol and the Liver

Edited by M. M. Fisher and J. G. Rankin

ALCOHOL AND THE LIVER

Edited by

M. M. Fisher
University of Toronto
Toronto, Ontario, Canada

and

J. G. Rankin
Addiction Research Foundation
Toronto, Ontario, Canada

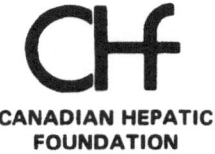

CANADIAN HEPATIC
FOUNDATION

PLENUM PRESS · NEW YORK AND LONDON

Library of Congress Cataloging in Publication Data

Main entry under title:

Alcohol and the liver.

(Hepatology—research and clinical issues; v. 3)
Includes index.
1. Liver—Diseases—Congresses. 2. Alcohol—Physiological effect—Congresses. I.
Fisher, Murray M., 1934-   II. Rankin, James G. III. Canadian Hepatic Founda-
tion. [DNLM: 1. Alcohol, Ethyl—Metabolism—Congresses. 2. Alcoholism—Complica-
tions—Congresses. 3. Liver—Metabolism—Congresses. 4. Liver diseases—Etiology—
Congresses. 5. Metabolism—Drug effects—Congresses. W1 HE913 v. 3/WI700 A352
1976]
RC846.A4   616.3'62   77-8648
ISBN-13:978-1-4613-4186-4   e-ISBN-13:978-1-4613-4184-0
DOI: 10.1007/978-1-4613-4184-0

Proceedings of the Third International Symposium
of the Canadian Hepatic Foundation, held in Toronto,
Ontario, Canada, May 14—15, 1976

© 1977 Plenum Press, New York
Softcover reprint of the hardcover 1st edition 1977

A Division of Plenum Publishing Corporation
227 West 17th Street, New York, N.Y. 10011

PREFACE

Alcohol abuse is this culture's most important drug problem. Statistics indicate that it is exacting a great and relentlessly increasing toll of human suffering. It is clear that the problem is not being dealt with in any effective manner.

At the invitation of the Canadian Hepatic Foundation, many of the world's experts gathered in Toronto, May 14-15 1976, to focus attention on one of the most important aspects of the alcohol problem - alcohol induced liver damage.

The epidemiology of alcohol induced liver disease was discussed and current views on the pathogenesis of the problem were reviewed. New insight into the pathological alterations of the liver was presented and some of our current therapeutic capabilities were discussed. Dr. Hans Popper summarized the Symposium and presented some of his views on those aspects of the problem which will require early attention by the research community.

The Symposium achieved its immediate objective - that of bringing together the committed experts of various disciplines for an updating of our understanding of alcohol and the liver and for a discussion of new approaches to the problem. As a backdrop to the Symposium, however, was large writing on the wall to the effect that we are expending our research talents and efforts on a totally unnecessary problem. Right now we probably know enough and have sufficient resources at our disposal to solve the problem. The less immediate, but more important, objective of the Symposium was to raise the general level of awareness that the time is long overdue for our culture to adopt a much more aggressive and organized approach to the prevention of alcohol induced liver disease.

The Canadian Hepatic Foundation believes that this was an important and successful Symposium and it is particularly grateful to the members of the Faculty who insured that success.

NOTE FROM THE EDITORS

Editing is a challenging way of life! Many helped reduce the particular challenge presented by "Alcohol and the Liver".

We appreciate the authors who submitted high quality manuscripts within the time requested.

We appreciate Louise Amantea who typed the manuscripts in an expert manner.

We appreciate Valerie Price who more or less did all the work.

Murray M. Fisher

James G. Rankin

CONTENTS

THE EPIDEMIOLOGY OF CIRRHOSIS OF THE LIVER: A STATISTICAL ANALYSIS OF MORTALITY DATA WITH SPECIAL REFERENCE TO CANADA

W. Schmidt

Addiction Research Foundation

Toronto, Ontario

This presentation will describe trends and regional variation in cirrhosis mortality, examine the relationship between these temporal and spatial variations and the general level of alcohol use, and provide estimates of the contribution of alcohol-related cirrhosis to total cirrhosis mortality. The statistics employed all refer to death from this cause, which is the most accessible and reliable measure of the impact of cirrhosis. Estimating the incidence or prevalence of cirrhosis in general populations is not easy and, to the best of my knowledge, has never been attempted.

Mortality rates from cirrhosis vary greatly from country to country. As can be seen in Table 1, in a recent year the rates of death from this disease in Western countries have ranged from 5.7 to 57.2 per 100,000 of the adult population - a tenfold difference. The Canadian rate lies in the middle of this range - it is about one-third of the French rate, which is the highest among Western countries, and roughly three times that in low ranking countries such as the United Kingdom, the Netherlands, Finland or Norway.

Regional variations in cirrhosis mortality within a country are usually less marked. The rates for the 10 Canadian provinces illustrate this point. The highest rates are in the three most populous provinces, Ontario, Quebec and British Columbia. The remaining provinces show no apparent regional patterns - with the Maritimes and the Prairies having quite similar rates.

Since World War 2, cirrhosis mortality has been increasing at a steady and rapid rate. Graphs 1 and 2 illustrate this increase for Canada as a whole and for the province of Ontario.

Table 3 provides indices of change for the 10 provinces separately.

TABLE 1

DEATHS ATTRIBUTED TO CIRRHOSIS PER 100,000 POPULATION
25 YEARS OF AGE AND OLDER IN VARIOUS COUNTRIES
1971, 1972

Country	Rate	Country	Rate
France	57.2	Hungary	20.7
Portugal	55.1	Belgium	20.5
Italy	52.1	Canada	19.6
Austria	49.1	Poland	17.2
West Germany	39.6	Denmark	16.2
Spain	38.3	Sweden	15.6
Roumania	34.6	Bulgaria	10.5
United States	28.6	New Zealand	8.2
Czechoslovakia	28.1	Norway	7.6
Greece	26.8	Finland	7.5
Yugoslavia	25.2	Netherlands	7.4
Switzerland	24.6	South Ireland	7.0
Japan	21.8	United Kingdom	5.7

The primary data were taken from the World Health Statistics Annual (1). The data for the U.S.A. and Belgium refer to 1971; for all other countries to 1972.

Evidently the rates in the adult population more than doubled over the last 22 years in Canada as a whole and showed a three- to five-fold increase in some provinces. The largest relative increases are found in provinces which had the lowest rates in the early post-war period (1946-50). As a result of this trend, regional differences in cirrhosis mortality have tended to become less marked over the past 20 years.

The rate of increase was generally greater in males than in females. As a consequence, the sex specific rates tend to diverge through time. The sex ratios in cirrhosis mortality for the last 30 years in Table 4 further illustrate this point. If these ratios represent genuine long-term tendencies we would predict that the existing preponderance of males among persons with cirrhosis will become even more pronounced in the future.

TABLE 2

DEATH ATTRIBUTED TO CIRRHOSIS OF THE LIVER PER 100,000
POPULATION AGED 25 AND OLDER, CANADA AND PROVINCES
1972

Province	Rate of Death		
	Total	Male	Female
Newfoundland	9.2	11.1	7.2
Prince Edward Island	15.2	19.7	10.7
Nova Scotia	15.5	23.7	7.4
New Brunswick	13.8	19.7	7.9
Quebec	19.9	28.8	11.5
Ontario	21.5	28.3	13.9
Manitoba	17.7	25.0	10.7
Saskatchewan	12.2	16.2	8.2
Alberta	15.2	19.4	10.8
British Columbia	22.7	28.2	17.3
Canada	19.5	26.7	12.5

The primary data were taken from Vital Statistics, Canada (2); death
rates are based on centred two-year moving averages.

Cirrhosis death rates are sensitive to the age distribution. The rates
are quite insignificant up to early adulthood, then rise continuously up to 60
years of age and decrease thereafter. Tables 5 and 6 indicate changes in the
age specific rates that have occurred over the post-war period. The rise
between 1950 and 1972 in Canada and Ontario has been largest in the rates
for ages 35 to 49 and smallest for those over 65 years. As a consequence,
the mean age of death has decreased. For Ontario, this decrease was from
60.4 for the five-year period 1946-1950 to 56.9 for the five years 1970-1974
($p < 0.01$). This trend becomes particularly relevant if the impact of the
disease is judged from the loss of life span or the reduction of working life it
causes. In this sense, the importance of a chronic or fatal disease is
inversely related to the age of its occurrence.

The urban-rural difference in mortality from this cause was fairly large
in the pre-war period but decreased considerably over the past thirty years
(Table 7). The latest available data indicate that the urban-rural ratio tends
to approach one.

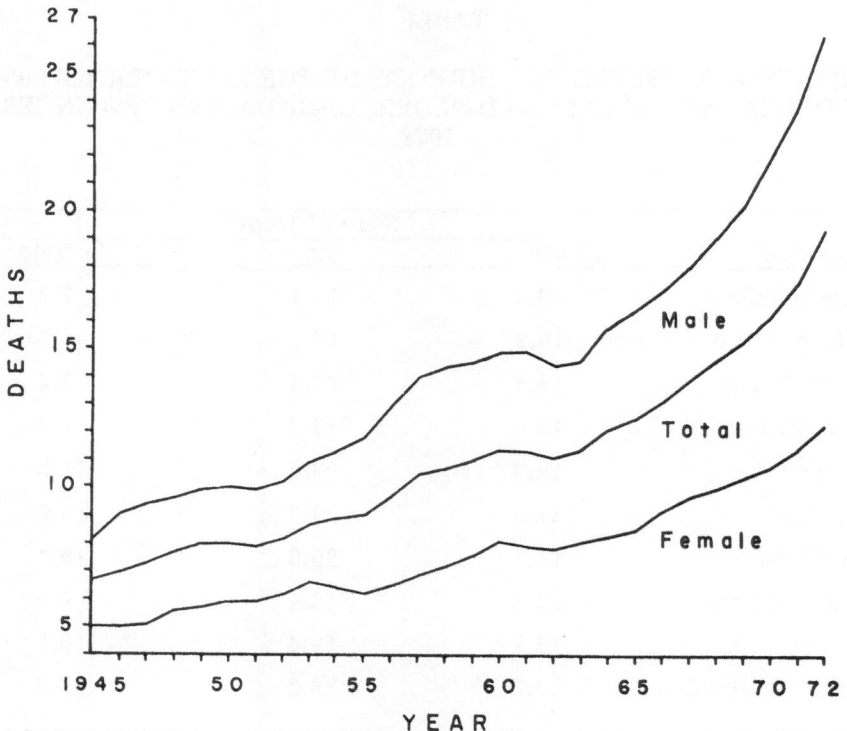

Graph 1   *Cirrhosis mortality per 100,000 population 25 years of age and*
             older, Canada 1945-1972 (2). Death rates are based on centred
             two-year moving averages corrected to allow for the effects of
             the 6th revision of the I.L.D.C.D.

In Graphs 3 and 4, the trend in cirrhosis mortality rates in Canada and Ontario is compared with the trend in death rates from all causes combined in the adult population. Clearly, the increases in cirrhosis rates are peculiar to this cause of death rather than a reflection of general mortality trends. For example, in 1944, there were fewer than five cirrhosis deaths for every 1,000 deaths from all causes in the male adult population of Ontario; by 1973, this ratio increased more than four-fold to 22 cirrhosis deaths per 1,000 deaths (Table 8). Changes in this ratio are particularly striking among middle-aged males. In 1945, among men 40-49 years of age, there was one cirrhosis death for 115 deaths from all causes; in 1972, one out of 18 deaths in this age group was attributable to cirrhosis, or, expressed differently, 5.6% of total mortality in 40-49 year old males is now attributable to cirrhosis.

It is also noteworthy that, in Canada in recent years, cirrhosis has been the most rapidly increasing cause of death in the population over 25 years of age, followed by cancer of the lung and bronchus and suicide. In Table 9, the

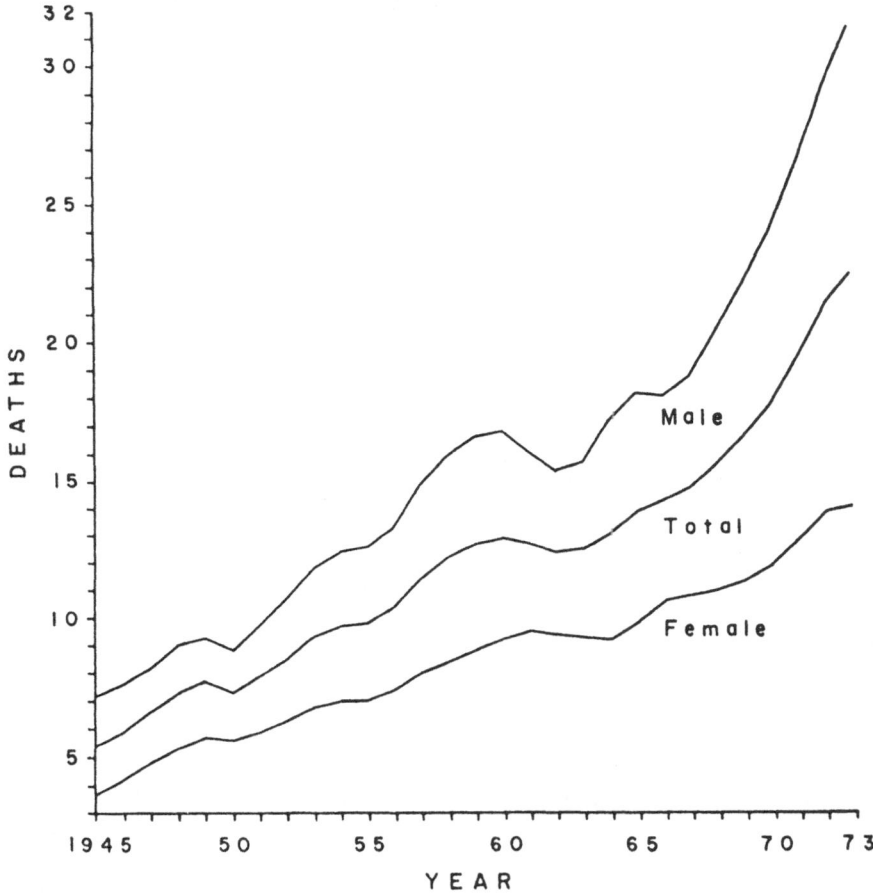

*Graph 2   Cirrhosis mortality per 100,000 population 25 years of age and
               older, Ontario 1945-1972 (3). Death rates are based on centred
               two-year moving averages corrected to allow for the effects of
               the 6th revision of the I.L.D.C.D.*

time trends in rates of death from these causes are shown for Ontario.
Apparently the two causes of death in the adult population which have risen
most rapidly are also potentially the most preventable diseases.   Lung
cancer is as closely related to smoking as cirrhosis is to drinking – both being
behaviours we may term "self-indulgent". In this regard, a characteristic of
mortality in Canada and more generally in the Western World during the last
20 years has been lack of improvement and even some increase in the
general mortality of middle-aged men, in contrast to the mortality of other
segments of the population which has shown improvement. The explanation

TABLE 3

RATIO OF LAST TO FIRST YEAR DEATH-RATE FROM CIRRHOSIS AND
AVERAGE ANNUAL RATES OF CHANGE IN THESE DEATH RATES,
CANADA AND PROVINCES, 1950-1972

Region	Ratio			Rate of Change in %		
	Male	Female	Total	Male	Female	Total
Canada	2.56	1.89	2.32	7.10	4.14	5.99
Newfoundland	3.54	4.45	4.00	11.54	15.68	14.59
Prince Edward Island	1.90	1.67	1.72	4.14	3.00	3.27
Nova Scotia	4.47	1.86	3.13	15.76	4.01	9.69
New Brunswick	2.69	1.79	2.45	7.67	3.69	6.58
Quebec	2.21	1.56	1.96	5.50	2.56	4.39
Ontario	3.00	2.24	2.40	9.15	5.75	6.40
Manitoba	3.69	1.84	2.81	12.23	3.82	8.25
Saskatchewan	2.12	1.63	1.82	4.42	2.96	3.72
Alberta	2.54	2.59	2.56	7.00	7.24	7.11
British Columbia	2.12	2.82	2.34	5.06	8.23	6.10

The primary data were taken from Vital Statistics, Canada (2); death rates
are for the population 20 years of age and older and are based on centred
two-year moving averages.

for this trend lies largely in the rapid increase of diseases related to alcohol
and tobacco use which have affected men of this age range more than any
other group.

The question now arises - what accounts for the temporal and spatial
variation in the rates of death from cirrhosis? The following clarifications
will aid in the examination of this question: 1) Clinical and experimental
research has firmly established the etiological importance of long-term
heavy alcohol intake in the development of cirrhosis. 2) The general level
of alcohol consumption in a population is closely related to the prevalence of
heavy use, which implies that the rate of drinkers of cirrhogenic quantities
rises and falls with the average per drinker consumption in a population.
This relationship has been confirmed in many empirical investigations (4).

TABLE 4

RATIO OF MALE TO FEMALE DEATH-RATE FROM CIRRHOSIS IN THE POPULATION 20 YEARS OF AGE AND OLDER, CANADA AND ONTARIO, 1946-1974

Year	Sex Ratio	
	Canada	Ontario
1946 - 1950	1.77	1.67
1951 - 1955	1.74	1.78
1956 - 1960	1.95	1.84
1961 - 1965	1.89	1.75
1966 - 1970	1.92	1.84
1971 - 1974	2.15	2.16

The primary data were taken from Vital Statistics, Canada (2); death rates are based on centred two-year moving averages.

TABLE 5

RATIO OF LAST TO FIRST YEAR DEATH-RATE FROM CIRRHOSIS AND AVERAGE ANNUAL RATES OF CHANGE IN THESE DEATH RATES BY AGE AND SEX, CANADA, 1950-1972

Age	Ratio			Rate of Change in %		
	Male	Female	Total	Male	Female	Total
20 - 34	1.80	1.58	1.71	3.63	2.27	3.24
35 - 49	4.01	2.76	3.52	13.72	8.00	11.45
50 - 64	2.70	2.23	2.49	7.73	5.60	6.76
65+	1.88	1.28	1.57	4.01	1.34	2.59

The primary data were taken from Vital Statistics, Canada (2); death rates are based on centred two-year moving averages.

TABLE 6

RATIO OF LAST TO FIRST YEAR DEATH-RATE FROM CIRRHOSIS
AND AVERAGE ANNUAL RATE OF CHANGE IN THESE DEATH
RATES BY AGE AND SEX, ONTARIO, 1950-1972

Age	Ratio			Rate of Change in %		
	Male	Female	Total	Male	Female	Total
20 - 34	2.83	1.29	2.17	8.33	1.30	5.30
35 - 49	3.84	3.09	3.72	12.91	9.49	12.37
50 - 64	3.31	2.22	2.85	10.50	5.60	8.39
65+	2.30	1.60	1.93	5.92	2.72	4.50

The primary data were taken from Ontario Vital Statistics (3); death
rates are based on centred two-year moving averages.

TABLE 7

RATIO OF URBAN TO RURAL DEATH-RATE FROM
CIRRHOSIS IN THE POPULATION 20 YEARS OF AGE
AND OLDER, ONTARIO, 1951-1971

Year	Cirrhosis Ratio		
	Male	Female	Total
1951	1.45	1.60	1.48
1961	1.42	1.28	1.35
1971	1.13	1.21	1.15

The primary data were taken from Ontario Vital
Statistics (3); "urban" refers to boroughs and cities of
50,000 population or more; death rates are based on
centred two-year moving averages.

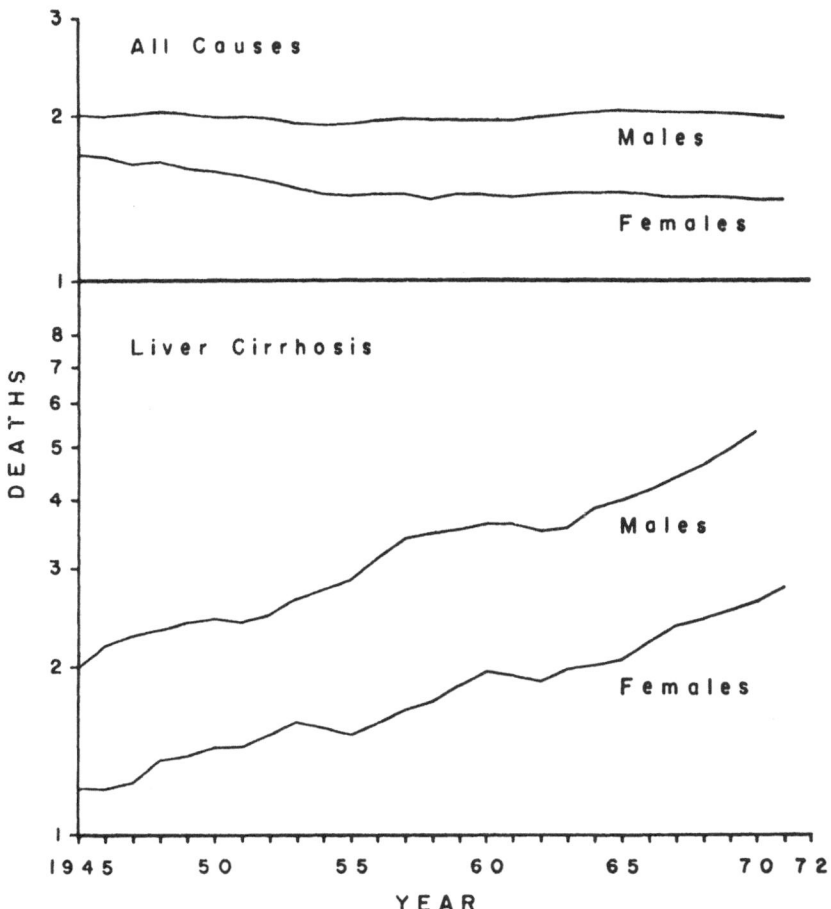

Graph 3   *Rate of death from all causes and cirrhosis in the population 25 years of age and older, Canada 1945-1972 (2). Death rates are based on centred two-year moving averages corrected to allow for the effects of the 6th revision of the I.L.D.C.D.*

Theoretically, therefore, variation in cirrhosis mortality rates, either from one region to another, through time in the same regions, or among segments of the population should be accompanied by similar variation in per capita consumption of alcoholic beverages. As Graphs 5 and 6 show, this expectation emerges clearly in the geographic comparisons shown earlier: international and regional differences in cirrhosis mortality rates are closely associated with differences in the apparent consumption of alcohol.

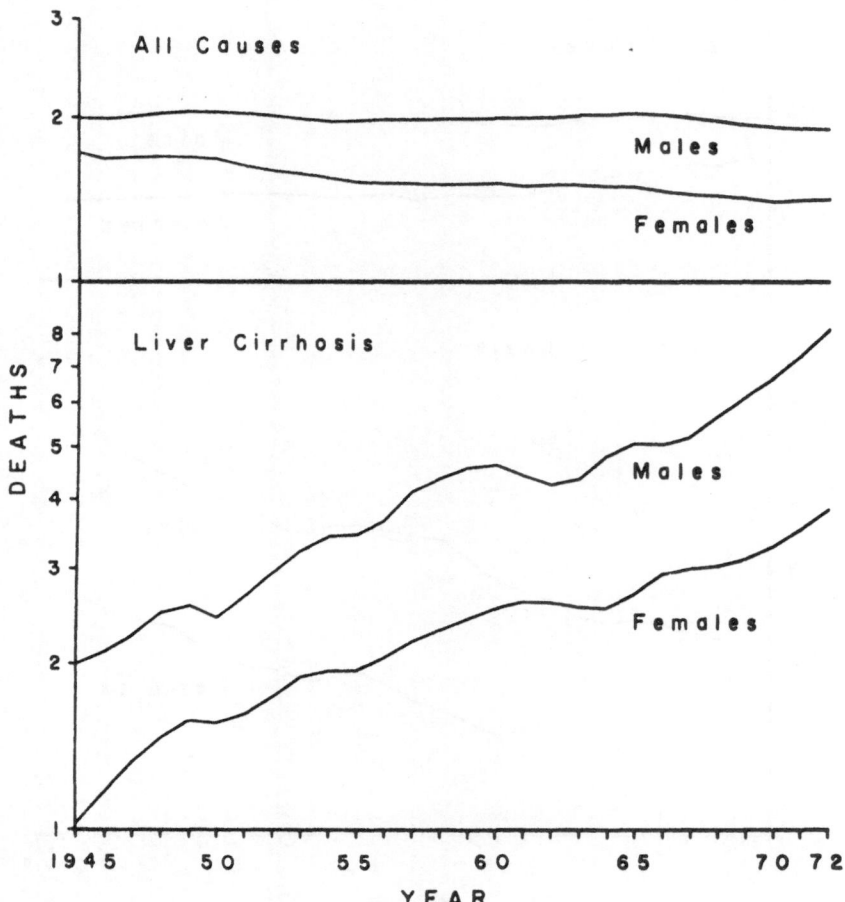

Graph 4   *Rate of death from all causes and cirrhosis in the population 25*
           years of age and older. Ontario 1945-1972 (3). Death rates are
           based on centred two-year moving averages corrected to allow
           for the effects of the 6th revision of the I.L.D.C.D.

This expected correlation with per capita consumption is further
illustrated by the very high coefficient in the spatial comparison of the
Eastern United States illustrated in Graph 7. Moreover, high coefficients of
correlation are also obtained in temporal series as shown for Ontario (Graph
8). Evidently, these data provide a consistent picture: the rate of death
from cirrhosis rises and falls with the level of alcohol consumption in
general populations.

TABLE 8

DEATHS ATTRIBUTED TO CIRRHOSIS PER 1,000
DEATHS FROM ALL CAUSES IN THE POPULATION
25 YEARS OF AGE AND OLDER, ONTARIO,
1944-1973

Year	Cirrhosis Ratio		
	Male	Female	Total
1944	4.95	3.34	4.20
1950	6.72	5.57	6.21
1955	8.33	5.42	7.07
1960	11.00	7.87	9.59
1965	11.68	8.13	10.16
1970	16.30	10.91	13.97
1973	21.77	13.05	17.91

The primary data were taken from Ontario Vital
Statistics (3); cirrhosis deaths are based on centred
two-year moving averages.

An objection to the inference that these correlations reflect a cause-
effect relationship is that the temporal series shown here, as well as most of
those reported in the literature (8), involve gradual and unidirectional trends
which do not permit us to distinguish spurious correlations. It is generally
accepted that abrupt and decisive changes in the independent variable
involving shifts in both directions provide a better opportunity to test such
associations (9). Such instances have occurred during and shortly after
World War 1 in several countries due to severe reductions in the supply of
alcohol. These reductions were always accompanied by a remarkably rapid
and very substantial drop in the cirrhosis death rates (10, 11, 12). In France,
extreme shortages occurred during both World Wars with particularly
dramatic effects on the mortality trend as shown in Graph 9 (13).The data in
this graph have been questioned on the grounds that deaths from a chronic
disease would not be expected to drop so suddenly when the aetiological
agent became less accessible. However, it has been pointed out (14) that
such sharp changes in cirrhosis mortality are not inconsistent with the
clinical course of the disease. Often the cirrhotic process can be halted by
abstinence and conversely a previously established liver pathology can be
reactivated in a short time when drinking is resumed.

TABLE 9

RATE OF DEATH PER 100,000 POPULATION 25 YEARS OF AGE AND OLDER, RATIO OF
LAST TO FIRST YEAR DEATH-RATE AND ANNUAL RATE OF CHANGE IN DEATH RATES
FROM CIRRHOSIS, LUNG CANCER AND SUICIDE, ONTARIO, 1950, 1972

Cause of Death	Rate of Death		Ratio			Rate of Change in %		
	1950	1972	Male	Female	Total	Male	Female	Total
Cirrhosis	7.6	21.4	3.32	2.47	2.81	10.59	6.69	8.25
Cancer of Lung	19.2	51.0	2.63	3.20	2.65	7.44	10.53	7.53
Suicide	13.6	21.2	1.38	2.18	1.55	1.76	5.39	2.54

The primary data were taken from Ontario Vital Statistics (3); death rates are based on centred
two-year moving averages.

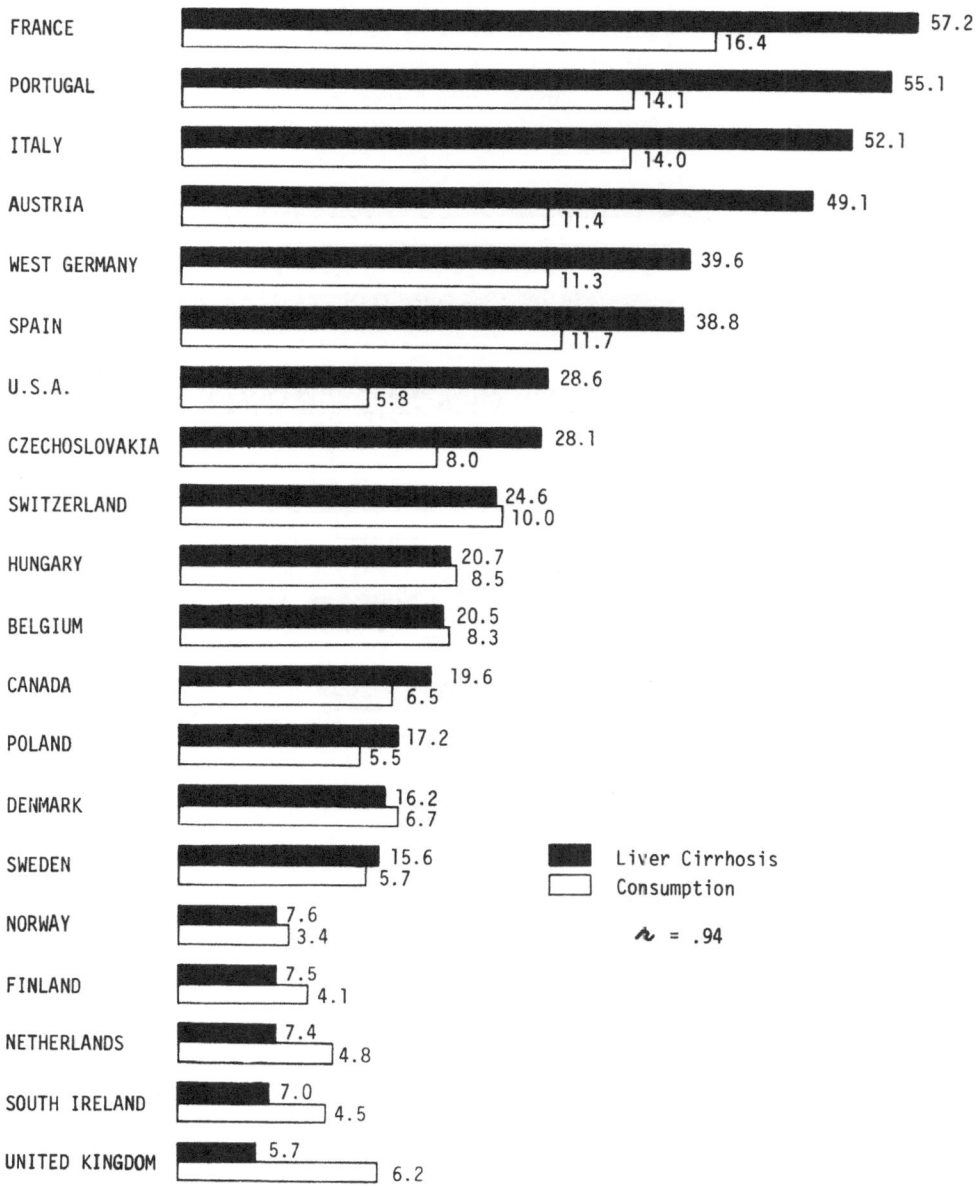

FRANCE	57.2
	16.4
PORTUGAL	55.1
	14.1
ITALY	52.1
	14.0
AUSTRIA	49.1
	11.4
WEST GERMANY	39.6
	11.3
SPAIN	38.8
	11.7
U.S.A.	28.6
	5.8
CZECHOSLOVAKIA	28.1
	8.0
SWITZERLAND	24.6
	10.0
HUNGARY	20.7
	8.5
BELGIUM	20.5
	8.3
CANADA	19.6
	6.5
POLAND	17.2
	5.5
DENMARK	16.2
	6.7
SWEDEN	15.6
	5.7
NORWAY	7.6
	3.4
FINLAND	7.5
	4.1
NETHERLANDS	7.4
	4.8
SOUTH IRELAND	7.0
	4.5
UNITED KINGDOM	5.7
	6.2

■ Liver Cirrhosis
□ Consumption

$\hbar = .94$

Graph 5   *Cirrhosis mortality per 100,000 population 25 years of age and older (1) and alcohol consumption per capita (5). Death rates are for 1972 except the U.S.A. and Belgium (1971); consumption figures are the 1968-1970 average consumption.*

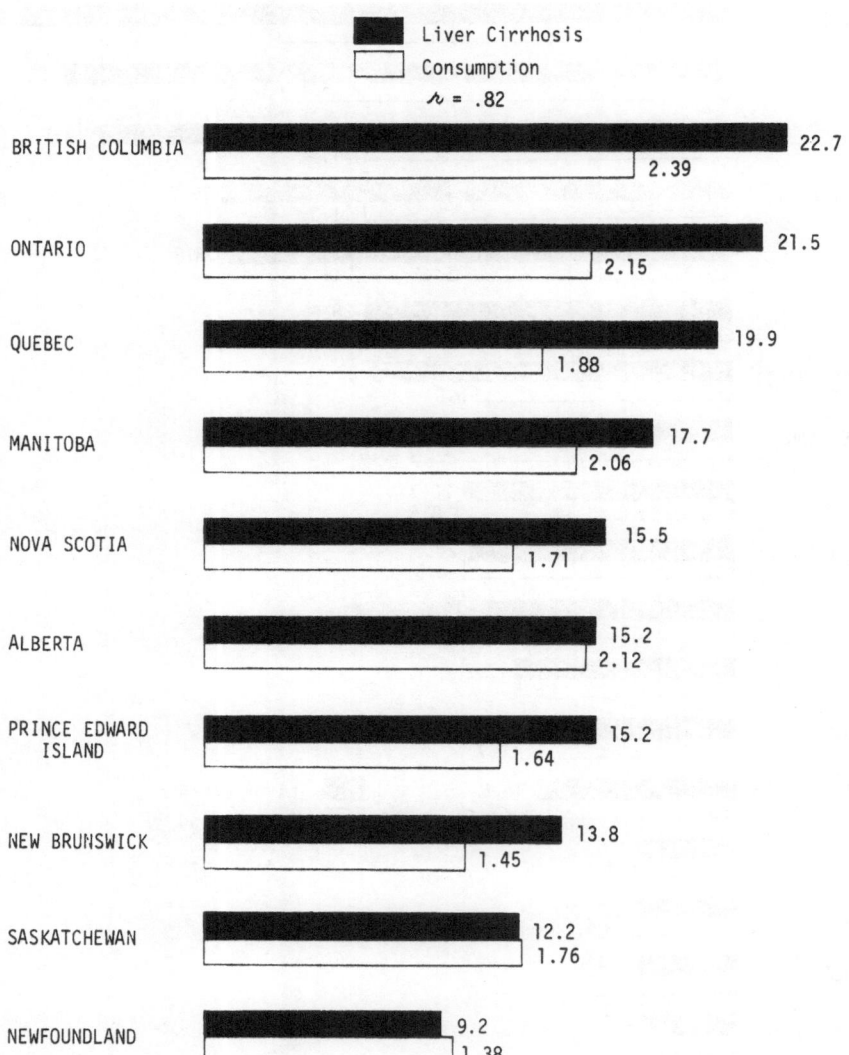

Graph 6   *Cirrhosis mortality per 100,000 population 25 years of age and older (2) and alcohol consumption per capita 15 years of age and older, 1971 (6) for the Provinces of Canada.*

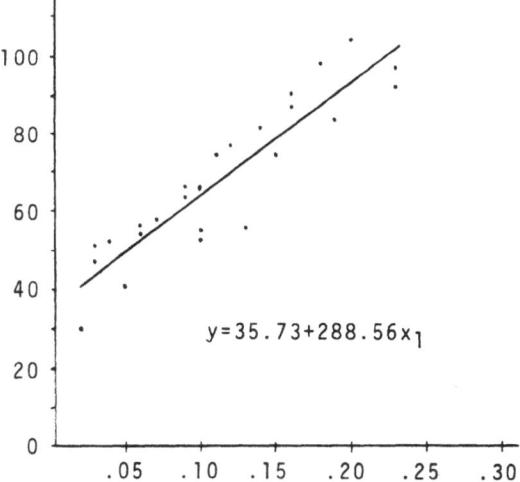

$$y = 35.73 + 288.56x_1$$

Graph 7   *The regression of cirrhosis mortality on wine consumption in the eastern United States - 1950. Based on data in Schmidt and Bronetto (7).*

Our earlier observation on the age and sex distribution of these deaths is also consistent with the hypothesis that variation in alcohol consumption rates explains variation in cirrhosis death rates. Adult males in Canada have higher death rates and higher alcohol consumption rates than adult females. Up to the age of 25, on the other hand, there is no consistent sex difference in mortality (Table 10).   The data shown in this table also indicate that, in this age group, the rates for both sexes and the sex ratios have remained quite stable over the past 30 years. This is due to the fact that mortality from cirrhosis among infants, children and young adults is caused by factors other than alcohol use. Apparently these factors have varied little over time.

The higher death rates in urban areas and the decrease in the urban-rural difference in Ontario between 1950 and 1970 noted earlier (Table 7) also coincide with alcohol consumption trends. A comparison of Ontario survey data from the 1950's with more recent data shows that urban-rural differences in alcohol use are far less marked now than they were 20 years ago (15, 16). In sum, there exists strong evidence for a dependence of the cirrhosis mortality level on the amount of alcohol consumption in general populations.

The mortality data described so far comprise all aetiological variants of cirrhosis and hence do not reveal to what extent alcoholic cirrhosis contributes to the mortality experienced from cirrhotic disease generally.

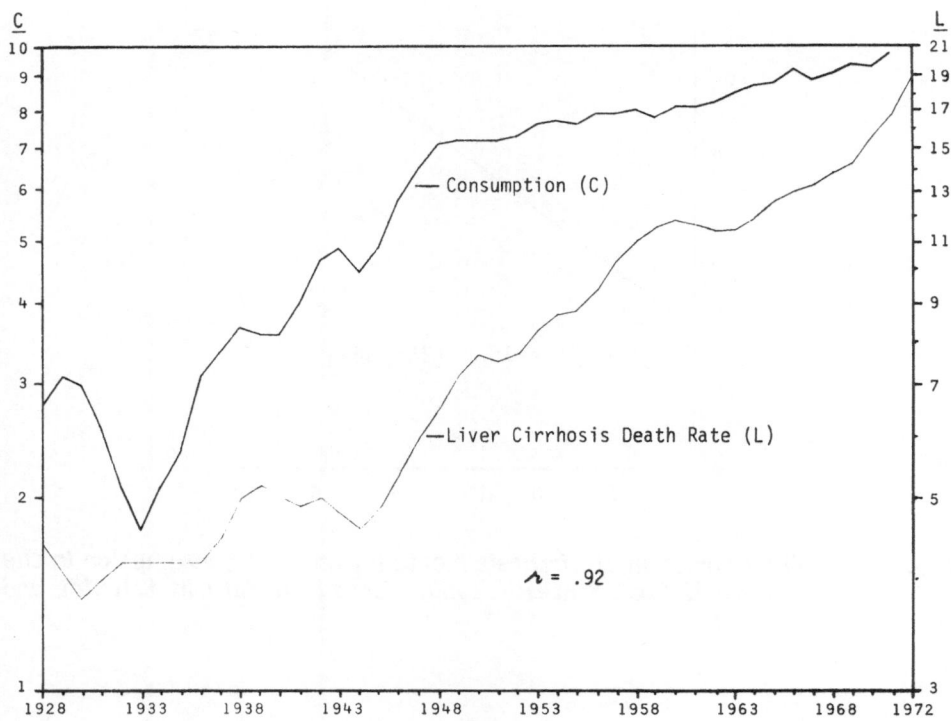

*Graph 8   Cirrhosis mortality per 100,000 population 20 years of age and
            older (3) and alcohol consumption per capita population 15 years
            of age and older (6),   Ontario 1928-1972.   Death rates were
            corrected to allow for the effects of the 6th revision of the
            I.L.D.C.D.*

This question becomes crucial in the interpretation of rate variations in
cirrhosis death rates. For example, are the very dramatic increases in these
deaths in Ontario over the past 30 years entirely attributable to increases in
alcoholic cirrhosis or have other aetiological types also contributed to the
increase?   To explore this question, methods have been devised for
estimating the alcohol caused proportion out of all cirrhosis deaths in
general populations.

    One method which is illustrated in Graph 10 consists of plotting the
cirrhosis death rates against the per capita consumption through time and
fitting a line of regression to these data. The point at the vertical axis
where this line intersects at a hypothetical zero alcohol-consumption marks
the rate of cirrhosis death that would be expected in the absence of any
alcohol use, or, in other words, the rate of death from non-alcoholic
cirrhosis. This point is marked '0' on the opposite scale which represents
estimates of the proportions of cirrhosis deaths that are attributable to
alcohol use. By this method, we would estimate that, in Ontario in 1973,
about 79% of all cirrhosis deaths were due to alcohol.

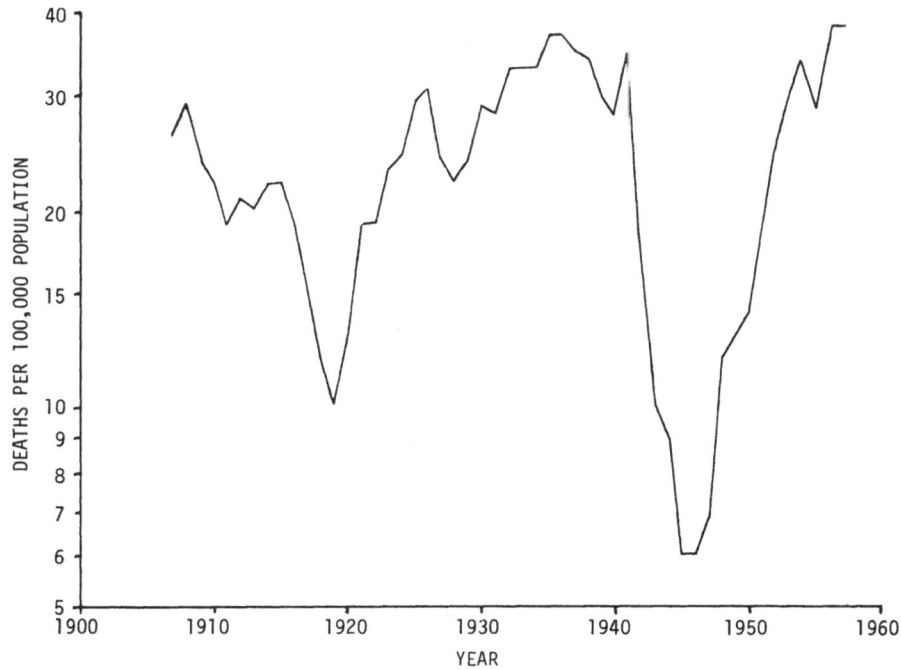

Graph 9   *Cirrhosis mortality rates: Paris 1907-1956. Based on data in Ledermann (13).*

TABLE 10

DEATHS ATTRIBUTED TO CIRRHOSIS PER 100,000
POPULATION UNDER AGE 25, ONTARIO, 1944-1974

| Year | Rate of Death | | |
	Males	Females	Total
1944–49	2.8	2.2	2.5
1950–54	2.6	1.8	2.2
1955–59	2.6	2.3	2.4
1960–64	2.1	2.8	2.6
1965–69	2.2	1.8	2.0
1970–74	1.3	1.2	1.3

The primary data were taken from Ontario Vital
Statistics (3).

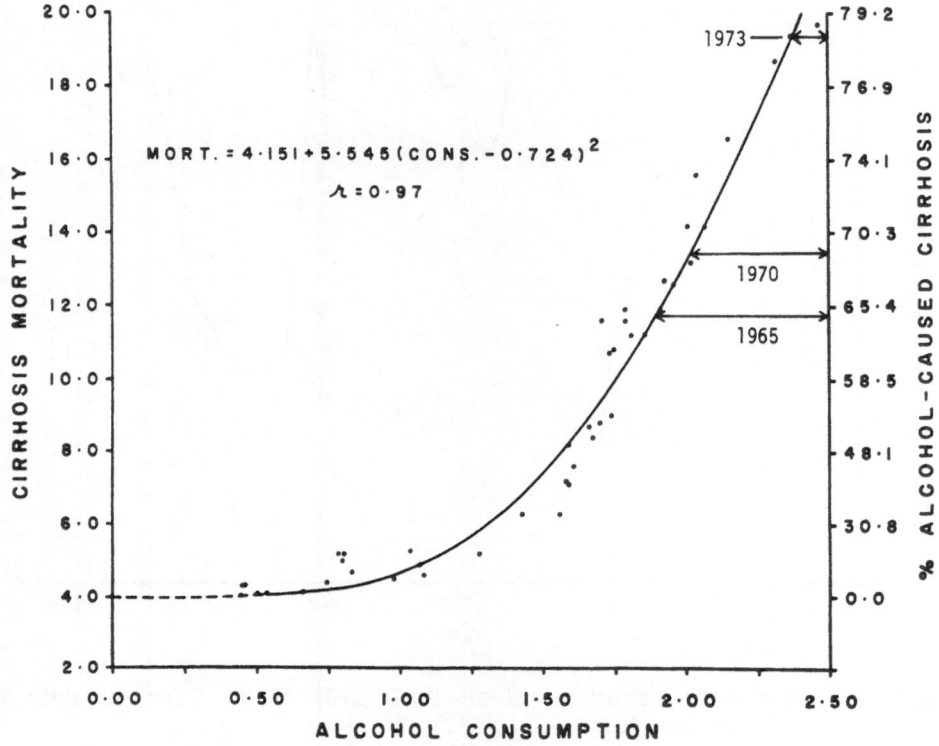

Graph 10   *The regression of cirrhosis mortality per capita 20 years of age and older (3) on alcohol consumption per capita 15 years of age and older (6),   Ontario 1932-1973 and estimates of the proportion of alcoholic cirrhosis. Death rates were corrected to allow for the effects of the 6th revision of the I.L.D.C.D.*

A second approach is based on a quite different set of data: cirrhosis deaths are reported on the death certificates as "with" or "without" mention of alcoholism and are classified accordingly in Vital Statistics. As Graph 11 indicates, this "reported" alcohol-related rate has increased more rapidly than the combined rate from all other aetiological types of cirrhosis. However, it is known that physicians often fail to report the contribution of alcoholism in such cases which precludes the use of these data as estimates of the true proportion of alcohol-caused cirrhosis deaths. An opportunity to determine the extent of this underreporting was provided in a recent mortality study of known alcoholics who resided in Ontario (17, 18). It was found that, out of a total of 181 deaths from cirrhosis that had occurred in this group between 1960 and 1972 99 or 54% were listed on the death

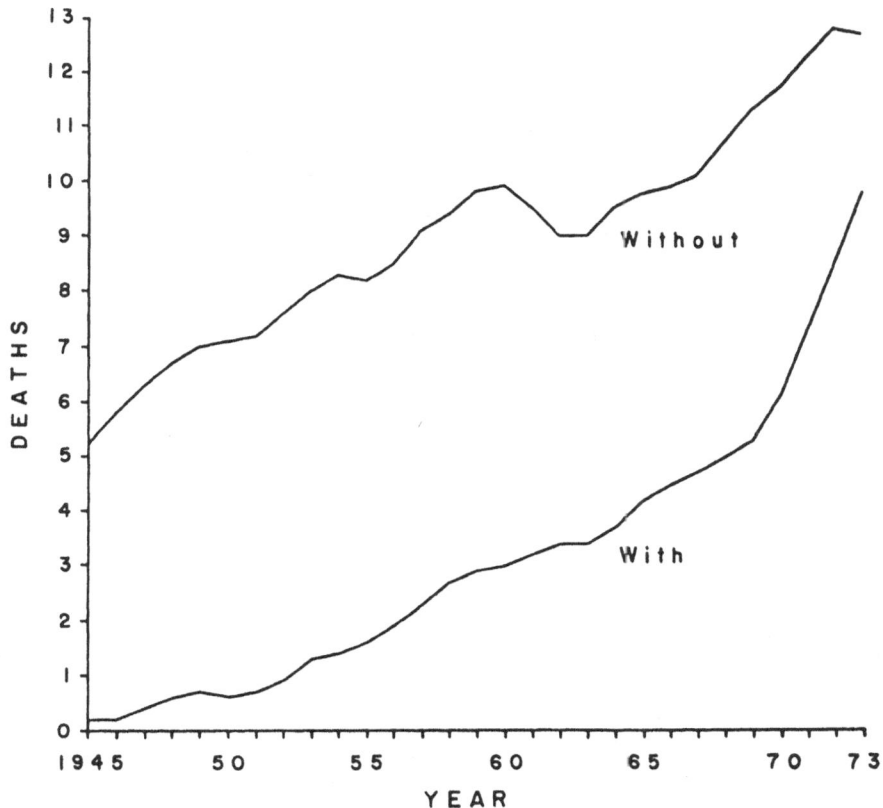

Graph 11   *Cirrhosis mortality "with" and "without" mention of alcoholism*
            per 100,000 population 25 years of age and older, Ontario 1945-
            1973 (3).   Death rates are based on centred two-year moving
            averages corrected to allow for the effects of the 6th revision
            of the I.L.D.C.D.

certificates as attributable to alcoholism.[1] Evidently the true proportion of
alcohol-caused cirrhosis among these alcoholics must have been close to 1.
If we correct the reported Provincial rates accordingly by applying the
factor 1/54 to the data in Graph 11 (the reported mortality from cirrhosis
with mention of alcoholism), we obtain the estimates shown in Table 11,
column 1.   Column 2 of this table shows corresponding estimates which
were obtained by the regression method discussed above (Graph 10).

---

[1] The proportion was relatively stable over time amounting to 52% for the
period 1960-1965 and 55% for the period 1966 to the present.

TABLE 11

ESTIMATES OF THE PROPORTION OF ALL
CIRRHOSIS DEATHS CAUSED BY HEAVY ALCOHOL
USE, ONTARIO

Year	Correction Method	Regression Method
1965	58%	62%
1970	64%	68%
1973	78%	78%
1974	81%	79%

Evidently these two methods - although employing quite different sets of data - produced very similar results thereby enhancing confidence in the estimates. It would appear then that the increase in cirrhosis mortality that has occurred in Ontario over the past 30 years was largely, if not entirely, attributable to increases in alcoholic cirrhosis. Currently, about 80% of all cirrhosis deaths in the adult population of this Province would be expected to be the result of heavy alcohol use. This proportion is even higher in certain segments of the population. For example, for males in the age range 35 to 60, the estimate of this proportion for 1973 is 94%.

Recently, it has been said that the use of other psychoactive substances, in conjunction with heavy drinking, may also contribute to the trends in cirrhosis mortality (19). While it is known that excessive drinkers tend to misuse drugs of this type (20), it is not clear whether any of these substances is significantly hepatotoxic, nor what part they may play in the aetiology of cirrhosis in heavy drinkers. The question whether such combinations influence the frequency of death from cirrhosis in alcoholics was explored by comparing the cirrhosis death rates of treated alcoholics for the period 1950 to 1959 with rates for the period 1964 to 1971 (17, 18). These two time spans represent roughly a "before" and "after" period with respect to the onset of the use of tranquilizers in the treatment of alcoholism and a wide range of other problems. If the use of these psychoactive substances has heightened the risk of hepatic disease in heavy drinkers, we would expect the cirrhosis death rate of alcoholics in the "after" period to be higher than in the "before" period. Clearly, the data do not support this expectation (Table 12). This finding constitutes additional support for the hypothesis that the trends in cirrhosis mortality over the post-war period are fully attributable to a rise in alcoholic cirrhosis resulting from increases in the general level of alcohol use in the population.

TABLE 12

DEATHS FROM CIRRHOSIS IN TWO SAMPLES OF ALCOHOLICS

Period of Follow-up	Man Years of Exposure to the Risk of Death	Number of Deaths	Age Adjusted Rate of Death per 10,000 Man Years
1950-1960	41,149	79	19.2
1964-1971	22,476	45	20.0

In conclusion, we may ask what the future holds with respect to the incidence of alcohol-related liver disease. Earlier I have shown a statistical dependence of the rate of death from cirrhosis on per capita consumption of alcohol. Accordingly, one would expect that future trends in alcohol use may also serve as a basis for predicting the incidence of cirrhosis. There exist many methods to forecast the demand of a commodity but, by and large, they are based on the interpretation of statistical data of past movements of relevant variables. The factors known to have a bearing on the demand of alcoholic beverages are: 1) personal disposable income, 2) real price of beverages in question and prices of related commodities that serve as substitutes or complements, and   3) changes in taste as reflected in trends in beverage preference. Recently a set of forecasting equations have been developed which performed very well over a historical sample period (1956-1972) as shown in Graph 12 (23). The dotted line from 1972 to 1984 represents a forecast of the demand which utilizes these equations and projections of the aforementioned three variables as generated by a National Forecast Service (Informetrica Limited (24)).

The forecast depicted in the graph indicates that the consumption per adult in Canada will continue to increase at roughly the same rate of growth experienced during the period 1956 to 1972 with minor variations from year to year. Over the entire forecast period, consumption is seen to reach 3.95 gallons per adult which represents a 73% increase over the level of 1972. Studies of the distribution of consumption have shown that the relationship between per capita consumption and the prevalence of heavy drinkers is parabolic, i.e., changes in the rate of heavy drinkers will, on the average, be proportional to the square of the increase in per capita consumption. Accordingly, we would expect that the rate of users of potentially cirrhogenic quantities will more than double by 1985. Obviously forecasts rely, to a large extent, on historical data. No matter how sophisticated the methods used, there is always the possibility that new factors may come into

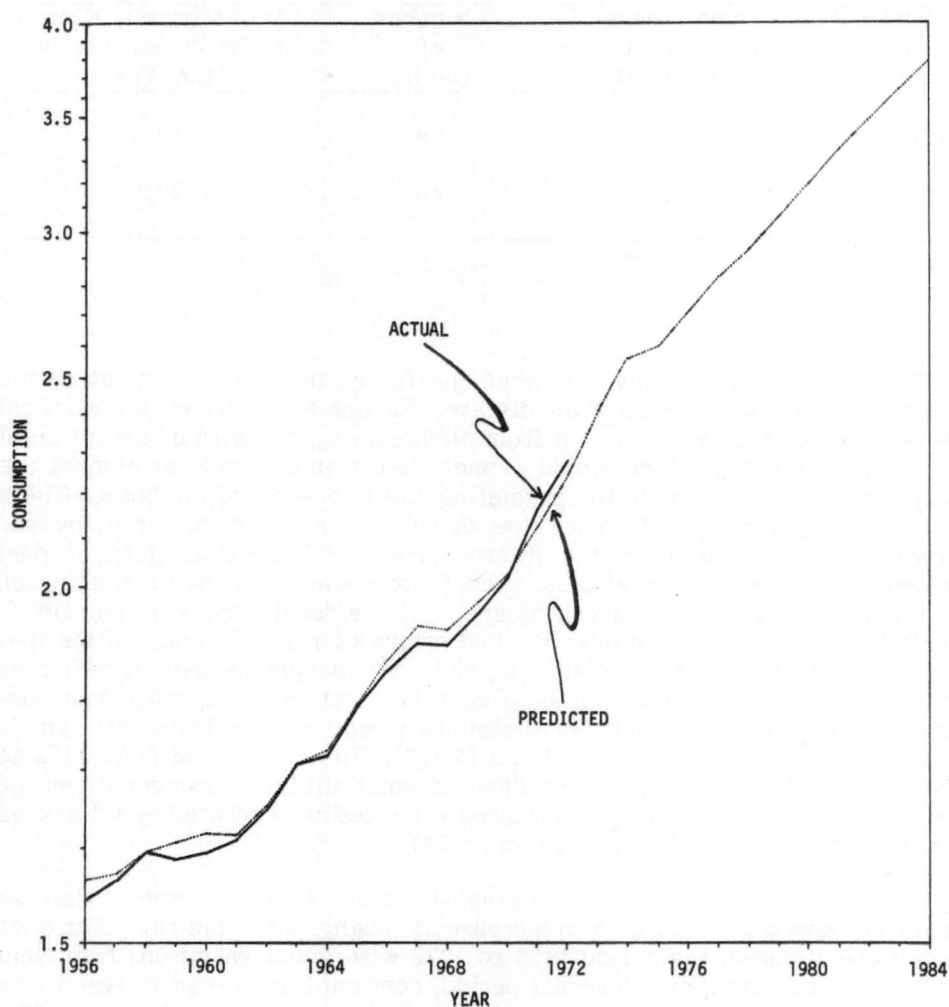

Graph 12   Predicted and actual Canadian consumption of alcoholic beverages. (Gallons of absolute alcohol per adult).

play that could affect consumption one way or the other.[1] However, econometric analysis has generally proved very successful in making predictions and it may well be that the predicted levels of alcohol use will actually occur. In this case we would predict that cirrhosis, which is now the 5th leading cause of death for men in the productive years from 25 to 64, will become the 3rd leading cause after heart disease and cancer.

It is now generally accepted that, for a program of prevention to be effective, controls will have to play a significant part. The potential usefulness of the many diverse restrictions through which control can be exercised has recently been examined in great detail (4, 25).   The conclusions reached can be summarized as follows: There is strong evidence that, whenever beverage alcohol becomes more readily available because of a relaxation in control laws, levels of consumption and rates of alcohol problems tend to increase. Furthermore, alcoholic beverages tend to behave in the consumer market like many other commodities so that their consumption is affected by their price level.

Accordingly, the Addiction Research Foundation has recently made the following recommendations to Government:

1. A taxation policy which maintains a reasonably constant relationship between the price of alcohol and levels of disposable income (income after taxes) in the Province. For example, if disposable income per capita rose 5% in a year, then the price of each alcoholic beverage offered for sale would be increased by that percentage.

2. A moratorium on further relaxation of alcohol control measures and the adoption of a health-oriented policy with respect to such measures. Essentially, this would mean that future proposals to change legislative or other provisions governing the marketing and distribution of alcoholic beverages would be tested against a health objective, namely the prevention of further increases in the prevalence of alcohol problems. The relevant question would become: Are the proposed changes likely to contribute to higher consumption levels and, therefore, to an increase in health costs?

3. An education program designed to increase public awareness of the personal hazards of heavy alcohol consumption, the economic and other consequences for society of high consumption levels, and the potential public health benefits of appropriate control measures. On this final point I can do no better than quote Edwards' views (26): "The reason why a person drinks

---

[1] For example, a study of the anticipated impact of the recently introduced wage and price guidelines indicated that, as a result of these measures, consumption will be somewhat lower than previously forecast. These calculations were based on the assumption that the guidelines will be completely successful (23).

abnormally are connected with both his personality and with his environment; his drinking will, in fact, result from an interaction of the two, so that, for example, an anxious person living where alcohol is cheap and attitudes to drinking are permissive will be more likely to become an excessive drinker than an anxious person who finds alcohol more difficult to obtain and attitudes less approving. Since we are not able to manipulate personality and produce a race with no neuroses, the only realistic method of exerting a benign influence on the prevalence of chronic alcohol problems is by control of environmental conditions of drinking and it is the availability element that remains the prime candidate for control."

REFERENCES

1.   World Health Statistics Annual Volume 1:   Vital Statistics and Causes of Death. Geneva: World Health Organization, 1972

2.   Statistics Canada Annual Reports: Vital Statistics. Ottawa: Queen's Printer, 1945-1974

3.   Province of Ontario Annual Reports: Vital Statistics. Toronto: Queen's Printer, 1944-1974

4.   BRUUN K, EDWARDS G, LUMIO M, MAKELA K, OSTERBERG E, PAN L, POPHAM RE, ROOM R, SCHMIDT W, SKOG OJ, SULKUNEN P: Alcohol Control Policies and Public Health.   Report of an International Working Group.   Helsinki, Finnish Foundation for Alcohol Studies, 1975

5.   SULKUNEN P: Drinking patterns and the level of alcohol consumption: an international overview. In Research Advances in Alcohol and Drug Problems, Volume 3. Y Israel et al, (eds.). New York, Wiley and Sons, in press, 1976

6.   Statistics Canada Annual Reports: Control and Sale of Alcoholic Beverages in Canada. Ottawa: Queen's Printer, 1945-1974

7.   SCHMIDT W, BRONETTO J: Death from liver cirrhosis and specific alcohol beverage consumption. Amer J Publ Hlth 52: (9) 1473-1482, 1962

8.   POPHAM RE: Indirect methods of alcoholism prevalence estimation: a critical evaluation. In Alcohol and Alcoholism. RE Popham (ed.). Toronto, University of Toronto Press, 1970. pp. 294-306

9.   CAMPBELL DT: Reforms as experiments. Amer Psychol 24: 409-421, 1968

10. POPHAM RE, JELLINEK EM: Alcohol estimation formula and its application to Canadian data. Quart J Stud Alc 17: 559-593, 1956

11. BRUUN K, KOURA E, POPHAM RE, SEELEY JR: Liver cirrhosis as a means to estimate the prevalence of alcoholism. Publ No. 8, Finnish Foundation for Alcohol Studies, Helsinki, 1960

12. JOLIFFE N, JELLINEK EM: Cirrhosis of the Liver. In Effects of Alcohol on the Individual, Volume 1. EM Jellinek (ed.). New Haven, Yale Univ Press, 1942. pp. 273-234

13. LEDERMANN S: Alcool, Alcoolisme, Alcoolisation: Mortalité, Morbidité, Accidents du Travail. Instit Nat d'Etudes Dém, Paris Trav Doc Cah 41. Paris: Presses Universitaires de France, 1964

14. TERRIS M: Epidemiology of cirrhosis of the liver. National mortality data. Amer J Publ Hlth 57: 2076-2088, 1967

15. POPHAM RE, SCHMIDT W: Statistics of Alcohol Use and Alcoholism in Canada 1871-1956. Toronto, University of Toronto Press, 1958

16. DE LINT JE, SCHMIDT W, PERNANEN K: The Ontario Drinking Survey: A Preliminary Report. A.R.F. Substudy 1 - 10&4&37 - 70, Toronto, 1970. (Mimeograph).

17. SCHMIDT W, DE LINT JE: Causes of death of alcoholics. Quart J Stud Alc 33: 171-185, 1972

18. SCHMIDT W: In preparation

19. RANKIN JG, SCHMIDT W, POPHAM RE, DE LINT JE: Epidemiology of alcoholic liver disease: Insights and problems. In Alcoholic Liver Pathology: JM Khanna, Y Israel and H Kalant (eds.). Toronto: Addiction Research Foundation, 1975. pp. 31-41

20. DEVENYI P, WILSON M: Barbiturate abuse and addiction and their relationship to alcohol and alcoholism. Can Med Assoc J 104: 215-218, 1971

21. RAVNSBORG IS: Medikamentmisbruk blant alkoholikere. Tidsskr norske Laegeforen 84: 617-619, 1964

22. GLATT MM: The abuse of barbiturates in the United Kingdom. Bulletin on Narcotics 14: 19-38, 1962

23. LAU HH: Forecasting of Canadian Consumption of Alcoholic Beverages. Addiction Research Foundation Substudy No. 758: Toronto, 1976. (Mimeograph)

24. The National Forecast Service Informetrica Limited, Ottawa, Canada. Candide Model 1.1 - July 11, 1975

25. POPHAM RE, SCHMIDT W, DE LINT JE: The effects of legal restraint on drinking. In Biology of Alcoholism, Volume 4: Social Biology. B Kissin and H Begleiter (eds.). New York, Plenum, in press, 1976

26. EDWARDS G: Public health implications of liquor control. The Lancet ii: 424-425, 1971

DISCUSSION

CHAIRMAN: J.G. RANKIN

POPPER: I have three questions concerning this most interesting unique presentation.   1)   What is the incidence of Hepatitis B Surface Antigenemia in the Canadian population? I think it is most important to put this into the context of what we have just heard so well developed.   2)   What is the relative amount of alcohol consumed as beer, wine and spirits? This has some important implications in many parts of the world.   3)   Italy and Greece both have a very high incidence of Hepatitis B Surface Antigenemia and apparently very little alcoholic hepatitis.   They have steatosis but no alcoholic hepatitis. Some Italian experts claim that most of their cirrhosis and hepatocellular carcinoma are related to viral hepatitis B and not to alcohol. I would like to get for the record what is really the Italian and Greek situation.   What is the incidence of cirrhosis in these countries and is there any difference between Southern Italy with its extremely high carrier rate for Hepatitis B Surface antigen and Northern Italy with its much lower carrier rate?

SCHMIDT: I am afraid that I cannot answer your first question. Your second question related to the contribution of the three main types of alcoholic beverage to the total consumption of alcohol and to the possible role that they play in the incidence of liver disease.   In Canada at the moment exactly 50% of the alcoholic beverages sold are sold as beer, 35-38% as distilled spirits and the remainder as wine. The role which the type of beverage may play in the variations of death rate from cirrhosis is a very difficult one. In general the contribution of the type of beverage does not seem to be all that important. It appears that the volume and duration of consumption rather than the specific type of beverage consumed is the best predictor of liver pathology. With respect to your third question, the regional break-downs are available for Italy but off-hand I cannot provide them.

JOLY: In partial answer to Dr. Popper's first question I might mention that Dr. Richer in our Liver Disease Unit has found that the incidence of Hepatitis B Surface Antigenemia in the Quebec population is five times higher than its average incidence in the rest of Canada. Therefore if there were a relationship between alcohol consumption and Hepatitis B one would expect to have a much greater incidence of cirrhosis in Quebec than in the rest of Canada. This I don't think is the case.

SCHMIDT: That is correct, Quebec's cirrhosis rate is exactly where one would predict it to be on the basis of its level of alcohol consumption compared to the other Provinces in Canada. In terms of beverage preference and drinking patterns, the Quebec population drinks very much like other North Americans drink - the preferred beverage is beer. There appears to be nothing unusual in the mortality pattern of the province of Quebec.

FISHER: The relative increase of alcoholic liver disease in the female in the United States and some other cultures is greater than that in the male. Is the Canadian female a hardier breed or is she not drinking as much? How do you explain the inconsistency of your data?

SCHMIDT: That is a very interesting question because there is an inconsistency. The information on alcohol consumption clearly indicates that females are drinking more and more like males in Ontario and in Canada as a whole. Accordingly we would expect that the mortality from cirrhosis or the incidence of liver disease should tend to become more and more similar to the male picture. There are two considerations which help explain this inconsistency. The first is the time lag involved. In Canada the population alcohol consumption data precede the mortality data by 5-10 years. The second important consideration is that if one works with total cirrhosis mortality one has to adjust for the proportion that has another etiology and that proportion is much smaller in females than in males. Mortality from cancer of the lung is a somewhat similar situation. It involves a large female/male difference, and a probable most important single etiological factor - smoking. But there is one crucial difference and this relates to the tendency of patterns of consumption to become more and more similar between males and females. The smoking situation precedes the drinking situation by about 10 years. This means that there was a similarity in the smoking behaviour of females and males ten years ago that we are only now beginning to approach in drinking. This means that the mortality sex ratios from cancer of the lung may predict what one will experience 10 to 15 years from now with respect to the sex ratios in liver cirrhosis. In fact the sex ratio in mortality from cancer of the lung increased until about five years ago, then it began to decrease. I predict that this divergence which we see now in liver cirrhosis mortality will level off within the next five years.

ISRAEL: Are those people who develop cirrhosis different from those who do not, in terms of their relative rates of ethanol metabolism?

SCHMIDT: There may be information available on this but I am not sufficiently informed to answer. It may be of some interest that there are clear sex differences involved. Females apparently develop cirrhosis while drinking a smaller amount of alcohol over a shorter period of time.

ISRAEL: Some drinks have a much higher congener content than others. Is the congener content of various alcoholic beverages important in terms of the production of liver disease?

SCHMIDT: The evidence indicates that the congeners are not important on the population level. The variation in the congener content among beverages would not be expected to produce a rate variation in the general population, the effect is too small.

FOX: Did you make the point that you think that one of the main routes of control is to control the availability of alcohol?

SCHMIDT: It is the most promising in view of the available data. There may be other routes which haven't been explored as fully.

FOX: The thing that disturbs me about this conclusion is that man has had access to alcohol for centuries and there is evidence that the rigid control of the availability of alcohol doesn't solve the problem of alcoholic cirrhosis or alcoholism. We can compare it to the drug situation, where rigid controls don't seem to be solving the problem of drug addiction or drug abuse.

SCHMIDT: Controlling the availability of alcohol won't solve the problem. But it may reduce it to an acceptable rate. I would argue that if you removed all the controls on drugs the drug problem would be much larger than it is. I would also add that the degree of alcohol availability has varied vastly over the centuries and in general the evidence indicates that those countries which exert the most rigid controls have the lowest rates of chronic alcohol problems.

SIMON: How close is the relationship between the cost of alcohol in relation to per capita income and the incidence of cirrhosis. I gather the data on this are equivocal.

SCHMIDT: There is a very close relationship between cost and consumption, and there is a very close relationship between consumption and cirrhosis mortality.

SIMON: Are there not areas of the world where the cost of alcohol is low and the incidence of cirrhosis is low?

SCHMIDT: I could give you dozens of examples of the opposite. There may be a country such as you describe, possibly Israel, where the rate of cirrhosis doesn't seem to be high and the cost of alcoholic beverages also doesn't seem to be high.   But one looks for consistency. One evaluates the totality of evidence and sees in which direction it points.

SASS-KORTSAK: In your graphs you correlated alcohol consumption and cirrhosis mortality. All of the countries fit the pattern very nicely except the United States where the incidence of cirrhosis appeared to be higher than would be expected. Furthermore there were discrepancies within Canada. In Saskatchewan for example, the incidence was lower than would be predicted from the alcohol consumption. Can you explain these observations?

SCHMIDT: If you break down the States of the Union into North, East, South and West you get very very good correlations. However if you put all the data in one bag the picture is not all that convincing. I believe that the inconsistency in the case of the United States is attributable to the extreme heterogeneity of the population. With respect to Saskatchewan I'm afraid I can't answer that.

METABOLISM OF ETHANOL AND THE EFFECT OF ETHANOL ON METABOLISM

Frank Lundquist

Department of Biochemistry A, The Panum Institute

University of Copenhagen, DK-2200, Copenhagen

It may appear surprising in view of the spectacular advances made in biology in recent years that the chemically simple process, the oxidation of ethanol via acetaldehyde to acetate, is still not sufficiently known with regard to biochemical mechanisms, localization in the body, and effects on the metabolism of other substances. In 1919, Mellanby showed that the concentration of ethanol in the blood of human subjects after a single dose decreased in a linear way for many hours (1). Widmark later made a careful study of the absorption, distribution and elimination kinetics of alcohol, which led to the extensive use in Scandinavia of blood alcohol determinations for forensic purposes (2). Lundsgaard showed that the liver is by far the most important organ for elimination of ethanol (3). Moreover, he faced the fact that ethanol is a nutrient which on average provides a considerable proportion of the energy needed for the human body, 10-15% in the case of Danish population. He also pointed out that only about 40% of the total metabolism can be met by the oxidation of alcohol. In the last decade or so interest in various aspects of alcohol metabolism has been increasing, partly because of the practical importance, but also because it involves some biochemically fundamental problems.

Metabolism of Ethanol in the Liver

Free acetate, the major end-product of ethanol oxidation in the liver, leaves the liver and is further metabolized in other tissues, especially muscles. Some acetate is also metabolized in the liver, the amount depending on the species and nutritional state of the animal. The oxidation occurs in two steps, ethanol to acetaldehyde, and acetaldehyde to acetate. The enzyme alcohol dehydrogenase (ADH) is present in all vertebrates so far studied. It catalyzes the reaction shown in Fig. 1. The enzyme, especially that isolated from horse liver, has been extensively studied. It consists of

CYTOSOL:

Ethanol + NAD$^+$ $\longrightarrow$ Acetaldehyde + NADH + H$^+$

(Consequences: Cytosol NADH/NAD increases 3-4
times. Acetaldehyde concentration in blood
increases to 10-20 μM).

MITOCHONDRIA:

Acetaldehyde + NAD$^+$ $\longrightarrow$ Acetate + NADH + H$^+$

(Consequences: Mitochondrial NADH/NAD
increases 2-3 times. Acetate concentration in
blood increases to about 1 mM).

Fig. 1   *Metabolism of ethanol at low concentrations.*

two peptide chains, which may be identical or slightly different, and in the
human liver at least nine different isoenzymes have been demonstrated.

In order to keep the oxidation of ethanol to acetaldehyde going
efficiently it is necessary to remove the two products, NADH and
acetaldehyde. The latter is oxidized preferentially in the mitochondria via
an enzyme with a very low K_m (less than 1 μM). This keeps the acetaldehyde
concentration low, while the acetate concentration increases to about 1 mM.
The considerable production of NADH in the cytoplasm poses some very
general questions. NADH cannot just pass into the mitochondria and be
oxidized via the respiratory chain. The concentration of NADH increases up
to the point where the ADH reaction is slowed down sufficiently to ensure
removal of all the NADH formed. In general this concentration is 3-4 times
the normal level.

ADH is not the only enzyme catalyzing the oxidation of ethanol to
acetaldehyde (Fig. 2). At higher concentrations, above about 20 mM,
oxidation by means of catalase and MEOS may play a role. In rat liver cells
it has been shown that at 80 mM ethanol the non-ADH ethanol oxidation
(measured after inhibition with 4-methylpyrazole) is about 2 μmole/g/min,
approximately the total rate observed at 5 mM ethanol. But the relative
magnitude of the two reactions was not determined (4). The rate of the
three systems in vivo might be evaluated by determination of the isotope
effect with tritium labelled ethanol, provided there are suitable differences
in the magnitude of this effect. The splitting of a hydrogen-carbon bond is
highly dependent on the hydrogen isotope involved. In the case of tritium

1. Catalase

$$(NADPH + H^+ + O_2 \longrightarrow H_2O_2 + NADP^+)$$

$$H_2O_2 + \text{ethanol} \longrightarrow \text{acetaldehyde} + H_2O$$

2. MEOS

$$NADPH + O_2 + \text{ethanol} + H^+ \longrightarrow NADP^+ +$$

$$\text{acetaldehyde} + 2H_2O$$

*Fig. 2   Additional reactions of ethanol metabolism at higher
concentrations.*

the rate is theoretically about 18 times slower than for protium. However,
the splitting reaction is rarely totally rate limiting in an enzymatic process.
Therefore the isotope effect, defined as the ratio of the velocity constants
for hydrogen and tritium, may be different for similar overall reactions
catalyzed by different enzymes. We have initiated a program to determine
the isotope effect under physiological conditions for the three reactions
already mentioned. We have confirmed the findings of Gang et al. that the
specificity of the three reactions is the same, i.e. the hydrogen atom split
off from ethanol has the same steric position in all three cases, tritium
being liberated when present in the R-position of ethanol but not when
present in the S-position (5). In the case of ADH, Damgaard found an
isotope effect of about four when initial conditions were used, in agreement
with the findings of some other workers (6, 7, 8, Fig. 3). However, when
acetaldehyde was added in concentrations near those found in vivo the
isotope effect decreased to about 1.2, (Figure 4). The reason for this is that
in the presence of acetaldehyde the back reaction proceeds at a considerable
rate and preferentially involves the unlabelled NADH. The latter reacts
with acetaldehyde and the specific radioactivity of the NAD ^{3}H increases.
In experiments with the perfused rat liver, we also found isotope effects of
this order at low ethanol concentrations (9).

Damgaard has studied both rat liver and ox liver catalase by means of a
number of different techniques (6). In the experiment shown in Fig. 5,
H_2O_2 was generated by means of glucose oxidation at a known rate. The
rate of the overall reaction was measured by having ADH and NADH in the
cuvette so that the rate of aldehyde formation could be directly followed
spectrophotometrically. The isotopic reaction was measured by the tritium
liberated into water. An isotope effect of 2.3 was found under different
conditions with both rat and ox liver catalase. The kinetics of this reaction
are quite complex, as the velocity depends on both ethanol concentration
and the ratio of hydrogen peroxide formation per molecule of catalase heme.
Table I shows the results obtained with rat liver catalase, when these factors
are changed within the physiological range. Similar studies on MEOS are in
progress but it is too early to say whether this approach can be made into a
practically useful method.

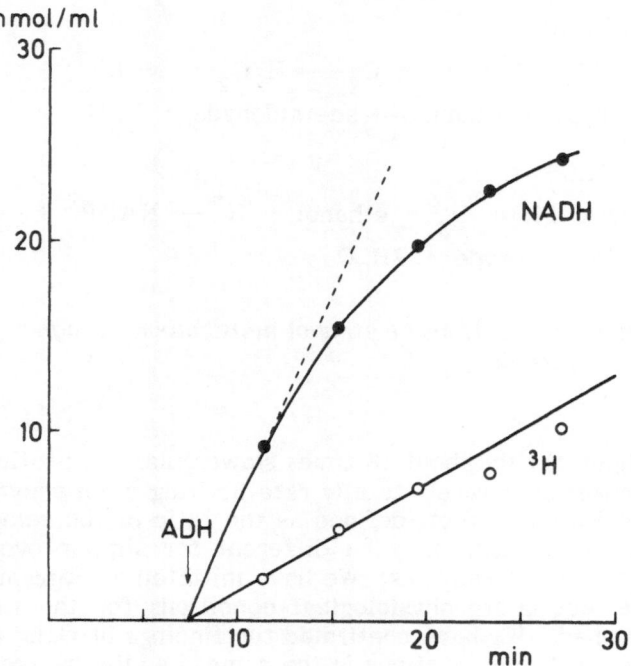

Fig. 3   *Isotope effect with horse liver alcohol dehydrogenase. $R-1-^3H-$*
              ethanol was used at a concentration of 7 mM. Temperature 37^0,
              pH 7.0. The reaction was started by addition of the enzyme.
              Filled circles: NADH production; Open circles: tritium present
              in NADH; measured after paper chromatography on samples to
              which excess 4-methyl pyrazole was added. $NADH/^3H = 3.83$
              (S. Damgaard).

Oxygen Uptake

The supplementary pathways for alcohol metabolism may be expected
not to give rise to the same number of ATP molecules as the ADH pathway,
as neither catalatic peroxidation, nor MEOS appears to be coupled to ATP
formation. A number of nutrients are compared with regard to the yield of
ATP in Table II. Provided that the need for ATP governs the O_2 uptake one
would expect a considerable thermic effect (specific dynamic action) of
ethanol. Especially at high concentrations an effect of the same order of
magnitude as for amino acids would be expected. There are indeed some
indications in the literature that an increased metabolism may be observed
after ingestion of ethanol. For instance Stoke and Stuart found a 13%
increase in oxygen uptake when whisky was taken together with a light meal
(10). When based on the rate of alcohol metabolism this would correspond to
an effect of 32%. A significant effect was also observed in the rat by these
authors and by others (11).

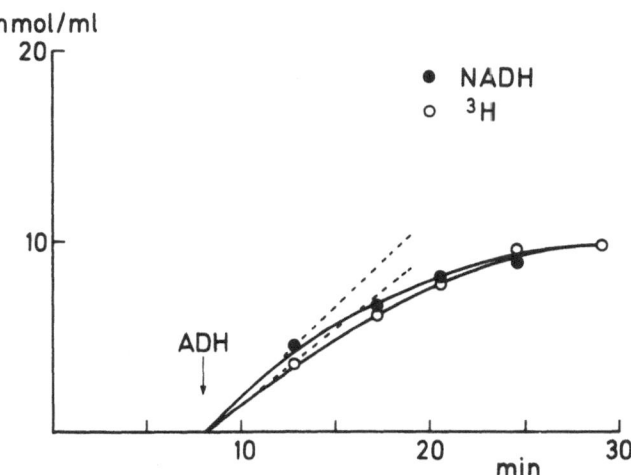

Fig. 4   Same procedure as in Fig. 3, but acetaldehyde was present at a
            concentration of 70 μM.   (S. Damgaard).

Variation of the Rate of Ethanol Metabolism

Fate of Reducing Equivalents

The reoxidation of NADH produced in the cytosol has been a major
problem in the more academic studies on alcohol metabolism. In general
those processes in the cytosol will not be sufficient to account for the actual
NADH oxidation. Oxidation of NADH via the respiratory chain located in
the mitochondria must also be involved. In order to account for such a
process several transport (shuttle) systems have been postulated. The
principle is that the substrate is reduced by NADH in the cytosolic
compartment to a substance which can penetrate the mitochondria and be
oxidized intramitochondrially. A simple system is the glycerol phosphate
cycle in which dihydroxyacetone phosphate is reduced by NADH in the
cytosol to glycerol phosphate which can penetrate the mitochondria and be
reoxidized intramitochondrially to dihydroxyacetone phosphate, which is
returned to the cytosol. The intramitochondrial enzyme has a rather high
K_m towards glycerol phosphate but the concentration of glycerol phosphate
increases very markedly during alcohol metabolism. Another mechanism is
the malate shuttle, in which oxaloacetate is the metabolite reduced by
cytosolic NADH.   As the transport of oxaloacetate through the mitochondrial membrane appears to be slow a transaminase step is probably
inserted as an intermediate process. In this case aspartate will be the
substance actually passing through the membrane.   A third somewhat
complex mechanism involves elongation of fatty acids by acetyl-CoA in the
mitochondrial membrane by means of extramitochondrial NADH, and
subsequent partial oxidation within the mitochondria to the original

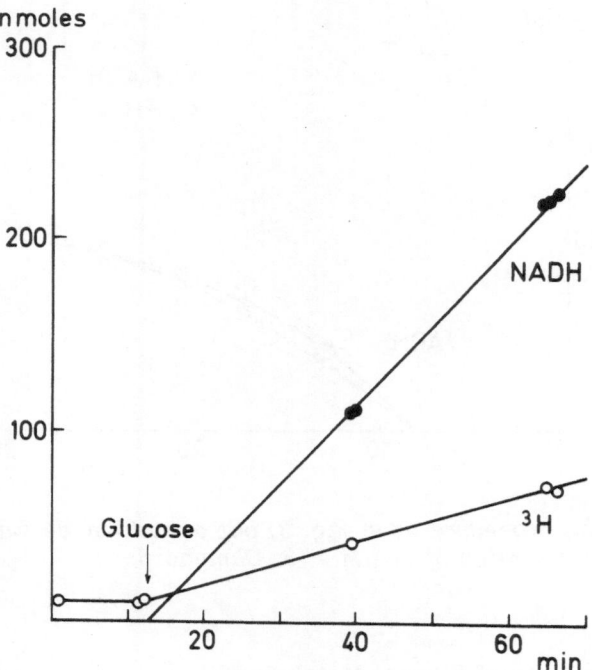

Fig. 5   *Isotope effect in the peroxidation of ethanol by rat liver catalase. R-1-^{3}H-ethanol was used at a concentration of 7 mM. Hydrogen peroxide was generated by glucose oxidase. Acetaldehyde production was measured by means of ADH and NADH (filled circles). Tritium liberation was measured in the water (open circles). NADH/^{3}H = 2.55 (S. Damgaard).*

TABLE I

RAT LIVER CATALASE

ETHANOL CONC.	H_2O_2/e	k_H/k_T
(mM)		
0.5	25	2.55
0.6	0.6	2.1
7	7	2.46
85	1	2.29
	AVERAGE	2.35

(S. DAMGAARD)

TABLE II

YIELD OF ATP IN OXIDATION OF
ETHANOL AND OTHER NUTRIENTS

SUBSTRATE	ATP PRODUCTION	
	mol/mol	mmol/kcal
GLUCOSE	38	56
TRIPALMITIN	409	54
AMINO ACIDS (mean of 11)		45
ETHANOL, MAX.	16	49
ETHANOL, MIN.	13	40

chainlength. Apparently this system works in a model system with isolated mitochondria (12). The relative importance of these systems is difficult to evaluate but starvation induced deficiency of some of the metabolites involved (malate, oxaloacetate, pyruvate) can reduce the rate of alcohol oxidation. Isolated liver cells prepared from rats fasted for 48 hours oxidize ethanol at a rate which is about half that measured in cells from fed rats. Characteristically, the addition of fructose, which provides a high intracellular concentration of pyruvate and other intermediary metabolites, causes the rate of ethanol oxidation to increase in the fasted, but not in the fed hepatocytes. Meijer et al. have suggested that in fasted rats the rate limiting factor for ethanol oxidation is the capacity of the shuttle mechanism(s), while in fed rats it is the availability of ADP for oxidative phosphorylation (13). In agreement with this theory, uncouplers of oxidative phosphorylation have no effect on the ethanol consumption of cells from starved rats, but do have a significant effect in the case of hepatocytes from fed rats. It should be kept in mind however that there are considerable differences between species with regard to the proportion of the total hepatic ADH activity which is actually used for alcohol oxidation. If this proportion is high there will be little room for increasing alcohol metabolism by this pathway.

The question has been raised whether shuttle mechanisms are always required (14). The presence of MEOS and to some extent the catalase pathway should reduce the need for transfer of reducing equivalents into mitochondria (Fig. 2). As the coenzyme used in these processes is NADPH, a mechanism is required for transhydrogenation from NADH to $NADP^+$. A possibility is the cycle shown in Fig. 6 in which the malic enzyme is involved. The transhydrogenation requires expenditure of one molecule of ATP for the carboxylation of pyruvate. Evidence for such a situation has been obtained by Selmer and Grunnet in isolated hepatocytes (4). These

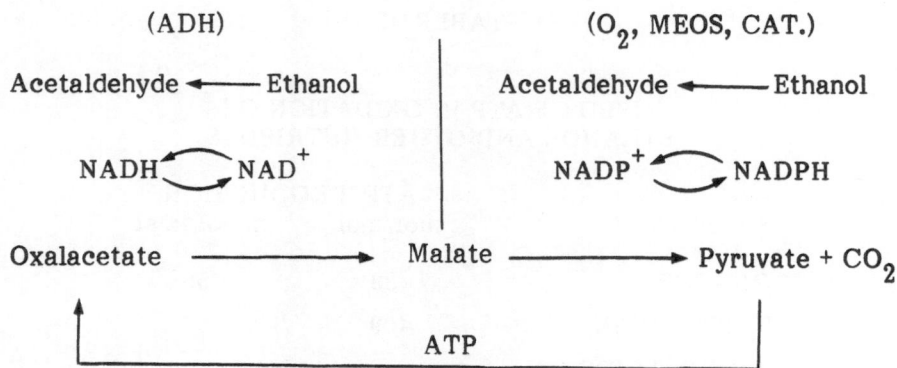

Fig. 6   Simultaneous oxidation of ethanol by ADH (NAD⁺) and NADH requiring pathways. If the two reactions proceed at identical rates no net transport of reducing equivalents from or to the mitochondria is required.

authors demonstrated a net transfer of hydrogen from mitochondria to cytosol at high ethanol concentrations (80 mM), when the ADH pathway was inhibited by 4-methylpyrazole. Another outlet for the excess cytosolic hydrogen is fatty acid synthesis. Grunnet has calculated that in the case of fed rats fatty acid synthesis requires an amount of reducing equivalents, which is of the same order of magnitude as that produced from ethanol at low concentrations (14). However, in fasted rats there does seem to be a definite need for shuttle mechanisms which can transfer hydrogen from the cytosol into mitochondria.

INCREASED NADH CONCENTRATION CAUSES

Increased metabolite ratio: red/ox.

- glycerol phosphate concentration
- glutamate concentration
- glucose production from fructose

Decreased gluconeogenesis from lactate

- glycerol uptake
- galactose uptake

Fig. 7

Effect of Ethanol on Metabolic Processes in the Liver

An increased NADH/NAD ratio in the liver induces a variety of metabolic effects (Fig. 7). The primary observation is that redox processes mediated by NAD/NADH are displaced in favour of the reduced component. This is the case both in the cytosol and in the mitochondrial compartment. For instance, the pyruvate concentration falls and that of glycerol phosphate rises. The fall in pyruvate concentration in turn influences the rate of gluconeogenesis from lactate, as the compulsory step, carboxylation of pyruvate, is dependent on the pyruvate concentration (15). This is believed to be the cause of alcoholic hypoglycemia in starved individuals.

Similarly, the increased concentration of glycerol phosphate may increase the esterification of fatty acids. Kondrup has studied the metabolism of labelled palmitate in the perfused rat liver (16). Table III shows that the uptake of palmitate is increased significantly by ethanol. This increase is the result of increased palmitate esterification, oxidation of the fatty acid to CO_2 and ketone bodies being reduced to about one-half (Table IV). The extent of these changes seems to be independent of the ethanol concentration. Release of triglycerides into the perfusate was apparently not influenced at low ethanol concentrations, but at 80 mM was reduced considerably, (Table V). The reasons for this are quite complicated and will not be discussed here.

In the case of carbohydrate metabolism the situation seems to be more clear. Thus glycerol uptake is inhibited by ethanol, largely as a consequence of glycerol kinase inhibition by the high glycerol phosphate concentration.

TABLE III

^{14}C-1 PALMITATE UPTAKE IN PERFUSED RAT LIVER

(μmol/min/liver)

ETHANOL CONC.	0	10 mM	80 mM
PALMITATE CONC.			
0.2 mM (3)	0.74	0.70	0.78
1.0 mM (6)	3.42	3.93*	3.87*

*$P < 0.05$

(J. KONDRUP)

TABLE IV

ESTERIFICATION AND OXIDATION OF ^{14}C-PALMITATE
IN PERFUSED RAT LIVER

(μmoles/min/liver)

ETHANOL	0	10mM		80 mM	
0.2 mM PALMITATE (3)					
ESTERIFICATION	0.76	0.75		0.72	
OXIDATION	0.05	0.02*		0.02	
1.0 mM PALMITATE (6)					
ESTERIFICATION	2.71	3.47*	(+0.76)	3.67*	(+0.96)
OXIDATION	0.68	0.37*	(−0.31)	0.27*	(−0.41)
UPTAKE	3.42	3.93*	(+0.51)	3.87*	(+0.45)

*P < 0.05

(J. KONDRUP)

TABLE V

RELEASE OF TRIGLYCERIDE FROM RAT
LIVER PERFUSED WITH 1 mM PALMITATE

	GLYCERIDE–GLYCEROL
	(nmoles/min/liver)
CONTROLS (3)	41.6 ± 4.1
10 mM ETHANOL (6)	38.8 ± 6.4
80 mM ETHANOL (6)	26.2* ± 4.8

*P < 0.005

(J. KONDRUP)

$$\text{Galactose} + \text{ATP} \longrightarrow \text{Galactose-1-phosphate}$$

$$\text{Galact.-1-phosph.} + \text{UDP-G} \rightleftharpoons \text{Glucose-1-phosph.} + \text{UDP-Gal}$$

$$\text{UDP-Gal} \rightleftharpoons \text{UDP-G}$$

$$\text{NADH}$$

Fig. 8   Mechanism of inhibition of galactose metabolism by ethanol.

Galactose uptake is also inhibited and the mechanism well understood as illustrated in Fig. 8. The epimerase catalyzing the interconversion of UDP-glucose and UDP-galactose is inhibited by NADH. As the rate of galactose-1-phosphate formation is rather high this means that galactose-1-phosphate accumulates in the liver cells. This sugar phosphate is a strong inhibitor of galactokinase, so the first and irreversible step in galactose metabolism will be inhibited.

Ethanol metabolism also increases the concentration of AMP, possibly as a result of acetate activation, and some of the consequences of this for liver metabolism are shown in Fig. 9. AMP is an important regulatory factor in carbohydrate metabolism and is also the main precursor of uric acid, a subject to be discussed in other chapters.

In this review the metabolic consequences of prolonged alcohol intake or the pathological changes resulting from alcohol abuse have not been discussed as these subjects are treated in other chapters.

INCREASED AMP CONCENTRATION CAUSES

Decreased	-	glycerol uptake
	-	glycogen synthesis
Increased	-	uric acid synthesis
	-	glycogenolysis (?)

INCREASED ACETALDEHYDE CONCENTRATION CAUSES

Inhibition of oxidation of aldehydes

Changes in catecholamine metabolism.

Fig. 9

REFERENCES

1. MELLANBY E: Alcohol, its absorption into and disappearance from the blood under different conditions. Medical Research Committee, Special Report Series No. 31, London, 1919

2. WIDMARK EM: Die theoretischen Grundlagen und die praktische Verwendbarkeit der gerichtlich-medizinischen Alkoholbestimmung. Berlin, Urban and Schwarzenberg, 1932

3. LUNDSGAARD E: Alcohol oxidation as a function of the liver. C.R. Trav Lab Carlsberg, Ser Chim 22: 333-337, 1938

4. SELMER J, GRUNNET N: Ethanol metabolism and lipid synthesis by isolated liver cells from fed rats. Biochim Biophys Acta 428: 123-137, 1976

5. GANG H, CEDERBAUM AI, RUBIN E: Stereospecificity of ethanol oxidation. Bioch Biophys Res Comm 54: 264-269, 1973

6. DAMGAARD S: In preparation

7. SIMON H, PALM D: Isotopeneffekte in der organischen Chemie und Biochemie. Angewandte Chemie 78: 993-1028, 1966

8. GERSHMAN H, ABELES RH: Deuterium isotope effects in the oxidation of alcohols in vitro and in vivo. Arch Bioch Biophys 154: 659-674, 1973

9. DAMGAARD S, SESTOFT L, LUNDQUIST F: The use of tritium and ^{14}C labelled ethanol in studies of ethanol metabolism at high ethanol concentrations. In Alcohol Intoxication and Withdrawal II. MM Gross (ed.). New York, Plenum Press, 1975. pp. 111-119

10. STOKE MJ, STUART JA: Thermic effects of ethanol in the rat and man. Nutr and Metab 17: 297-305, 1974

11. PIROLA RC, LIEBER CS: Energy wastage in rats given drugs that induce microsomal enzymes. J Nutr 105: 1544-1548, 1975

12. GRUNNET N: Oxidation of extramitochondrial NADH by rat liver mitochondria. Possible role of acyl-SCoA elongation enzymes. Bioch Biophys Res Comm 41: 909-917, 1970

13. MEIJER AJ, VAN WOERKOM GM, WILLIAMSON JR, TAGER JM: Rate-limiting factors in the oxidation of ethanol by isolated rat liver cells. Biochem J 150: 205-209, 1975

14. GRUNNET N: Mechanism for transfer of reducing equivalents (as NADH) from the cytosol to mitochondria and the need for such transfer in ethanol metabolism. In <u>Regulation of Hepatic Metabolism.</u> F Lundquist, N Tygstrup (eds.). Copenhagen, Munksgaard 1974. pp. 520-529

15. KREBS HA, FRIEDLAND RA, HEMS R, STUBBS M: Inhibition of hepatic gluconeogenesis by ethanol. <u>Biochem J 112</u>: 117-124, 1969

16. KONDRUP J: In preparation

THE ROLE OF ETHANOL METABOLITES IN HEPATIC LIPID PEROXIDATION

N. R. Di Luzio and T. E. Stege

Department of Physiology, Tulane University School of Medicine

New Orleans, Louisiana 70112

INTRODUCTION

The spectrum of alcoholic liver injury comprises three major disorders, namely fatty liver, alcoholic hepatitis and cirrhosis (1). Because the fatty liver is readily inducible in both patients and experimental animals, and is the initial event in alcohol-induced hepatic pathology, it has been the most extensively studied aspect of alcoholic liver disease. The increased lipid is primarily in the form of triglycerides and it is entirely reversible upon discontinuation of alcohol abuse (2). In spite of intensive investigative efforts, the pathogenesis of the alcohol-induced fatty liver has not yet been fully resolved (1, 3).

In the early 1960's our laboratory demonstrated that the ethanol-induced fatty liver could be prevented by the administration of antioxidants which inhibit lipid peroxidation (4). The hypothesis was advanced at that time that hepatic injury from ethanol might be due to lipid peroxidation. Since then the occurrence of lipid peroxidation in liver homogenates following ethanol administration has been reported by a number of laboratories (5, 6, 7, 8). The lipid peroxidation concept of ethanol-induced fatty liver predicates a free radical event associated with ethanol metabolism rather than ethanol per se as the mechanism of hepatic injury. In an effort to evaluate this concept, pyrazole, an inhibitor of alcohol dehydrogenase, has been recently employed to block ethanol metabolism (9, 10). The administration of ethanol to pyrazole treated rats resulted in sustained elevations in blood ethanol and gross intoxication (9), but the classical ethanol-induced fatty liver did not occur (11, 12). These results stress that metabolites of ethanol oxidation such as acetate or acetaldehyde, or alterations induced by ethanol metabolism such as the redox changes imposed on the liver cell may contribute to the ethanol-induced liver injury, as reflected by fatty liver development.

TABLE I

BLOOD ETHANOL AND ACETALDEHYDE LEVELS IN ANIMALS PRETREATED WITH DISULFIRAM OR PYRAZOLE PRIOR TO ETHANOL ADMINISTRATION[a,b]

Pretreatment	Six Hours Following Ethanol		Sixteen Hours Following Ethanol	
	Blood Acetaldehyde (mg%)	Blood Ethanol (mg%)	Blood Acetaldehyde (mg%)	Blood Ethanol (mg%)
Saline	0.36 ± 0.05	375 ± 45	0.20 ± 0.03	153 ± 29
Pyrazole	0.44 ± 0.03	$512 \pm 38*$	0.32 ± 0.10	$491 \pm 32*$
Disulfiram	$0.86 \pm 0.06*$	$553 \pm 40*$	$0.77 \pm 0.07*$	$274 \pm 26*$

[a]Disulfiram (60 mg/100 g body wt) orally, or pyrazole (50 mg/100 g body wt) intraperitoneally was administered 16 hours prior to the oral administration of ethanol (6 g/kg body wt).

[b]All data represent the mean ± standard error of 9 animals. Determinations were made in duplicate. Ethanol and acetaldehyde concentrations were determined using a gas chromatograph.

*Indicates significance $p < 0.05$ over saline–ethanol animals.

In the present study ethanol metabolites were assessed in vivo for their role in the development of both a fatty liver and the induction of lipid peroxidation by employing pyrazole, an inhibitor of alcohol dehydrogenase, and disulfiram, and inhibitor of aldehyde dehydrogenase. Acetate was also administered in vivo to evaluate its ability to induce a fatty liver as well as hepatic lipid peroxidation. Additionally, acetate, ethanol and acetaldehyde were further assessed for their capacity to induce lipid peroxidation in vitro by incubation with liver homogenates. Finally, hepatic lipid peroxidation was evaluated in animals with impaired liver function resulting from a chronic ethanol diet.

METHODS

Female Sprague-Dawley rats previously maintained on Purina lab chow and water ad libitum were fasted overnight prior to treatment. Animals were pre-treated with disulfiram (Ayerst, 60 mg/100 g body weight) in saline orally, or pyrazole (K&K Laboratories, 50 mg/100 g body weight) in saline intraperitoneally 16 hours prior to ethanol. Ethanol (131 mM/kg or 6 g/kg body weight) in a 40% saline solution was administered orally and animals sacrificed 2, 6, or 16 hours later. Blood alcohol and acetaldehyde levels were measured with a Carle flame ionization gas chromatograph using a modification of the method of Druitz and Truitt (13). Thiobarbituric acid (TBA) assays for malonaldehyde (MDA) were carried out according to Comporti et al (6). Lipid peroxidation measurements using chemiluminescence were performed on the supernatant from 30% wt/vol liver homogenates which were centrifuged at 500 x g at $0°C$ for ten minutes. Two ml of the resulting supernatant plus 5 ml of 0.15 M potassium phosphate buffer (pH 7.4) and 3 ml of 0.15 M potassium chloride were incubated in scintillation vials under air at $37°C$ in a Dubnoff Shaker. Chemiluminescence, as a reflection of lipid peroxidation, was evaluated using a Nuclear-Chicago Mark I liquid scintillation spectrophotometer in the out-of-coincidence mode at $10°C$ (14).

Female Sprague-Dawley rats with an average initial body weight of 120 g were maintained for 3 weeks on a chronic ethanol diet of liquid Metrecal (15) in which 50% of the total calories were derived from either sucrose, laboratory ethanol or Old Crow bourbon (86 proof). This diet was supplemented with sodium caseinate to insure a protein content of 22% of the total calories.

Plasma BSP retention was determined using a modification of the technique of Casals and Olitsky (16). Rats were administered 5 mg/100 g body weight BSP in the tail vein and blood samples were taken from the inferior vena cava 30 minutes later. Liver triglycerides were determined by the method of Van Handle and Zilversmit (17) and protein concentrations were determined according to the method of Lowry et al (18). Lipid soluble antioxidants were determined following the methods of Glavind (19).

Data are expressed as the mean ± standard error and group means were compared using the Student's test at 95% level of confidence.

RESULTS

As expected, animals pretreated with pyrazole or disulfiram showed blood ethanol levels which were significantly increased over control values 6 hours following ethanol (Table I). Sixteen hours following ethanol the blood ethanol levels of the pyrazole pretreated animals remained elevated. However, at 16 hours following ethanol, animals pretreated with disulfiram showed blood ethanol levels which, although significantly elevated over ethanol controls, were markedly reduced when compared to 6 hour levels of animals pretreated with disulfiram.

Animals pretreated with disulfiram had blood acetaldehyde levels which were 2-fold greater than ethanol and pyrazole-ethanol treated animals at 6 and 16 hours. Sixteen hours following ethanol, the blood acetaldehyde level of the ethanol control animals was reduced to 50% of its 6 hour level.

Animals administered ethanol developed significant increases in liver triglycerides over saline controls at both the 6 and 16 hour intervals (Table II). The fatty liver induced by ethanol was prevented by pretreatment with pyrazole. Animals pretreated with disulfiram, on the other hand, developed significant increases in liver triglycerides whether subsequently treated with either ethanol or saline. Liver triglycerides at the 6 hour and 16 hour intervals in disulfiram pretreated animals were increased 2-fold over saline controls.

Liver homogenates from rats pretreated with saline, pyrazole or disulfiram and sacrificed 2 or 6 hours following ethanol administration were evaluated for lipid peroxidation via the thiobarbituric acid (TBA) assay (Table III). Liver homogenates prepared from animals which received ethanol alone manifested a significant 2-fold increase in the production of malonaldehyde (MDA) over saline controls at the two hour interval. Six hours following ethanol treatment, however, the 50% increase in MDA in the ethanol animals was not statistically significant over saline controls.

Animals pretreated with disulfiram and later treated with saline showed no significant difference in MDA production from saline controls at both 2 and 6 hour intervals. However, animals receiving disulfiram and subsequently administered ethanol exhibited significantly increased MDA production over disulfiram controls at both the 2 and 6 hour intervals. Six hours following ethanol, animals pretreated with disulfiram had MDA increases 3-fold greater than controls.

Animals which received pretreatment with pyrazole and subsequently with saline developed significant increases in hepatic MDA levels over saline controls at both the 2 and 6 hour intervals. Livers from animals which were pretreated with pyrazole and later administered ethanol demonstrated marked decreases in MDA production at the 2 and 6 hour interval when compared to pyrazole-saline treated animals. TBA assays of the pyrazole-ethanol animals at the 6 hour interval were comparable to results from saline-saline control animals.

TABLE II

LIVER TRIGLYCERIDES OF ANIMALS PRETREATED WITH DISULFIRAM OR PYRAZOLE PRIOR TO ETHANOL ADMINISTRATION[a,b]

Pretreatment	Treatment	N	Six Hours Following Ethanol mg/g	mg/liver	N	Sixteen Hours Following Ethanol mg/g	mg/liver
Saline	Saline	27	4.5 ± 0.5	30.3 ± 4.0	19	3.9 ± 1.0	24.4 ± 6.2
Saline	Ethanol	30	7.8 ± 0.7*	64.4 ± 6.0*	23	12.4 ± 1.7*	86.0 ± 10.9
Pyrazole	Saline	16	4.4 ± 0.8	35.8 ± 7.2	17	2.5 ± 0.4	19.2 ± 2.3
Pyrazole	Ethanol	17	5.7 ± 0.9	40.9 ± 6.4	18	3.1 ± 0.5	23.6 ± 3.0
Disulfiram	Saline	25	8.1 ± 0.9*	72.5 ± 10.1*	17	11.8 ± 1.9*	86.5 ± 13.9*
Disulfiram	Ethanol	27	10.5 ± 1.1*	89.8 ± 8.5*	18	9.3 ± 1.1*	71.8 ± 8.6

[a]Disulfiram (60 mg/100 g body wt) orally, and pyrazole (50 mg/100 g body wt) intraperitoneally were administered 16 hours prior to the oral administration of ethanol (6 g/kg).

[b]Data are expressed as the mean of N animals ± standard error.

*Indicates significance ($p < 0.01$) over saline – saline controls.

TABLE III

LIPID PEROXIDATION IN LIVER HOMOGENATES MEASURED BY
THE THIOBARBITURIC ACID (TBA) ASSAY[a,b]

Pretreatment	Treatment	N	Two Hours Following Ethanol μg Malonaldehyde/g	N	Six Hours Following Ethanol μg Malonaldehyde/g
Saline	Saline	12	15.0 ± 1.7	9	16.8 ± 2.7
Saline	Ethanol	11	37.0 ± 8.9*	9	26.6 ± 5.1
Disulfiram	Saline	6	29.0 ± 5.9	10	20.0 ± 3.8
Disulfiram	Ethanol	7	41.5 ± 15.3	11	69.9 ± 17.9*
Pyrazole	Saline	5	54.6 ± 22.7*	8	45.3 ± 13.6*
Pyrazole	Ethanol	5	34.7 ± 16.5	7	19.4 ± 6.5

[a]All data are expressed as the mean of N experiments run in duplicate ± standard error and represent malonaldehyde (MDA) production in liver homogenates after 120 minutes of incubation at 37°C.

[b]Disulfiram (60 mg/100 g body wt) orally and pyrazole (60 mg/100 g body wt) intraperitoneally were administered 16 hours prior to the oral administration of ethanol (6 g/kg body wt).

*Indicates significance ($p < 0.05$) over saline-saline controls.

Recently a more convenient and sensitive method to measure lipid peroxidation employing photon emissions or chemiluminescence has been developed in our laboratory (14). Since Baumgartner et al (20) have demonstrated that acetaldehyde can interfere with the determination of malonaldehyde as analyzed by the TBA assay, inherent limitations exist in the use of the TBA assay in studies of possible ethanol induced peroxidation processes. For these reasons lipid peroxidation measurements on animals pretreated with disulfiram and subsequently treated with ethanol were re-evaluated using this newly developed chemiluminescence procedure. Liver homogenates were centrifuged at 500 x g for ten minutes and the resulting supernatant was incubated with a phosphate buffer in a scintillation vial at 37°C. Photon emission measurements were made on a Nuclear-Chicago Mark I liquid scintillation spectrophotometer operated in the out-of-coincidence mode and results are expressed as cpm/mg protein (Table IV).

TABLE IV

LIPID PEROXIDATION OF LIVER HOMOGENATES
AS MEASURED BY CHEMILUMINESCENCE (cpm/mg Protein)
SIX HOURS FOLLOWING ETHANOL[a]

Treatment[b]	N	Incubation Time		
		0 min	30 min	60 min
Saline	7	35 ± 6	546 ± 371	1,166 ± 699
Ethanol	6	38 ± 10	1,284 ± 446	2,462 ± 764
Disulfiram + Saline	7	60 ± 22	784 ± 364	2,401 ± 811
Disulfiram + Ethanol	7	62 ± 20	1,608 ± 473*	3,554 ± 867*

[a]All data are expressed as the mean of N experiments run in duplicate ± standard error. Each scintillation vial contained 2 ml of liver homogenate supernatant in a final volume of 10 ml incubated under air at 37°C.

[b]Disulfiram (60 mg/100 g) was administered orally to fasted rats 16 hours prior to the oral administration of ethanol (6 g/kg).

*Indicates significance of $p < 0.05$ over saline control.

Animals treated with ethanol alone showed increases in chemiluminescence, although not statistically significant, of greater than 100% over saline controls at both 30 and 60 minute intervals. In agreement with TBA results, liver homogenates from animals pretreated with disulfiram and subsequently administered ethanol demonstrated significantly enhanced chemiluminescence at the 30 and 60 minute incubation intervals over saline controls. Chemiluminescence values of animals pretreated with disulfiram alone were equivalent to saline controls.

Since acetate is one of the major metabolites of hepatic ethanol metabolism, and since Richards et al (21) have implicated acetate as a factor in the ethanol-induced fatty liver, rats were administered acetate in vivo in an effort to evaluate the ability of acetate to induce increased liver triglycerides as well as increased lipid peroxidation. Saline or equimolar sodium acetate or ethanol was administered in 3 doses at four hour intervals. The divided doses of acetate were required due to its toxicity. The animals were sacrificed 16 hours after the final dose and the livers were analyzed for triglyceride content (Table V-A). Animals administered ethanol developed nearly a 4-fold increase in liver triglycerides over saline controls.

TABLE V

A. LIVER TRIGLYCERIDES FROM ANIMALS TREATED WITH ACETATE, ETHANOL OR SALINE[a,b]

Treatment	N	mg/g Liver	mg/Total Liver
Saline	10	1.9 $\pm$ 0.5	11.5 $\pm$ 3.2
Acetate	14	3.9 $\pm$ 0.7*	25.8 $\pm$ 4.6*
Ethanol	14	7.7 $\pm$ 1.1*	46.4 $\pm$ 6.0*

B. CHEMILUMINESCENCE OF LIVER HOMOGENATES FROM RATS TREATED WITH ACETATE OR SALINE[a,b]

Treatment	N	0 min	30 min	60 min
Saline	8	52 $\pm$ 15	277 $\pm$ 96	609 $\pm$ 98
Acetate	8	91 $\pm$ 19	453 $\pm$ 93	846 $\pm$ 98

[a] Ethanol (131 mM/kg or 6 g/kg), sodium acetate (131 mM/kg) or saline were given orally as three equal doses four hours apart. Animals were then sacrificed 16 hours following the last dose for triglyceride analysis or 2 hours following last dose for chemiluminescence measurements (cpm/mg protein). For chemiluminescence, 2 ml of liver homogenate supernatant was incubated at $37^\circ C$ in a total volume of 10 ml.

[b] All data are expressed as the mean of N animals $\pm$ standard error.

[c] Indicates significance $p < 0.05$ over saline control.

Acetate administration also resulted in a significant increase in liver triglycerides over the saline control. However, the acetate-induced increase in liver triglycerides was only half as great as that induced by an equimolar dose of ethanol. Hepatic lipid peroxidation measurements using chemiluminescence were made on animals treated with 3 doses of saline or acetate and sacrificed 2 hours following the final dose (Table V-B). Animals administered acetate exhibited no significant difference in levels of hepatic lipid peroxidation over saline controls.

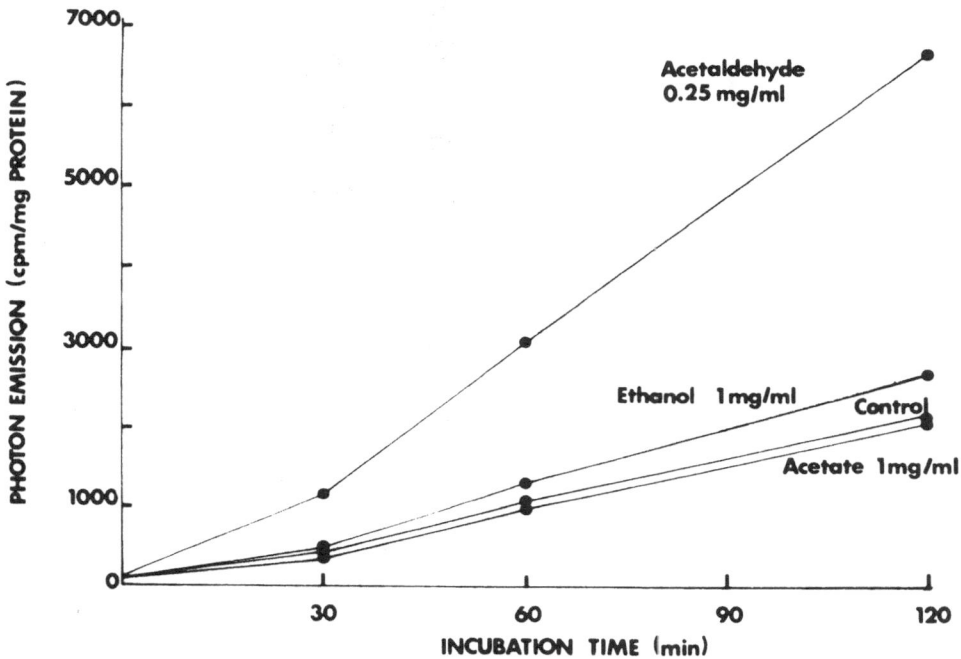

Fig. 1   *In vitro* chemiluminescence in liver homogenates incubated with
          ethanol, sodium acetate or acetaldehyde. Data are expressed as
          the mean of three experiments run in duplicate. Each vial
          contained two ml of liver homogenate supernatant in a total
          volume of 10 ml. Ethanol, sodium acetate, or acetaldehyde
          were added at the start of the incubation and the vials sealed.
          Incubation temperature was $37^{\circ}C$.

The lipid peroxidation capacity of ethanol, acetate and acetaldehyde
was also assessed in vitro using chemiluminescence. When either ethanol
(100 mg%) or sodium acetate (100 mg%) was incubated with liver
homogenates, no significant difference from control values resulted at any
time period, (Figure 1). However, when acetaldehyde (25 mg%) was
incubated with liver homogenates, significant increases ($p < 0.05$) in
chemiluminescence resulted at the 60 and 120 minute intervals.

When varying concentrations of acetaldehyde were incubated for 60
minutes with liver homogenates, increases in chemiluminescence (expressed
as the change in cpm/mg protein over control) were directly related to
increasing concentrations of acetaldehyde (Figure 2). This enhanced
chemiluminescence could be significantly blocked by glutathione, an
antioxidant which inhibits lipid peroxidation. When glutathione (100 mg%)
was added to liver homogenates containing acetaldehyde (25%), chemiluminescence was significantly reduced (Table VI).

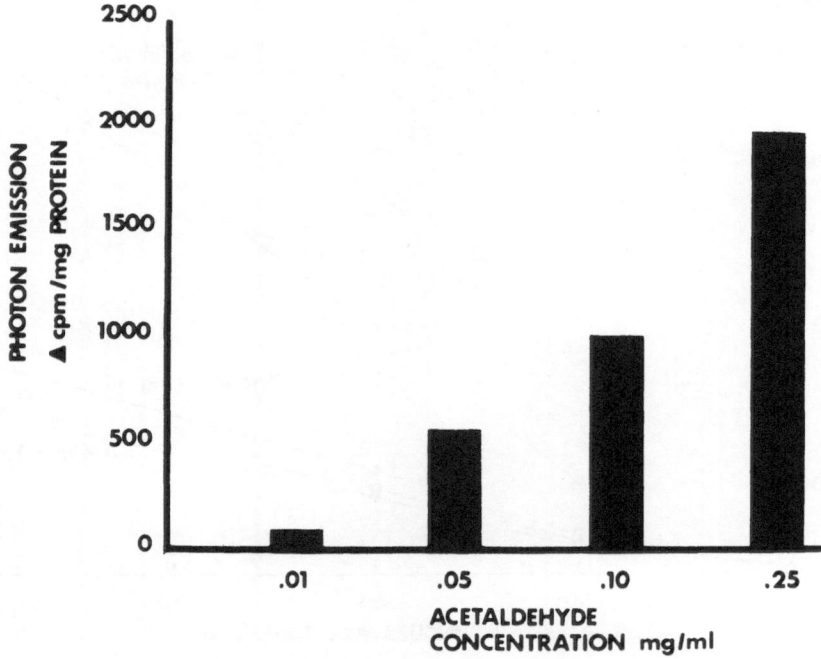

Fig. 2   *Increased chemiluminescence in liver homogenates after 60*
minutes incubation with various concentrations of acetaldehyde.
Data are expressed as the mean difference (Δ) in cpm from
control liver homogenates in 3 separate experiments run in
duplicate.   Each scintillation vial contained 2 ml of liver
homogenate supernatant in a total volume of 10 ml. Acetalde-
hyde concentrations were added at the start of incubation and
the vials sealed. Incubation temperature was 37°C.

Central to the concept of ethanol-induced liver injury is the chronic abuse of ethanol (1, 3, 22). Therefore, a chronic ethanol diet was evaluated for its ability first to induce liver damage and secondly to induce hepatic lipid peroxidation. The chronic ethanol diet employed consisted of a liquid Metrecal diet (15) in which 50% of the calories were derived from sucrose, laboratory ethanol, or bourbon (86 proof). Animals on the sucrose diet grew in 3 weeks to a mean weight of 200± 5 g. Animals on the ethanol or bourbon diet grew to a mean body weight of 140 ± 4 g. Over the last 2 weeks of the diet, the ethanol intake per rat averaged 15± 2 g/kg/day. Evaluation of liver function revealed significant alterations in both the ethanol and bourbon groups (Table VII). BSP retention was four times greater in the bourbon and ethanol animals than in the sucrose controls. Liver triglycerides were also significantly elevated in the chronic ethanol and bourbon groups. Further, both plasma GOT and GPT enzyme levels were increased significantly in the ethanol and bourbon groups. Blood lactate/ pyruvate ratios, an indicator of

TABLE VI

INHIBITION BY GLUTATHIONE OF ACETALDEHYDE-INDUCED
CHEMILUMINESCENCE[a]

Homogenate[b]	Incubation Time	
	0 min	60 min
Control	11 ± 3	510 ± 84
Control + Glutathione	23 ± 10	71 ± 18*
Acetaldehyde	177 ± 25*	2,461 ± 980*
Acetaldehyde + Glutathione	198 ± 13*	73 ± 12*

[a]All data are expressed as the mean cpm/mg protein of four
experiments run in duplicate ± standard error.

*Indicates statistical significance ($p < 0.05$) over control.

[b]Acetaldehyde (25 mg%) and/or glutathione (Sigma reduced form, 100
mg%) were added at the start of incubation to normal liver
homogenates.   Each scintillation vial contained 2 ml of liver
homogenate supernatant in a total volume of 10 ml. Incubation was
at 37°C in an air atmosphere.

metabolic alterations often found following ethanol administration (3, 23)
were also elevated in the ethanol and bourbon groups.   Animals on the
ethanol or bourbon diets also had significantly decreased levels of hepatic
lipid soluble antioxidants.   No significant difference was observed between
the ethanol and bourbon groups.

Animals on the chronic ethanol, bourbon and sucrose diets were also
evaluated for levels of hepatic lipid peroxidation (Figure 3).   Liver
homogenates from animals on ethanol and bourbon diets demonstrated
significantly ($p < 0.05$) higher chemiluminescence over the sucrose controls
at the zero, 30 and 60 minute incubation periods. Enhanced chemiluminescence at the zero time period is suggestive of in vivo hepatic peroxidation
in the ethanol or bourbon groups.

DISCUSSION

Pyrazole pretreatment caused a significant decrease in the ethanol-
induced fatty liver as previously reported (11, 12, 24). In contrast disulfiram

TABLE VII

CHRONIC ETHANOL-INDUCED LIVER ALTERATIONS[a,b]

	Sucrose	Ethanol	Bourbon
Plasma BSP (mg%)	1.6 ± 0.2	6.4* ± 1.4	5.7* ± 1.2
Liver triglycerides, mg/g liver	7.2 ± 1.4	14.8* ± 2.6	14.8* ± 3.6
Liver triglycerides, mg/total liver	49.3 ± 9.0	94.6* ± 13.6	92.1* ± 20.4
Plasma SGOT's (Sigma-Frankle Units)	58 ± 3	78* ± 5	80* ± 6
Plasma SGPT's (Sigma-Frankle Units)	15 ± 1	46* ± 9	56* ± 8
Lactate/Pyruvate Ratios	15 ± 4	23 ± 9	24 ± 6
Hepatic lipid soluble antioxidants (μg antioxidants/g liver)	0.73 ± 0.05	0.58* ± 0.03	0.59* ± 0.04

[a]Diet consisted of Metrecal (Mead Johnson) plus sodium caseinate (to increase protein calories to 22% of total) plus either sucrose, laboratory ethanol, or bourbon (86 proof) as 50% of the total calories. Animals were maintained on the diet for 21 days.

[b]All data are expressed as the mean ± standard error of nine animals.

*Indicates significance $p < 0.05$ over sucrose control.

pretreatment with or without subsequent treatment with ethanol resulted in a fatty liver. Disulfiram induced hepatic lipid alterations may be acetaldehyde-induced. Krebs and Perkins (25) have demonstrated in rats that small but distinct amounts of ethanol are formed continuously by bacteria in the gut. The entrance of this small amount of ethanol into the portal vein alone with the inhibitory effects of disulfiram on acetaldehyde metabolism may result in a fatty liver. Truitt et al (26), using rats, as well as Siegers et al (27), using guinea pigs, have demonstrated that the acute administration of acetaldehyde in vivo results in significant increases in

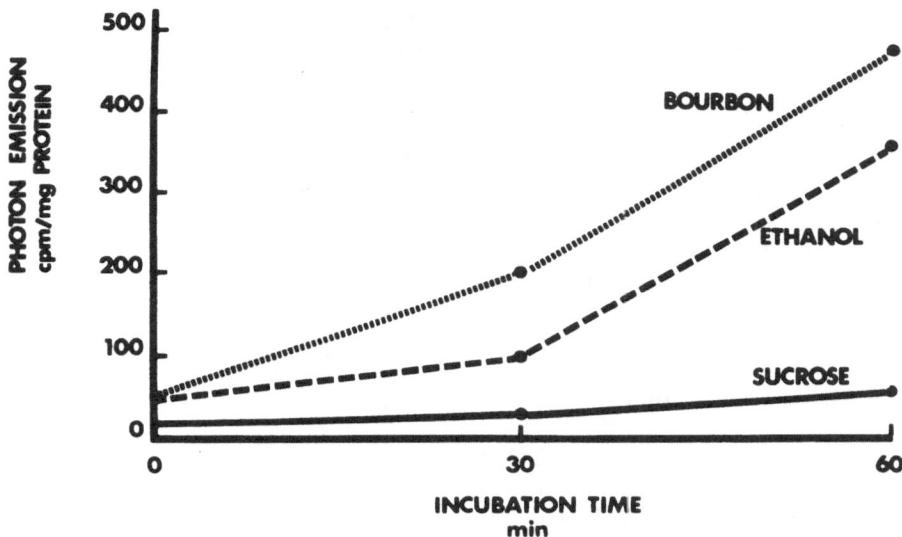

Fig. 3   Chemiluminescence of liver homogenates from animals on a
            chronic ethanol diet. Each point represents the mean of at
            least four experiments run in duplicate. Two ml of liver
            homogenate supernatant was incubated in a total volume of 10
            ml at $37^{\circ}C$. Animals were on the protein supplemented chronic
            ethanol-Metrecal diet for 21 days in which 50% of the calories
            were derived from ethanol, bourbon or sucrose.

liver triglycerides. Richards and co-workers (21), on the other hand,
reported that chronic administration of both disulfiram and ethanol in rats
did not affect liver triglycerides.

The in vivo administration of acetate was also found to increase liver
triglycerides. This is in agreement with previously reported results by
Richards et al (21) who demonstrated a 2-fold increase in liver triglycerides
over saline controls in rats sacrificed 16 hours following oral acetate
administration. Although a major fraction of the acetate derived from
ethanol can be recovered in hepatic venous blood (28), there is evidence that
acetate, like ethanol can inhibit fatty acid oxidation in the liver (29). The
findings suggest that acetate can induce elevated triglycerides and that the
acute ethanol-induced fatty liver may result, at least in part, from acetate
formed via ethanol oxidation.

Our results appear to indicate that acetaldehyde and acetate both
contribute to the ethanol-induced fatty liver. However, this effect may be a
result of the metabolism of acetaldehyde and acetate (i.e. redox changes)
rather than acetaldehyde or acetate per se.

    The enhancement of lipid peroxidation following ethanol administration has been confirmed by other investigators (5, 6, 7, 8, 30). Since pyrazole pretreatment by itself enhanced lipid peroxidation, lipid peroxidation results from pyrazole–ethanol treated animals were inconclusive. The administration of disulfiram, as evaluated by either the TBA or chemiluminescence procedures, had no effect on lipid peroxidation. However, the disulfiram plus ethanol treated animals manifested significantly enhanced hepatic lipid peroxidation, suggesting the possibility that lipid peroxidation may be due to an elevation in acetaldehyde levels. Indeed, acetaldehyde, when incubated in vitro with liver homogenates, resulted in enhanced lipid peroxidation. In contrast, acetate, whether administered in vivo or in vitro, did not demonstrate any capacity for the induction of hepatic lipid peroxidation. These results implicate acetaldehyde to be a major factor in hepatic lipid peroxidation induced by ethanol.

    When hepatic lipid peroxidation levels were measured in rats with liver injury induced by chronic ethanol or bourbon diets, they were signficantly increased over sucrose controls. Liver antioxidant levels were also markedly reduced in the animals on the chronic ethanol or bourbon diets. Studies by Di Luzio (30) have demonstrated that ethanol can modify the antioxidant balance of the liver so that enhanced peroxidation may occur. Thus, following ethanol administration, cellular antioxidants may not normally be present in sufficient quantity to protect the liver from prooxidants which conceivably exist after ethanol metabolism. Studies by Hartman and Di Luzio (15) indicate that the antioxidant DPPD, which is distributed with intracellular lipids, is capable of altering the kinetics of chronic ethanol-induced lipid peroxidation as well as triglyceride accumulation.

    Consistent with our results indicating acetaldehyde to be the major mediator of ethanol-induced hepatic lipid peroxidation injury, other research groups have also recently implicated acetaldehyde as a factor in ethanol-induced liver injury. Recent studies by Cederbaum et al (31, 32) have demonstrated that acetaldehyde may inhibit mitochondria energy production and utilization by inhibiting respiration. Hasumura et al (33) have also recently demonstrated that prolonged consumption of ethanol will significantly reduce the capacity of rat liver mitochondria to oxidize acetaldehyde. Significantly, mitochondria have high concentrations of polyunsaturated fatty acids (34) and several powerful peroxidative catalysts such as iron and hemeproteins making them particularly susceptible to peroxidative injury. Di Luzio (35) has previously demonstrated that ethanol-induced hepatic lipid peroxidation appears to selectively affect the mitochondria.

    Our composite results suggest the hypothesis that the oxidation of ethanol resulting in a significant elevation in hepatic parenchymal cell acetaldehyde concentrations would initiate lipid peroxidative injury to the mitochondria. Mitochondrial injury would decrease acetaldehyde metabolism resulting in more peroxidative injury. The net result of chronic ethanol abuse, therefore, would be the progressive liver cell injury so often found in alcoholism.

SUMMARY

Lipid peroxidation has been implicated as a possible mechanism of ethanol-induced hepatic cell injury. In an effort to further evaluate this concept, hepatic lipid peroxidation and triglyceride measurements were determined in vivo in acute ethanol treated rats pretreated with either pyrazole, an inhibitor of alcohol dehydrogenase, or disulfiram, an inhibitor of aldehyde dehydrogenase. Additionally, acetate, the end product of ethanol metabolism, was administered equimolar to rats in vivo to determine its role in hepatic lipid peroxidation and triglyceride accumulation. Peroxidative events were measured in vitro using rat liver homogenates incubated with either ethanol, acetaldehyde or acetate. A newly developed method was employed to assay the degree of induced peroxidation by measuring photon emission by means of a scintillation spectrophotometer operated in the out-of-coincidence mode. These composite experiments demonstrated acetaldehyde to be a major source of the ethanol-induced hepatic lipid peroxidation. Since the in vivo administration of acetate resulted in elevated liver triglycerides, the ethanol-induced fatty liver appeared to be related not only to acetaldehyde but acetate as well. In addition to acute ethanol studies, rats were maintained on a liquid ethanol diet for three weeks in which ethanol provided 50% of the calories. Maintenance on this diet resulted in significant liver dysfunction as denoted by elevations in plasma BSP, GOT and GPT levels. Animals maintained on the chronic ethanol diet also demonstrated increased liver triglycerides and enhanced hepatic lipid peroxidation. Our composite results indicate that chronic ethanol abuse leading to liver injury may possibly be mediated by acetaldehyde-induced lipid peroxidation.

ACKNOWLEDGEMENTS

This work was supported, in part, by USPHS grant AA00209.

REFERENCES

1. RUBIN E, LIEBER CS: Relation of alcoholic liver injury to cirrhosis. Clin Gastroenterol 4: 247-272, 1975

2. RUBIN E, LIEBER CS: Ethanol metabolism in the liver. In Progress in Liver Diseases, vol 4. H Popper, F Schaffner (eds.). New York, Grune and Stratton, 1972. pp. 549-566

3. MIDDLETON HM, DUNN GD, SCHENKER S: Alcohol-induced liver injury: pathogenic considerations. In The Liver: Normal and Abnormal Functions. FF Becker (ed.). New York, Marcel Dekker, Inc., 1975. pp. 647-678

4. DI LUZIO NR: A mechanism of acute ethanol-induced fatty liver and the modification of liver injury by antioxidants. Lab Invest 15: 50-63, 1966

5. COMPORTI M, BENDETTI A, CHIELI E: Studies on the in vitro peroxidation of liver lipids in ethanol-treated rats. Lipids 8: 498-502, 1973

6. COMPORTI M, HARTMAN AD, DI LUZIO NR: Efect of in vivo and in vitro ethanol administration on liver lipid peroxidation. Lab Invest 16: 616-624, 1967

7. KOES M, WARD T, PENNINGTON S: Lipid peroxidation in chronic ethanol treated rats: in vitro uncoupling of peroxidation from reduced nicotine adenosine dinucleotide phosphate oxidation. Lipids 9: 899-904, 1974

8. REITZ RC: A possible mechanism for the peroxidation of lipids due to chronic ethanol ingestion. Biochem Biophys Acta 380: 145-154, 1975

9. GOLDBERG L, RYDBERG V: Inhibition of ethanol metabolism in vivo by administration of pyrazole. Biochem Pharmacol 18: 1749-1762, 1969

10. BLOMSTRAND R, THEORELL H: Inhibitory effects of ethanol oxidation in man after administration of 4 methyl pyrazole. Life Sci 9: 631-640, 1970

11. MORGAN JC, DI LUZIO NR: Inhibition of the acute ethanol-induced fatty liver by pyrazole. Proc Soc Exp Biol Med 134: 462-466, 1970

12. BLOMSTRAND R, FORSELL L: Prevention of the acute ethanol-induced fatty liver by 4-methyl pyrazole. Life Sci 10: 523-530, 1971

13. DURITZ G, TRUITT EB, Jr: A rapid method for the simultaneous determination of acetaldehyde and ethanol in blood using gas chromatography. Q J Studies Alc 25: 498-510, 1964

14. STEGE TE, DI LUZIO NR: Ethanol-induced liver injury: the role of lipid peroxidation. I. Evaluation of lipid peroxidation by photoemission. Exp Mol Pathol (submitted), 1976

15. HARTMAN AD, DI LUZIO NR: Inhibition of the chronic ethanol-induced fatty liver by antioxidant administration. Proc Soc Exp Biol Med 127: 270-276, 1968

16. CASALS J, OLITSKY PK: Tests for hepatic dysfunction in mice. Proc Soc Exp Biol Med 63: 383-390, 1946

17. VANHANDLE E, ZILVERSMIT DB: Micromethod for the direct determination of serum triglycerides. J Lab Clin Med 50: 152-157, 1957

18. LOWRY OH, ROSEBROUGH NJ, FARR AL, RANDALL RJ: Protein measurements with the folin phenol reagent. J Biol Chem 193: 265-275, 1951

19. GLAVIND J: Antioxidants in animal tissue, Acta Chem Scand 17: 1635-1640, 1963

20. BAUMGARTNER WA, BAKER N, HILL VA, WRIGHT ET: Novel interference in thiobarbituric acid assay for lipid peroxidation. Lipids 10: 309-311, 1975

21. RICHARDS RG, MENDENHALL CL, TRICK T: The relationship of ethanol and its oxidation products to hepatic steatosis. Gastroenterol 66: 892, 1974

22. EGHOJE KN, JUHL E: Factors determining liver damage in chronic alcoholics. Scand J Gastroenterol 8: 505-512, 1973

23. KHANNA JM, KALANT H, LOTH J: Effect of chronic intake of ethanol on lactate/pyruvate and hydroxybutyrate/acetoacetate ratios in the rat liver. Can J Physiol Pharmacol 53: 299-303, 1975

24. KHANNA JM, KALANT H, LOTH J, SEYMORE F: Effect of 4-methyl pyrazole and pyrazole on the induction of fatty liver by a single dose of ethanol. Biochem Pharm 23: 3037-3043, 1974

25. KREBS HA, PERKINS JR: The physiological role of liver alcohol dehydrogenase. Biochem J 118: 635-644, 1970

26. TRUITT EB, DRUITZ G, MARKOWITZ E, TWARDOWICZ AH: Role of acetaldehyde in the action of alcohol on hepatic triglyceride content. Fed Proc 25: 657, 1967

27. SIEGERS CP, STRUBELT O, BREINING H: The acute hepatotoxic activity of alcoholic beverages and some of their congeners in guinea pigs. Pharmacology 12: 296-302, 1974

28. LUNDQUIST F, TYGSTRUP N, WINKLER K, MELLEMGAARD K, MUNCK-PETERSEN S: Ethanol metabolism and production of free acetate in the human liver. J Clin Invest 41: 955-961, 1962

29. CEDERBAUM AI, RUBIN E: Differential effects of acetate on palmitate and octanoate oxidation; segregation of acetyl CoA pools. Arch Biochem Biophys 166: 618-628, 1975

30. DI LUZIO NR: Antioxidants, lipid peroxidation and chemical-induced liver injury. Fed Proc 32: 1875-1881, 1973

31. CEDERBAUM AI, LIEBER CS, RUBIN E: The effect of acetaldehyde on mitochondrial function. Arch Biochem Biophys 161: 26-39, 1974

32. CEDERBAUM AI, LIEBER CS, RUBIN E: Effect of acetaldehyde on
    fatty acid oxidation and ketogenesis by hepatic mitochondria. Arch
    Biochem Biophys 169: 29-41, 1975

33. HASUMURA Y, TESCHKE R, LIEBER CS: Acetaldehyde oxidation by
    hepatic mitochondria: decrease after chronic ethanol consumption.
    Science 189: 727-729, 1975

34. FLEISCHER S, ROUSER G: Lipids of subcellular particles. J Am Oil
    Chem 45: 588-607, 1965

35. DI LUZIO NR: The role of lipid peroxidation and antioxidants in
    ethanol-induced lipid alterations. Exp Mol Pathol 8: 394-402,
    1968

PYRIDINE NUCLEOTIDES AND ETHANOL

Ellen R. Gordon

McGill University Medical Clinic, Montreal General Hospital

Montreal, Quebec   H3G 1A4

It is well established that ethanol is oxidized to acetate in the liver, and that reducing equivalents are formed in the process (1, 2). During these reactions there is a marked shift in the oxidation-reduction level of the liver to a more reduced state, suggesting that reducing equivalents are being formed at rates which exceed the hepatocytes' capacity to handle them (3-11). Concomitant with this alteration in redox state there is a lack of any significant change in the oxygen consumption of the liver, an inability of the liver to store ethanol, and an apparent lack of any feed-back control mechanism for the regulation of ethanol oxidation (10-13). This suggests that ethanol is used as a preferred substrate, and the reducing equivalents formed during its oxidation therefore compete with the hydrogen ions produced in other metabolic pathways. Although the rate-limiting step in the oxidation of ethanol has not been precisely defined, it appears that, in vivo, the activities of the enzymes involved are not rate-limiting, but rather that the reactions are limited by the re-oxidation of NADH (14-16). Under these circumstances it is the cell's capacity to handle these reducing equivalents that regulates the rate of removal of ethanol, and determines the change in flux of substrates in other metabolic pathways. Recent data obtained in my laboratory agree with much of the literature and indicate that the hepatocytes' capacity to handle the excess reducing equivalents depends on the activity of systems involved in translocating these ions into the mitochondria and on the activity of the respiratory chain. These processes are affected not only by the dose but also by the mode of administration of ethanol (acute or chronic) as well as by the nutritional and hormonal status of the animal. These data will be reviewed here.

In the liver, under normal physiological conditions, the reducing equivalents required for the respiratory chain are supplied mainly by the oxidation of fatty acids (85%) and, to a lesser extent, by glycolysis and the activity of the citric cycle (17, 18). When ethanol is present, its oxidation supplies the major portion of the fuel for the respiratory chain and it has been shown experimentally that fatty-acid oxidation, glycolysis and the activity of the citric acid cycle are all depressed (5, 13). These reducing equivalents arise because the main pathway for ethanol disposition is through a NAD^+-linked alcohol dehydrogenase system located in the cytosol (1). During this reaction the 1-R-hydrogen of ethanol is transferred to the coenzyme NAD and acetaldehyde and NADH are formed. In the second step, which occurs in the mitochondria, acetaldehye is converted by a NAD^+-linked aldehyde dehydrogenase to acetate, and another NADH is formed (19). Thus, as one mole of ethanol is converted to a mole of acetate, two moles of NADH are produced. Recently, enzyme systems other than alcohol dehydrogenase have been shown to participate in the metabolism of ethanol (20, 21). Evidence has been presented for the involvement of the microsomal ethanol oxidizing system (20) and a catalase hydrogen peroxide system (21). Although the exact identity of the enzyme system involved is much disputed, investigations with inhibitors and tritiated ethanol indicate clearly that other pathways are involved (20-25). However, the quantitative contribution of these possible pathways has never been determined precisely. The interesting aspect of these alternative pathways is that the 1-R-hydrogen of ethanol is transferred to a OH ion, and water is formed. In these reactions then, the NADH is not produced in the cytoplasm, and one less NADH is formed as ethanol is converted to acetate.

Under normal physiological conditions, the hepatocytes' capacity to handle the reducing equivalents formed during a NAD^+-linked dehydrogenase reaction depends on: (a) the cytosolic requirements for NADH in other pathways such as gluconeogenesis, lipid synthesis, or desaturation etc.; (b) the activity of the shuttle systems, which are metabolic processes whereby reducing equivalents are translocated into the mitochondria (α-glycerol-phosphate, malate-asparate, and fatty acid shuttles), and (c) the activity of the respiratory chain which is governed by the availability of ADP and the energy requirements of the cell. Thus these systems become directly involved in the metabolism of ethanol and in turn may be affected by ethanol.

Following a single ingestion of ethanol, there is a sudden excess of reducing equivalents in the liver as indicated by the increased steady-state concentrations of the pyridine-nucleotide NADH. The change in redox state of the liver has been well documented, and has been shown to be a function of both the dose of ethanol and the length of time following administration (7, 11). However, as pointed out by Krebs (26), the total hepatic levels of NADH and NAD give little information because such measurements fail to differentiate between free and protein-bound nucleotides and give no information on the distribution of the nucleotides between various cell compartments. However, a small number of dehydrogenase systems can be used to assay the NAD^+/NADH ratio of various compartments of the cell, since in certain metabolic states the concentrations of their oxidized and reduced substrates are in near equilibrium with the nucleotides. Thus one can calculate the redox state of the cytoplasm utilizing the substrate levels of the NAD^+-linked lactate dehydrogenase system, and of the mitochondria utilizing the substrate levels of the NAD^+-linked β-hydroxybutyrate dehydrogenase system.

Measurements of these metabolites made following an acute ingestion of ethanol indicate that the redox state of both the cytoplasm and mitochondria is shifted to a more reduced level (4, 11). These changes are influenced to a significant extent by the nutritional and the hormonal status of the animal. Forsander noted that the hepatic L/P ratio was increased in the fed animal, as a result of a marked decrease in the hepatic concentration of pyruvate accompanied by little or no change in the lactate levels (11). On the other hand, in a starved animal, the ratio was shifted to an even more reduced level because the lactic acid levels rose while the pyruvate levels remained the same (11). The administration of pyruvate enhanced the rate of ethanol elimination in the starved animal, but had little effect in the fed animal (27). The administration of thyroxine to starved animals increased the redox state of the cytosol and enhanced the rate of removal of ethanol while a similar treatment in fed animals was much less effective (27). It is of interest to note that the activities of the systems which translocate hydrogen ions from the cytosol into the mitochondria would be enhanced by these treatments. The metabolism of pyruvate would provide substrates utilized in the malate-aspartate shuttle and the administration of thyroxine would cause an increase in the activity of the mitochondrial glycerol-3-phosphate dehydrogenase and thereby enhance the activity of the glycerol-3-phosphate cycle. It would then appear that in the starved animal a rate-limiting step in the metabolism of the ethanol is the translocation of reducing equivalents into the mitochondria.

In further support of this concept, Williamson's group (28) demonstrated that the oxidation of ethanol can be limited by the intracellular concentrations of the intermediates of the malate-asparate and α-glycerol-3-phosphate cycles (Table I). The addition of lactate to a suspension of hepatocytes isolated from starved rats increased the rate of ethanol oxidation by almost two-fold. This change was associated with a marked increase in the concentrations of the metabolites of the malate-aspartate and α-glycerol-phosphate shuttle systems. The addition of the same concentration of lactate to hepatocytes isolated from fed rats also increased the rate of ethanol oxidation but to a lesser degree, and the effect was largely inhibited by quinolinate, indicating that the stimulation by lactate was due solely to an increased requirement of ATP in gluconeogenesis.

The addition of substances which promote the oxidation of NADH by the mitochondrial electron chain also has been shown to enhance the rate of ethanol oxidation (Figure 1) (29). These substrates (fructose, lactate, ammonium salts, ornithine and dinitrophenol (DNP)) acted by increasing the turnover rate of adenine nucleotides, and thus accelerated the re-oxidation of NADH. However, during their metabolism, each of these substrates (with the exception of DNP) would not only require ATP but would also provide precursors for the substrates involved in the translocation of reducing equivalents into the mitochondria. Thus both the activity of the shuttle

TABLE I

ETHANOL OXIDATION IN LIVER CELLS FROM STARVED AND FED RATS

Conditions of animal	Additions	Metabolic changes (μmol/h per g dry wt. of cells)		Metabolite concentrations (μmol/g dry wt. of cells)		
		-ΔEthanol	Δ Glucose	Malate	Aspartate	Glycerol-3-phosphate
Starved	None	215±22 (4)	3.4±0.4(4)	0.6±0.15(3)	0.3;0.9 (2)	1.9±0.3 (3)
	Lactate	416±43 (4)	66±7 (4)	9.9±1.5 (3)	1.2;1.2 (2)	3.3±0.5 (3)
	Quinolinate	214±37 (4)	1.9±0.4(4)	0.9±0.1 (3)	–	1.3±0.4 (3)
	Quinolinate + lactate	317±37 (4)	7.5±0.8(4)	24.2±1.1 (3)	–	2.2±?.2 (3)
	Malate	303±18 (3)	9.4±0.8(3)	–		1.9;3.0 (2)
Fed	None	433±12 (3)	369±86 (3)	1.9;2.1 (2)	1.7;2.5 (2)	7.8;22.6 (2)
	Lactate	575±89 (3)	483±64 (3)	13.3;17.9(2)	5.5;5.9 (2)	3.9;26.5 (2)
	Quinolinate	443±29 (3)	358±80 (3)	1.1;2.5 (2)	2.4;3.8 (2)	5.3;19.3 (2)
	Quinolinate + lactate	490±50 (3)	394±84 (3)	18.4;41.4(2)	11.4;6.4 (2)	4.3;4.5 (2)
	Malate	470±28 (3)	346±75 (3)	–	–;7.2 (1)	–

Data from Biochem J 150:205-209, 1975.   Printed with permission of author and journal.

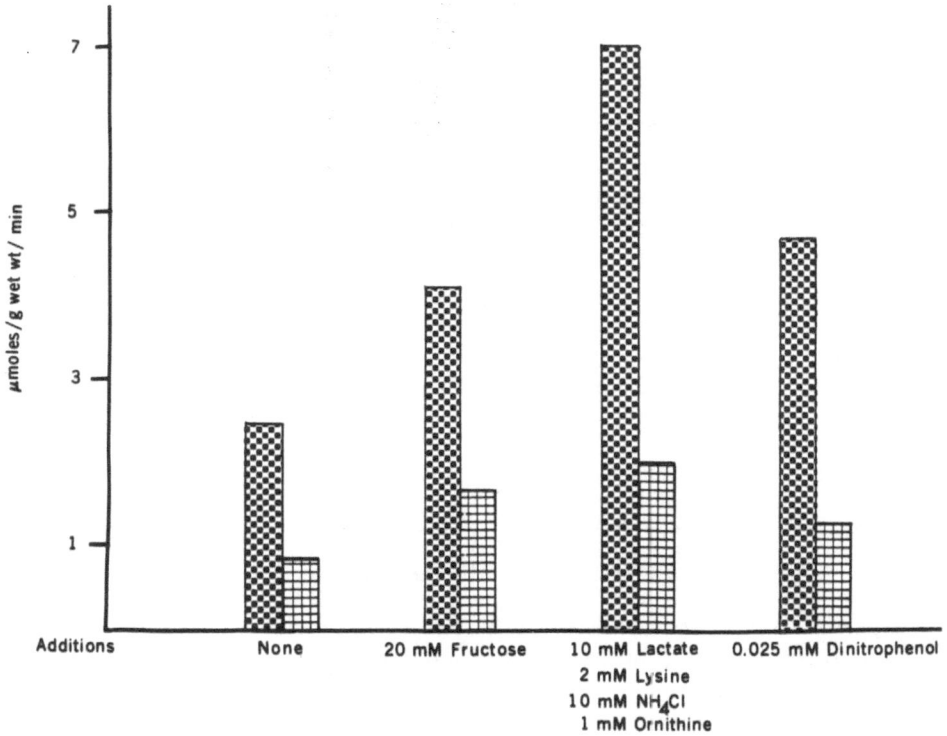

Fig. 1   *Effect of Various Substrates on Oxygen Uptake and Acetate*

Formation by Isolated Rat Liver Cells

▓ *OXYGEN UPTAKE*   ▦ *ACETATE FORMATION*

Data taken from Reference 29 and printed with the permission of Authors and Journal.

systems and the process of oxidative phosphorylation control the metabolism of ethanol following an acute dose.

An examination of metabolic patterns in the liver, following varying doses of ethanol, indicates that changes are dose-dependent. In data reported by Guynn's group the mitochondrial and cytosol-free $NAD^+/NADH$ ratios and the cytoplasmic-free NADP/NADPH were more reduced with lower doses of ethanol (0.69, 1.7 g/kg) and became progressively more oxidized with increasing doses (3.0 g/kg) (30). Similar changes were reported by Lundquist's group (31) who noted a marked drop in the L/P ratios of liver slices when the ethanol concentration of the media was increased from 40 to 80 mM (L/P ratio being 231 and 147 respectively). These changes are associated with an increased rate of ethanol oxidation (32), suggesting that pathways other than alcohol dehydrogenase may indeed be involved in the oxidation of this substrate.

TABLE II

NAD$^+$ AND NADH LEVELS IN ETHANOL-INDUCED FATTY LIVER[a]

Treatment	NAD$^+$ μmoles/g wet wt of liver	NADH μ moles/g wet wt of liver	NAD$^+$/NADH
Control	684 ± 28 (14)	92 ± 10 (13)	8.6 ± 1.1 (11)
Ethanol[b]	494 ± 15^c (7)	441 ± 34^c (8)	1.2 ± 0.1^c (7)
1 day off ethanol	594 ± 88 (6)	64 ± 7 (5)	10.1 ± 1.3 (5)

[a]Values ± S.E.M.   Figures in parentheses denote the number of animals in each group.

[b]Rats maintained for four weeks on a nutritionally adequate diet containing 36 cal % as ethanol.

[c]Statistically significant with respect to control ($p < 0.02$).

In animals consuming ethanol for prolonged periods of time, as a portion of a nutritionally adequate diet, the rate of ethanol uptake by the liver is also increased (22). This suggests that the cell's capacity to handle reducing equivalents has been enhanced. Of course other factors could be involved. The oxidation-reduction level of the liver in these animals is also shifted to a more reduced level (6, 9, 33) (Table II). However, it is difficult to correlate this change with that observed following an acute dose of ethanol since the associated diet also affects the redox level of the liver markedly (26). For a prolonged intake of ethanol, this change is associated with a decrease in the state of phosphorylation of the cytosol, accounted for by a sizeable drop in the ATP level and accompanied by no significant change in ADP or orthophosphate levels. Both an increased utilization and a decreased synthesis have been invoked to account for this change (33, 34). The cell's capacity to handle the reducing equivalents would be very different in these two situations. In the one instance, the activities of the systems translocating reducing equivalents into the mitochondria and the respiratory chain would be enhanced in a manner similar to that observed in a hypermetabolic state (34). On the other hand, a depression in ATP synthesis

TABLE III

CALCULATED REDOX STATE OF THE HEPATIC CYTOPLASM

NAD^+-linked dehydrogenase system	Control	Ethanol
I) Pyruvate : lactate	478	449
II) Dihydroxyacetone phosphate : α-glycerol phosphate	1016	425
III) Oxaloacetate : malate	1658	1218

Calculations were made from data obtained in Table II.

The pH of the system was assumed to be 7.0 and K values of 1.11×10^{-4}, 1.8×10^{-4} and 2.78×10^{-5} were used for the lactate, α-glycerol phosphate, and malate NAD^+-linked dehydrogenase systems respectively.

would indicate a decreased capacity of the cell to handle NADH. The explanation for the increased rate of ethanol oxidation would then require other metabolic processes.

In rats consuming ethanol as part of a nutritionally adequate diet, a reduced redox state was found in both the cytosol and mitochondria of the liver (Table III). However, it was noted that the NAD^+-linked dehydrogenase systems were not in equilibrium in the cytosol in either the control or experimental animals (Table III). In the ethanol-treated animals, the redox state of the NAD^+-lactate dehydrogenase system remained unchanged, while that of both the α-glycerol phosphate and malate dehydrogenase systems was shifted to a more reduced level. This lack of change in L/P ratio was unexpected. An infusion of 10 mM of ethanol into the portal vein produced a marked decrease in this ratio within 15 minutes. The change was caused by a sudden decrease in pyruvate levels rather than any marked increase in the level of lactic acid. These data and those of Tygstrup (35) indicate that changes in the redox state of the NAD^+-linked dehydrogenase systems are dependent in the concentration of ethanol present in the liver. The decrease in the redox level of the NAD^+-linked α-glycerol-phosphate and malate dehydrogenase systems probably reflects the increased flux of hydrogen ions through these systems.

The translocation of reducing equivalents from the cytosol into the mitochondria may well be affected by the chronic ingestion of ethanol and

TABLE IV

METABOLIC LEVELS OF SYSTEMS TRANSLOCATING REDUCING
EQUIVALENTS INTO THE MITOCHONDRIA[a]

A. Malate-Aspartate	Control	Ethanol[b]
Aspartate	0.742 ± 0.05 (14)	0.440 ± 0.035[c] (14)
Malate	0.471 ± 0.04 (7)	0.626 ± 0.045[d] (6)
Glutamate	4.46 ± 0.25 (9)	4.83 ± 0.37 (8)
Oxaloacetate	0.019 ± 0.002 (7)	0.023 ± 0.002 (7)
α-Keto-glutarate	0.081 ± 0.006 (14)	0.075 ± 0.005 (7)
B. α-Glycerol-phosphate		
α-glycerol phosphate	0.35 ± 0.02 (13)	0.79 ± 0.07[d] (8)
Dihydroxyacetone phosphate	0.064 ± 0.003 (7)	0.061 ± 0.005 (7)

[a]Metabolite concentrations are expressed in μmoles/g wet wt of liver. The number in parentheses denotes the number of animals in each group.

[b]Rats maintained for four weeks on a nutritionally adequate diet containing 36 cal % as ethanol.

[c]Statistically significant with respect to control (P < .001).

[d]Statistically significant with respect to control (P < .02).

requires consideration. Cederbaum and Rubin (36, 37) noted that the chronic consumption of ethanol did not abolish the permeability barrier of mitochondria to NADH. Also no significant difference was noted in the activity of reconstituted malate-aspartate, α-glycerol-phosphate and fatty acid shuttle systems between mitochondrial preparations from ethanol-fed rats and their pair-fed controls. Measurements of the hepatic levels of these metabolites indicated that the concentration of some of these substrates had increased and others decreased slightly (Table IV). The increased levels of malate and α-glycerol phosphate concomitant with the reduced state of the mitochondria suggest that the capacity of the respiratory chain to handle the reducing equivalents formed in the cytosol had been exceeded. The aspartate levels were significantly lowered in the ethanol-fed rats compared to those observed in the controls. These levels were not decreased to values observed in starved animals (15). Therefore it seems unlikely that the translocation of reducing equivalents into mito-chondria would be impeded by this change, but this remains to be proven. However these data suggest that the shuttle systems are not impaired by the chronic intake of ethanol.

Controversy surrounds the effect of chronic consumption of ethanol on the activity of the respiratory chain (33, 34, 39). One group of investigators has observed an enhanced activity (34), while others have noted a reduction (33, 38). In our experiments no evidence was found for an increased activity of the respiratory chain in the liver of ethanol-treated animals. The endogenous rates of oxygen consumption were similar in hepatocyte preparations from ethanol-treated animals and their respective controls (Table V). When the animals were starved for 18 hours before sacrifice, an increase in the rate of oxygen consumption was noted in cell preparations from both the ethanol-fed rats and their respective pair-fed controls, but not in preparations from fasted normal animals. The rates of oxygen consumption obtained in these latter experiments were 50% greater than those obtained utilizing preparations from fasted normals. The extent of this difference was the same as that observed by other investigators (34). In the fasted animals, the hepatic triglyceride levels were 18.0; 3.2; and 1.9 mg/g wet wt in the ethanol-treated, pair-fed controls and normal animals respectively. It is of interest to note that the hepatic lipid content of the pair-fed controls is in the same range as that reported by Israel's group in the ethanol-treated animals (3.8 mg/g wet wt of liver) (16). It appears that the availability of substrates may account for the different rates of oxygen consumption reported in these studies.

The activity of the adenine nucleotide translocase system was measured in these animals as this system, which translocates ADP into the inner membrane of the mitochondria, regulates the process of oxidative phos-phorylation. No significant change was noted in this carrier system until alterations were observed in the metabolism of long chain CoA derivatives of fatty acids. This occurred only after prolonged periods of ingesting ethanol at a level of 36 cal %. A decrease was found in this system which correlated well with an increase in the mitochondrial level of long chain CoA derivatives of fatty acids (known inhibitors of this system) and the

TABLE V

OXYGEN CONSUMPTION IN ISOLATED LIVER CELLS FROM STARVED AND FED RATS

Treatment	Fed	Starved
	μmoles of 0_2 consumed/min/g wet wt[a]	
Normal	2.54 ± 0.50	2.01 (2.11,1.90)
Ethanol - treated[b]	2.51 ± 0.46	3.10 (3.10,3.11)
Pair-fed controls	2.56 ± 0.15	3.77 (3.70,3.84)

[a]Mean values ± S.E.M. of 4 or 2 experiments.

[b]Sprague Dawley rats maintained for four weeks on a nutritionally adequate diet containing 36 cal % as ethanol.

decreased hepatic content of ATP (Table VI). These results suggest that, with time, the level of long-chain CoA derivatives of fatty acids in the mitochondria increases in animals consuming ethanol as part of their diet. This in turn impedes the translocation of ADP into the mitochondrial membrane, and thus limits the rate of oxidative phosphorylation and the hepatocytes' capacity to handle the reducing equivalents.

These changes could explain the reduced redox state of the mito-chondria. However it then becomes necessary to invoke mechanisms other than the re-oxidation of NADH to explain the increased rate of removal of ethanol in these ethanol-treated animals. Thus systems which do not form NADH may indeed be involved in the oxidation of this substrate.

In summary the rate of removal of ethanol appears to be regulated by the capacity of the hepatocyte to handle reducing equivalents formed during the oxidation of this substrate.   Thus the activity of the systems translocating reducing equivalents into the mitochondria, and the activity of the respiratory chain, both of which are governed by the nutritional and hormonal status of the animal, control the metabolism of ethanol. At high doses of ethanol and after chronic ingestion of ethanol other pathways are involved so that the re-oxidation of NADH plays a lesser role under these conditions.

TABLE VI

THE LEVEL OF LONG CHAIN CoA DERIVATIVES OF FATTY ACIDS, ATP, AND THE ACTIVITY OF THE ADENINE TRANSLOCASE SYSTEM IN RATS FED ETHANOL[a,b]

Treatment	ATP	Adenine Nucleotide Translocase Activity	Long Chain Acid CoA Derivatives of Fatty Acids	
			Total Liver	Mitochondria
	μmoles/g wet wt	units[c]	μmoles/g wet wt	μmoles/5.0 mg protein
Controls	2.62 ± 0.13 (17)	100 (22)	38.5 ± 2.6 (12)	2.11 ± 0.13 (12)
Ethanol	1.37 ± 0.08^d (10)	35.4 ± 5.5^d (14)	55.5 ± 2.7^d (8)	2.89 ± 0.15^d (8)

[a]Rats maintained on the liquid diet containing ethanol at a level of 36 cal % for 4 weeks.

[b]Values given are mean ± S.E.M., and the numbers in parentheses denote the number of animals in the group.

[c]Units — the activity was expressed in dpm per mg of mitochondrial protein. Since the radioactivity added to the system was not always the same in different experiments, the data were normalized by assigning a value of 100 to the activity obtained in the pair-fed liquid control group of the day and by expressing the data obtained for the experimental groups as a percentage of the control group's activity.

[d]Statistically significant with respect to Control, $P < 0.01$.

SUMMARY

An excess of reducing equivalents is formed in the liver when ethanol is oxidized to acetate by NAD^+-linked dehydrogenase systems. The capacity of the hepatocyte to handle these reducing equivalents is governed by both the activity of the shuttle systems, which translocate reducing equivalents from the cytosol into the mitochondria, and by the activity of the respiratory chain which itself is controlled by the availability of ADP and by the energy demands of the cells. These systems then control the rate of ethanol removal by the liver. The nutritional and hormonal status of the animal were shown to affect the activity of the shuttle systems, although the chronic consumption of ethanol as part of an adequate diet had little direct effect. Evidence is presented indicating that in starved animals, substrates which enhance the turnover of adenine nucleotides increase the rate of ethanol oxidation. No evidence was found in the ethanol-treated animals for a hypermetabolic state in the liver. Instead, the results suggest rather that with time, the level of long chain CoA derivatives of fatty acids in the mitochondria increases and that this in turn impedes the translocation of ADP into the mitochondrial membrane, and this limits the rate of re-oxidation of NADH in the process of oxidative phosphorylation. Changes in the metabolic levels at high doses of ethanol and after chronic consumption of ethanol indicate that a pathway other than alcohol dehydrogenase may be involved in the metabolism of ethanol.

ACKNOWLEDGEMENTS

This work was supported by the Canadian Hepatic Foundation, and Medical Research Council Grant MA-2341.

REFERENCES

1. JACOBSEN E: Metabolism of ethyl alcohol. Pharmacol Rev 4: 107-135, 1952

2. LUNDSGAARD E: Alcohol oxidation as a function of the liver. Compt R Trav Lab Carlsberg 22: 333-337, 1938

3. FORSANDER OA: Influence of the metabolism of ethanol on the lactate/pyruvate ratio of rat-liver slices. Biochem J 98: 244-247, 1966

4. RAWAT AK: Effects of ethanol infusion on the redox state and metabolite levels in rat liver in vivo. Eur J Biochem 6: 585-592, 1968

5. LUNDQUIST F: The metabolism of alcohol. In Biological Basis of Alcoholism. Y Israel and J Mardones (eds.). Wiley Interscience, New York, 1971. pp. 1-52

6. GORDON ER: The effect of chronic consumption of ethanol on the
    redox state of the rat liver. Can J Biochem 50: 949-957, 1972

7. CHERRICK GR, LEEVY CM: The effect of ethanol metabolism on
    levels of oxidized and reduced nicotinamide-adenine dinucleotide in
    liver, kidney and heart. Biochim Biophys Acta 107: 29-37, 1965

8. MAJCHROWICZ E, BERCAW BL, COLE WM, GREGORY DH: Nicotina-
    mide adenine dinucleotide and the metabolism of ethanol and
    acetaldehyde. Quart J Stud Alc 28: 213-224, 1967

9. KALANT H, KHANNA JM, LOTH J: Effect of chronic intake of ethanol
    on pyridine nucleotide levels in rat liver and kidney. Can J Physiol
    Pharmacol 48: 542-549, 1970

10. WALLGREEN H, BARRY H   III: Actions of Alcohol, Vol. I,
    Biochemical, Physiological and Psychological Effects.   Elsevier
    Publishing Co, Amsterdam, 1970. pp. 35-153

11. FORSANDER OH, RAIHA N, SALASPURO M, MAENPAA PH:
    Influence of ethanol on the liver metabolism of fed and starved
    rats. Biochem J 94: 259-265, 1965

12. MAJCHROWICZ E: The effects of ethanol on liver metabolism. In
    Alcohol Intoxication and Withdrawal. MM Gross (ed.). Adv Exper
    Med Biochem. Plenum Publishing Co, New York, 1975. pp. 79-104

13. HAWKINS RD, KALANT H, KHANNA JM: Effects of chronic intake
    ethanol on rate of ethanol metabolism. Can J Physiol Pharmacol
    44: 241-257, 1966

14. LINDROS KO, VIHMA R, FORSANDER OH: Utilization and metabolic
    effects of acetaldehyde and ethanol in the perfused rat liver.
    Biochem J 126: 945-952, 1972

15. WILLIAMSON JR, OH KAWA K, MEIJER AJ: Regulation of ethanol
    oxidation in isolated rat liver cells. In Alcohol and Aldehyde
    Metabolizing Systems. RG Thurman, T Yonetani, JR Williamson
    and B Chance (eds.). Academic Press, New York, 1974. pp. 365-
    382

16. VIDELA L, ISRAEL Y: Factors that modify the metabolism of ethanol
    in rat liver and adaptive changes produced by its chronic
    administration. Bioch J 118: 275-281, 1970

17. FRITZ IB: Factors influencing the rates of long-chain fatty acid
    oxidation and synthesis in mammalian systems. Physiol Rev 41:
    52-129, 1961

18. WILLIAMSON RJ, SMITH CM, LA NOUE KF, BRYLA J: Feedback control of the citric acid cycle in energy metabolism and the regulation of metabolic process in mitochondria. MA Mahlman and RW Hanson (eds.). Academic Press, New York, 1972. pp. 185-210

19. LINDROS KO: Acetaldehyde oxidation and its role in the overall metabolic effects of the liver. In Regulation of Hepatic Metabolism. F Lundquist and N Tygstrup (eds.). Academic Press, New York, 1974. pp. 417-431

20. LIEBER CS, DE CARLI LM: Hepatic microsomal ethanol-oxidizing system. In vitro characteristics and adaptive properties in vivo. J Biol Chem 245: 2505-2512, 1970

21. THURMAN RG, OSHINO M, CHANCE B: The role of hydrogen peroxide production and catalase in hepatic ethanol metabolism. Adv Exp Med Biol 59: 163-183, 1975

22. LIEBER CS, DE CARLI LM: The role of the hepatic microsomal ethanol oxidizing system (MEOS) for ethanol metabolism in vivo. J Pharm Exp Ther 181: 279-287, 1972

23. LIEBER CS, RUBIN E, DE CARLI LM, MISRA P, GANG H: Effects of pyrazole on hepatic function and structure. Lab Invest 22: 615-621, 1970

24. McCAFFREY JB, THURMAN RG: Mechanism of adaptive increase in ethanol utilization due to chronic prior pretreatment with alcohol. In Alcohol and Aldehyde Metabolizing Systems. RG Thurman, T Yonetani, JR Williamson and B Chance (eds.). Academic Press, New York, 1974. pp. 483-492

25. ROGNSTAD R, CLARK DG: Tritium as a tracer for reducing equivalents in isolated liver cells. Eur J Biochem 42: 51-60, 1974

26. KREBS HA, VEECH RL: Regulation of the redox state of the pyridine nucleotides in rat liver. In Pyridine Nucleotide Dependent Dehydrogenase. H Sund (ed.). Springer-Verlag, Berlin, 1970. pp. 413-434

27. LINDROS KO: Role of the redox state in ethanol-induced suppression of citrate-cycle flux in the perfused liver of normal, hyper-, and hypothyroid rats. Eur J Bioch 26: 338-346, 1972

28. MEIJER AJ, VAN WOERKOM GM, WILLIAMSON JR, TAGER JM: Rate-limiting factors in the oxidation of ethanol by isolated rat liver cells. Biochem J 150: 205-209, 1975

29. KREBS HA, STUBBS M: Factors controlling the rate of alcohol disposal by the liver. Adv Exp Med Biol 59: 149-161, 1975

30. GUYNN RW, PIEKLIK JR: Dependence on dose of the acute effects of ethanol on liver metabolism in vivo. J Clin Invest 56: 1411-1419, 1975

31. LUNDQUIST F, THIEDEN H, GRUNNET N: Ethanol as an energy producing substrate. In Metabolic Changes Induced by Alcohol. GA Martini and Ch Bode (eds.). Springer Verlag, New York, 1971. pp 108-114

32. GRUNNET N, QUISTORFF B, THIEDEN HID: Rate-limiting factors in ethanol oxidation by isolated rat-liver parenchymal cells. Effect of ethanol concentration, fructose, pyruvate and pyrazole. Eur J Biochem 40: 275-282, 1973

33. GORDON ER: Mitochondrial functions in an ethanol-induced fatty liver. J Biol Chem 248: 8271-8280, 1973

34. ISRAEL Y, VIDELA L, BERNSTEIN J: Liver hypermetabolic state after chronic ethanol consumption. Hormonal interrelation and pathogenic implication. Fed Proc 34: 2052-2059, 1975

35. TYGSTRUP N, RENECK L, ROMØE S, KEIDING S: Effect of submaximal ethanol elimination on hepatic redox levels in man. In Alcohol and Aldehyde Metabolizing Systems. RG Thurman, T Yonetani, JR Willamson, B. Chance (eds.). Academic Press, New York, 1974. pp. 469-481

36. CEDERBAUM AI, LIEBER CS, BEATTIE DS, RUBIN E: Characterization of shuttle mechanisms for the transport of reducing equivalents into mitochondria. Arch Biochem Biophys 158: 763-781, 1973

37. CEDERBAUM AI, LIEBER CS, TOTH A, BEATTIE DS, RUBIN E: Effects of ethanol and fat on the transport of reducing equivalents into rat liver mitochondria. J Biol Chem 248: 4977-4986, 1973

38. CEDERBAUM AI, RUBIN E: Molecular injury to mitochondria produced by ethanol and acetaldehyde. Fed Proc 34(11): 2045-2052, 1975

THE INFLUENCE OF ETHANOL ON ALBUMIN METABOLISM

Marcus A. Rothschild, M. Oratz and S.S. Schreiber

Radioisotope Service, New York Veterans Administration
Hospital, New York, New York 10010; Dept. of Medicine,
New York University, School of Medicine; and Dept. of
Biochemistry, New York University College of Dentistry

The mechanisms responsible for the production of protein within the liver cells are the subject of continued detailed investigations and the myriad of steps located between the initial turning on of the assembly line to the final extrusion of the completed molecule offer innumerable areas for regulation or modification and thus control. In attempting to outline the effects of any particular stress on the synthetic mechanism it will ultimately be necessary to delineate the steps as they proceed in the formation of the protein. Further, it will be necessary to use as specific an isolated system as possible so that the interplay of in vivo factors tending to dampen the effects of one stress or another can be eliminated.

Serum albumin has long been used as an index for health and disease and particularly has been considered to play an important role in prognosticating the effects of ethanol induced hepatic cirrhosis (1-9). Serum albumin is produced within the liver cells, transported through the cell, and extruded directly into hepatic plasma. Therefore, the albumin synthetic system is an excellent model for studying the effects of ethanol on the liver. In general, protein synthesis occurs via the following steps. Though the RNA synthesis necessary for protein production occurs within the nucleus, the protein synthetic pathways are located in the cytoplasm of the liver cell. In the liver cell there are two classes of ribosomes, one bound to the endoplasmic reticulum and the other free within the cytoplasm (10-12). The latter appears to play an important role in the early initiation of albumin production for these ribosomes appear to synthesize a peptide, possibly the signal peptide, of six amino acids, of which three are arginine (13-17). It is this signal peptide which somehow acts to notify the endoplasmic reticulum that a protein is to be made whose future is export from the cell (18). The ribosome is composed of two units - a smaller 40 S and a larger 60 S unit - and once the growing albumin molecule is attached to the endoplasmic reticulum it passes through the center of the larger ribosomal subunit to be inserted into the microtubular structure. The growing peptide anchors this larger subunit to the endoplasmic reticulum (19-22). Not only does protein synthesis have to be initiated but as each amino acid is accepted onto the ribosome it is translocated from one site to another and factors responsible for this elongation of the polypeptide have been isolated. For peptide elongation to continue translocation from one site to another has to occur with movement from one spot on the ribosome to another as well as from codon to codon on the messenger RNA. Eventually, through specific codes, the protein synthesis is terminated and the ribosomes are released from the mRNA in the form of subunits (23-33). There appear to be factors which interfere with the ability of these subunits to immediately recombine in the absence of other factors immediately available. Thus, with as complicated a system as this and with so many gaps in the available knowledge, it is clear that the specific effects of ethanol in terms of the mechanism of its action are still a long way off. But, we can summarize the effects of ethanol or its metabolic byproducts, and indicate certain gross effects on albumin synthesis.

The level of serum albumin in the body is obviously the rather complex end result not only of the synthetic mechanism which we have outlined above but also of distribution and degradation (8). However, low levels of serum albumin are frequently observed in patients with alcohol induced liver disease (8). And, even though the total exchangeable albumin pool has been found to be elevated in large numbers of cirrhotic subjects, particularly those with ascites, the depressed level of serum albumin has long been ascribed to defective synthesis. This observation was checked in patients with cirrhosis and ascites (34), and it was found that 7 of 19 subjects studied had elevated rates of albumin synthesis, 5 patients normal and 7 had depressed rates, even though the serum albumin level was low and the globulin level elevated in all subjects, (Table I). These studies were performed when the patients had been on an adequate diet for 2-3 days and had been removed from ethanol for that length of time. Thus, the effects that were seen in vivo could not necessarily be ascribed to the influence of

TABLE I

ALBUMIN SYNTHESIS, CIRRHOSIS AND ASCITES

NUMBER OF PATIENTS	ALBUMIN SYNTHESIS mg/kg/day	SERUM	
		ALBUMIN	GLOBULIN
		g/100 ml	
7	79	1.7	4.4
5	152	1.9	4.4
7	287	2.1	4.6

ethanol per se. Further, in vivo and in the isolated perfused liver, a short term fast for as limited a time as twenty-four hours results not only in a marked decrease in the rate of albumin synthesis but also in significant disaggregation of the endoplasmic membrane bound polysome, that subcellular organelle responsible for the synthesis of the albumin molecule (9, 35-38). In an attempt to separate the acute effects of ethanol administration from those possibly related to nutrition per se, studies with the isolated perfused rabbit liver were begun. The perfusate consisted of either washed rabbit red cells or rabbit blood with the albumin concentration adjusted to approximately 3 g/100 ml with either bovine or rabbit albumin and the amino acid contents adjusted to preset levels (39). Albumin synthesis in this preparation was determined either immunologically or by the ^{14}C carbonate technique (39). The viability of the liver preparation was monitored by measurements of urea synthesis, lactate and pyruvate levels, oxygen extraction and the lack of accumulation of intracellular enzymes in the perfusate. When the liver was derived from a fed donor and the standard perfusate employed, albumin synthesis averaged 18 mg/100 g wet liver wt/hr. (38, Table II). A decrease to 9 mg was noted when the liver was obtained from donors fasted either for 24 or 48 hours. In order to determine the specific effects of various amino acids on albumin synthesis the liver from a fasted donor was utilized and the perfusate was enriched methodically with 10 mM levels of essential amino acids. It was observed that tryptophan, arginine, ornithine, lysine, phenylalanine, glutamine, alanine, threonine and proline stimulated albumin production to values which approached or exceeded those seen in the liver derived from a fed donor (39), whereas leucine, valine, methionine and histidine failed to do so (39). These 4 amino acids failed to stimulate urea synthesis, the latter having been increased along with albumin production in the group of amino acids resulting in excess albumin production (Table III).

TABLE II

THE EFFECTS OF FASTING ON ALBUMIN SYNTHESIS
IN THE ISOLATED PERFUSED LIVER

DONOR	ALBUMIN SYNTHESIS mg/100 wet liver weight per hour	DEGREE OF POLYSOME AGGREGATION % of profile heavier than trisome*
FED	18 + 2	69 + 3
FASTED	9 + 1	49 + 4

*Degree of polysome aggregation was determined from the fraction of the total polysome profile heavier than the trisome peak (39).

TABLE III

ALBUMIN SYNTHESIS AND AMINO ACIDS

DONOR	PERFUSATE	UREA SYNTHESIS	ALBUMIN SYNTHESIS
FASTED	STIMULATING AMINO ACIDS ARG ORN* TRP LYS PHE ALA THR PRO GLU	INCREASED	INCREASED
FASTED	NON STIMULATING AMINO ACIDS LEU VAL MET HIS	UNAFFECTED	PERSISTED AT LOW RATE CHARACTERISTIC OF THAT FOUND IN LIVERS FROM DONOR

*ORNITHINE NOT FOUND IN ALBUMIN

TABLE IV

EFFECT OF ETHANOL ON ALBUMIN SYNTHESIS (39)

DONOR	PERFUSATE	UREA SYNTHESIS	ALBUMIN SYNTHESIS	DEGREE OF BOUND POLYSOME AGGREGATION
		mg/100g wet liver weight per hour		% of profile heavier than trisome
FED	ETHANOL	11 ± 2	6 ± 1	28 ± 3
FED	ETHANOL ARGININE	28 ± 4	12 ± 1	53 ± 4
FASTED	ETHANOL	20 ± 4	5 ± 1	$10 - 20$
FASTED	ETHANOL ARGININE	34 ± 7	6 ± 1	$5 - 10$

ETHANOL 200 mg%   ARGININE 10 mM

VALUES ARE MEAN ± S.E. OF MEAN

When ethanol at a level of 200 mg% was added to the perfusate of livers from fed donors, albumin synthesis fell to average only 6 mg/100 g wet liver wt/hr. As with the prior studies (with livers from fasted rabbits perfused without ethanol) the same amino acids resulted in a stimulation of albumin production in the face of continued exposure to this level of ethanol (39) (Table IV).

When the combined stresses of fasting and ethanol were studied, however, the amino acids which had formerly been effective in reversing the ethanol induced inhibition of albumin production were totally ineffective (39) (Table IV). In attempting to understand the mechanism of action of the stresses of fasting and ethanol and of the effects of the stimulating amino acids, ^{3}H uridine was added to the perfusion and the bound and free polysomes were isolated in the different groups (39). The polysome profiles were obtained by means of linear sucrose density gradient analysis and the isolated fractions were assayed for incorporation of ^{3}H uridine (39). The precursor specific activity of the uridine at the site of synthesis of the RNA was not known; thus it was only possible to compare the relative specific activity of the RNA isolated from the bound and free polysomes. Since the ribosomal subunits appear to be available for incorporation into either of

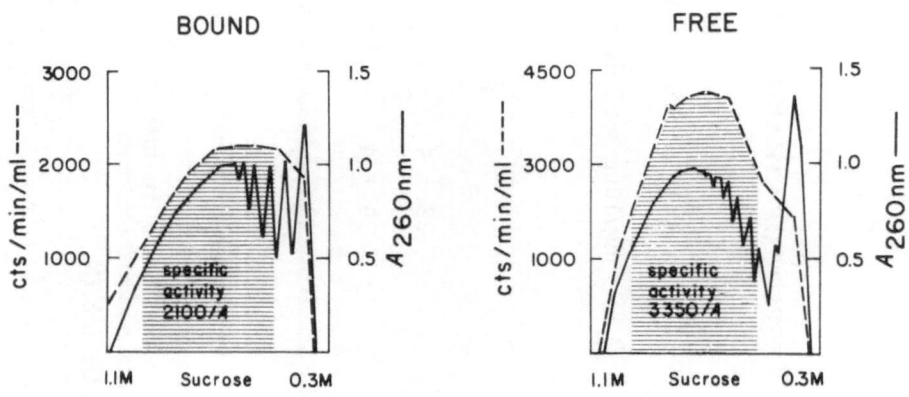

Fig. 1   Polysome profiles obtained from the liver of a fed donor perfused with the control perfusate.
Bound polysome profile on the left and the free polysome profile on the right.
Both polysome profiles show aggregation as indicated by the increased absorbance as the gradient increases towards the more concentrated sucrose levels. The hatched areas represent the portions of each gradient used to calculate the specific activity ^{3}H uridine/A, for each profile. The specific activity of each profile was obtained; the ratio of these activities (B/F) = 0.62.

these organelles, labeling of one polysome species higher than the other would indicate a decreased ability of the labeled ribosomal subunit pool to cycle through that particular polysome population (40, 41). In the fed control preparation, both the bound and the free polysomes were aggregated with some 69% of the polysome profile heavier than trisomes. Furthermore, the bound to free polysome ^{3}H uridine ratio averaged 0.6 (39) (Figure 1). Following a fast there was a marked loss of hepatic RNA and there was considerable disaggregation of the bound polysome, but the ^{3}H bound/free polysome ratio was unaltered. With the ethanol perfusates and perfusion for 2.5 – 3.5 hours, no loss of hepatic RNA was noted, but marked disaggregation of the bound polysome occurred with a significant decrease in the bound to free ^{3}H uridine ratio (Figure 2) suggesting that the effects of ethanol differed from that of fasting at least by two main points: first, there was no reduction in RNA during the acute exposure to the alcohol and second, there appeared to be an inhibition of newly synthesized labeled ribosomes cycling on to the endoplasmic reticulum bound polysome. Further, when the liver was obtained from a fasted donor and perfused with ethanol, albumin

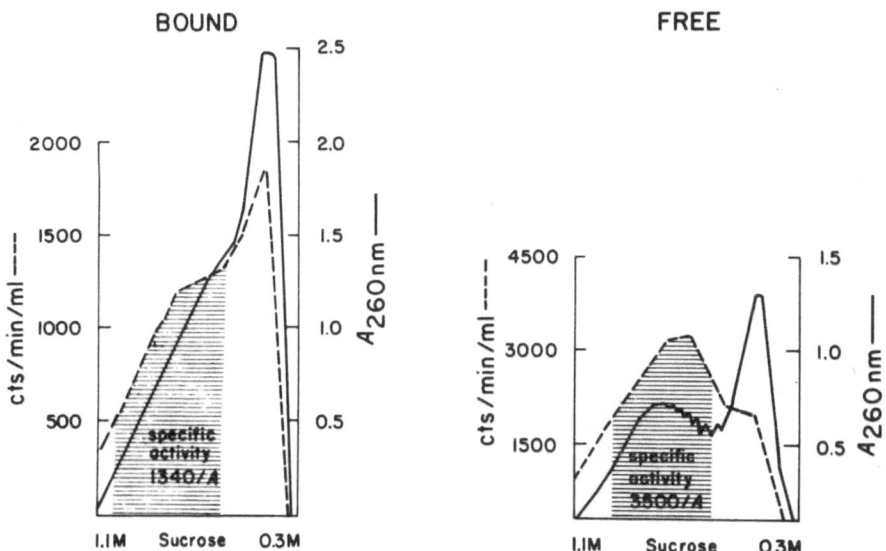

Fig. 2   *Polysome profiles obtained from the liver of a fed donor perfused with 200 mg% ethanol. (See Fig. 1) (39).*
   Bound polysome profile on the left and the free polysome profile on the right. Ratio of specific activities: B/F = 0.38.
   The found polysome is disaggregated with only a small fraction of the absorbance found in the heavier layers of the sucrose gradient. The free polysome is aggregated while the bound/free, ^{3}H uridine/ A , ratio is depressed, suggesting a decreased cycling of newly synthesized ribosomal RNA on to the bound polysome.

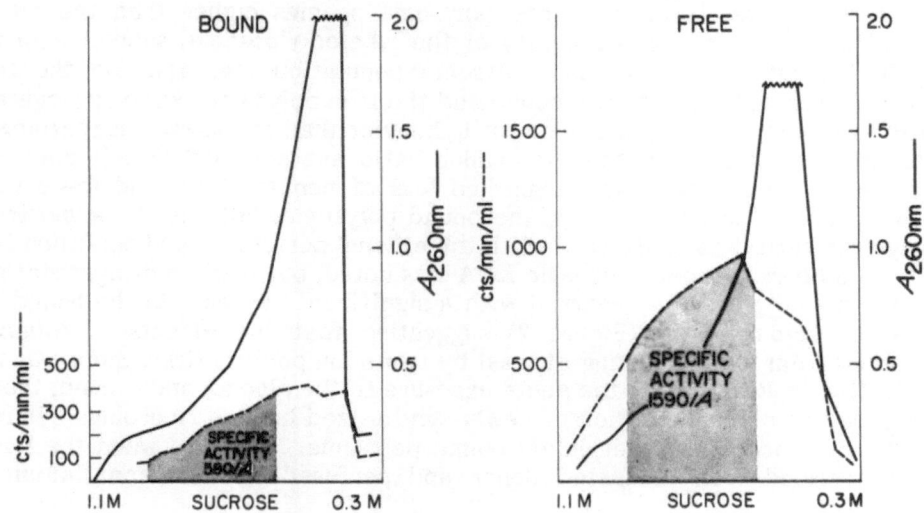

Fig. 3   Bound and free polysome profiles obtained from a liver from a
           fasted donor perfused with 200 mg% ethanol.
           Both profiles are disaggregated and the bound/free polysome ^{3}H
           uridine/ A . ratio is depressed. Ratio of specific activities: B/F =
           0.36.

synthesis was depressed even further and both the bound and free polysomes
were disaggregated (Figure 3) (39). In addition, when the liver was derived
from a fed donor, the stimulating amino acids were capable of causing
significant reaggregation of the bound polysome to values averaging 60 to 70
per cent of the degree of aggregation found in the fed control preparation.
These amino acids, however, were totally incapable of producing any degree
of aggregation of either the bound or free polysome when the combined
stresses of fasting and alcohol were investigated, (Figure 3, Table IV). These
results strongly suggest that the prior nutritional state and the presence of a
significant concentration of exogenous amino acids plays an important role
in preventing the acute effects of alcohol on the protein synthetic
mechanism.

      In attempting to unravel the mechanism whereby these exogenously
infused amino acids produced the reversal of both the alcohol and fasting
induced changes in albumin sythesis, our attention was focused on the
observation that one of the amino acids which was effective was ornithine,
an amino acid not incorporated into protein. However ornithine, while being
a key amino acid in the urea cycle, is also the direct precursor of the
polyamines, putrescine, spermidine and spermine (Figure 4). And it seemed
as if the last might be the important key in explaining the stimulating
effects that various amino acids showed in albumin production. In support of
this concept was the observation that all the amino acids which resulted in
the stimulus to albumin production, when fasting was used as the stress,

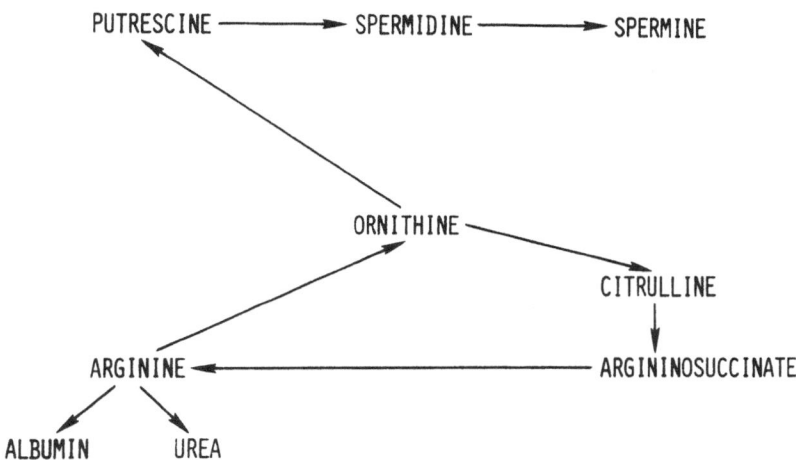

Fig. 4   Schematic representation of the synthetic pathways of the polyamines.

resulted not only in increments in albumin production but also in urea synthesis. This question was investigated utilizing the same system but enriching the perfusate, not with amino acids but with 1 mM spermine equivalent to the levels found in liver tissue in vivo (42). It was shown that whether the stress was fasting or ethanol the addition of spermine resulted in significant reaggregation of the endoplasmic membrane bound polysome (42). However, albumin synthesis remained relatively depressed in both these situations even though the basic organelle responsible for albumin synthesis was returned towards its normal state of aggregation (Table V). Since arginine is the amino acid with the shortest hepatic half-life, it was felt that this amino acid (which is also increased if the rate of urea synthesis is increased) might be rate-limiting. Thus, in addition to spermine, 10 mM arginine was added to the perfusates and now albumin synthesis equalled that found in the fed control state and the combination of ethanol, arginine and spermine, using a liver from a fasted donor, was not statistically different from the fed control preparation. Thus, arginine and spermine appeared synergistic in their ability not only to reaggregate the endoplasmic membrane bound polysome, aided by spermine, but also to supply the rate limiting amino acid, arginine, for albumin production. It is interesting to speculate that an additional role of arginine may be related to its presence in the proalbumin hexapeptide which may bind the growing albumin molecule to the endoplasmic reticulum and contains at least 3 arginine residues (13). Additional studies on the myriad steps in protein synthesis from initiation through elongation to termination will have to be performed before the specific role in these factors can be evaluated ultimately.

TABLE V

EFFECT OF SPERMINE ON ALBUMIN SYNTHESIS (42)

DONOR	PERFUSATE	UREA SYNTHESIS	ALBUMIN SYNTHESIS	DEGREE OF BOUND POLYSOME AGGREGATION
		mg/100g wet liver weight per hour		% of profile heavier than trisome
FASTED	SPERMINE	74 $\pm$ 7	10 $\pm$ 1	65 $\pm$ 3
FASTED	SPERMINE ARGININE	208 $\pm$ 38	16 $\pm$ 3	60 $\pm$ 2
FED	ETHANOL SPERMINE	20 $\pm$ 2	9 $\pm$ 1	46 $\pm$ 4
FED	ETHANOL SPERMINE ARGININE	54 $\pm$ 5	17 $\pm$ 2	53 $\pm$ 2

ETHANOL 200 mg%   ARGININE 10 mM   SPERMINE 1 mM

VALUES EXPRESSED AS THE MEAN $\pm$ S.E. OF MEAN

TABLE VI

EFFECTS OF ACETALDEHYDE ON ALBUMIN SYNTHESIS

DONOR	PERFUSATE	UREA SYNTHESIS	ALBUMIN SYNTHESIS	DEGREE OF BOUND POLYSOME AGGREGATION
		mg/100g wet liver weight per hour		% of profile heavier than trisome
FED	ETHANOL	11 ± 2	6 ± 1	28 ± 3
FED	ACETALDEHYDE	20 ± 2	11 ± 1	61 ± 3
FED	ARGININE	55 ± 4	12 ± 1	52
FASTED	ACETALDEHYDE	50 ± 3	11 ± 1	49 ± 2
FASTED	ACETALDEHYDE ARGININE	102 ± 16	14 ± 2	62 ± 6

ETHANOL 200 mg%   ARGININE 10 mM   ACETALDEHYDE 2 mg%

VALUES EXPRESSED AS THE MEAN $\pm$ S.E. OF MEAN

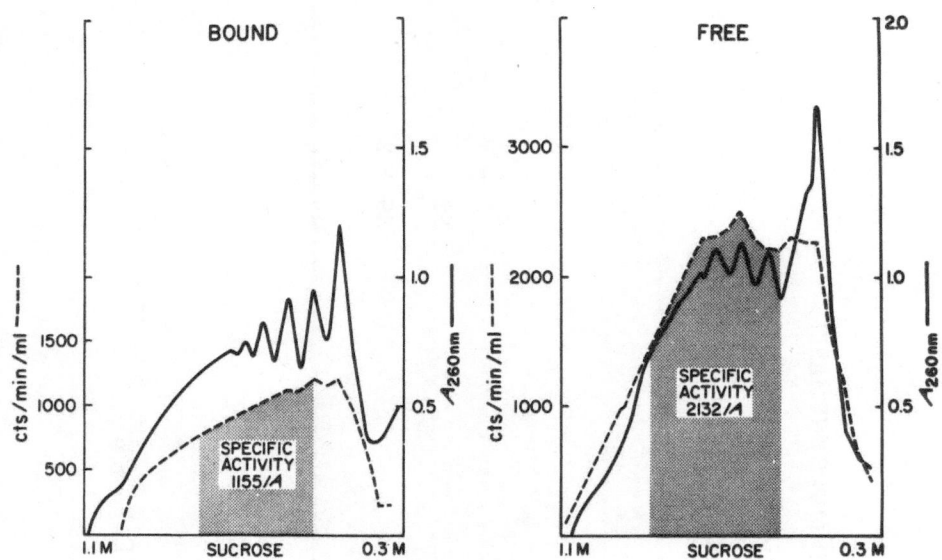

Fig. 5   *Bound and free polysome profiles from the liver of a fasted*
donor perfused with 2 mg% acetaldehyde.
Bound polysome profile to the left and the free polysome profile
to the right. Ratio of specific activities: B/F = 0.54.
Following perfusion with 2 mg% acetaldehyde for 3.5 hours,
significant polysome disaggregation was not observed and the
bound/free ^{3}H uridine/ A . ratio was not lowered.

In the production of specific lesions within the liver cell it has clearly been shown that alcohol per se causes a disruption of the endoplasmic reticulum. But the mechanism for this destructive phenomenon is clear. Recently much attention has been devoted to acetaldehyde, the primary metabolite of alcohol. For not only has acetaldehyde been shown to alter the intermediary metabolism within the liver cell (43-50), but acetaldehyde has been shown to result in a depression in cardiac muscle protein synthesis (51-52). In the perfusion studies with 200 mg% ethanol, acetaldehyde levels in the liver outflow have been observed to be about 2 mg%. Thus, studies were undertaken in which the livers were perfused continuously with 2-3 mg% acetaldehyde. When the liver was derived from a fed donor (Table VI) the infusion of acetaldehyde, while lowering albumin synthesis to 11 mg/100 g wet liver wt, a value double that seen with the alcohol perfusions, failed to cause any significant polysome disaggregation and did not lower the bound to free polysome ^{3}H uridine ratio. Further, when the liver was derived from a fasted donor, this level of acetaldehyde failed to lower albumin production more than that seen with fasting alone and again did not alter the degree of aggregation of the polysome (53) (Figure 5). In addition, excess arginine not only reversed the acute effects of acetaldehyde when the liver was derived from a fed donor but also completely reversed the acute effects of the combined stresses of fasting and acetaldehyde, a phenomenon which was not observed when alcohol was infused instead of acetaldehyde. Thus, while there are effects of acetaldehyde on albumin synthesis, namely a decrease in albumin production, the mechanism of action of this metabolic byproduct of alcohol does not appear to be the same as with alcohol per se as evidenced by the limited effect in the fed donor and by the lack of effect of acetaldehyde when the donor was fasted. While acetaldehyde per se may be toxic to some organs these present studies offer no support to the concept that the acute effects seen with the alcohol represent the influence of acetaldehyde.

DISCUSSION

In attempting to understand, at least in a preliminary fashion, the effects of ethanol exposure on protein synthesis, 3 major points must be considered: energy availability, availability of substrate, and the integrity of the protein synthesizing mechanism with the cell. It has been clearly shown that exposure to ethanol results in significant alterations in mitochondrial morphology and function and thus it may be expected to effect energy availability in terms of ATP production. Thus, it was not unreasonable to expect that these changes might have some influence on the protein synthetic mechanism. However, it has been shown that hepatic polysomes are extremely resistant to disaggregation caused by decreases in ATP levels (54). Further, since the levels of ATP found in acute alcohol exposure have not been shown to decrease (55), it is unlikely that these alterations, per se, are the major cause of the disruption of the hepatic subcellular mechanism for the synthesis of proteins seen following ethanol exposure.

A second and probably most important factor in maintaining the integrity of the polysomal system for the synthesis of serum albumin and other proteins appears to be an adequate supply of amino acids externally administered to the liver (9). Whereas a short term fast for 24 hours or less rapidly decreases albumin production and disaggregates the endoplasmic membrane bound polysome and is associated with a rapid loss of hepatic RNA, externally administered amino acids rapidly reverse these findings. Acute exposure to ethanol produces the same effects without the loss of hepatic RNA but inhibiting the cycling of newly synthesized RNA onto the bound polysome. Ethanol has been shown to influence the intestinal transport of amino acids (56), possibly by "interfering with energy generating processes coupled to the carrier mechanism" (57), and thus, even though an adequate diet was supplied the liver might be exposed to a situation equivalent to a pharmacologic fast. However, in the isolated perfused liver, no impediment to hepatic uptake of externally administered ^{14}C amino acids was noted in the presence of a concentration of ethanol of 200 mg% (58). The adequately fed liver is capable of withstanding an acute stress of ethanol much better than the liver derived from a fasted donor. For, in the latter situation, not only the bound but also the free polysomes are disaggregated and the liver from a fasted donor fails to respond to measures with which the fed liver can easily and rapidly reverse the acute toxic effects of ethanol on albumin synthesis. While it is clear that exposure to ethanol in experimental situations, even in the presence of an adequate diet (59-60), can produce the pathologic changes seen in cirrhosis of the liver adequate nutrition appears to be vital in preventing the acute effects of ethanol or its metabolites on the albumin synthesizing mechanism.

The integrity of the intracellular cytoplasmic polysomal system for the synthesis of albumin appears to be the primary target of the effects of ethanol in decreasing albumin production. Acute exposure to ethanol rapidly disrupts the endoplasmic reticulum and it is conceivable that alterations in this intracellular organelle could be the cause of the altered rates of albumin production. While the fractional rate of transferrin synthesis has also been observed to decrease, no effect of ethanol has been observed on fibrinogen synthesis, another protein destined for export and requiring a valid microtubular structure. Specific amino acids delivered to the liver through the portal vein play important roles in maintaining the integrity of the endoplasmic reticulum bound polysome.   Of these amino acids, ornithine and arginine appear to play critical roles. Not only is ornithine not found in serum albumin, but all the amino acids that stimulate albumin synthesis also stimulate urea synthesis - an observation which demands that increased quantities of ornithine and arginine will be available to the liver cell. It was this observation which suggested that the effects of specific amino acids in reversing the acute effects of alcohol might be related to a dual mechanism - the first involving arginine directly, and the second based upon the concept that ornithine is the immediate precursor of the polyamines, compounds which have been shown to be vital in maintaining the integrity of the polysome system. Arginine is the most rapidly turning over hepatic amino acid and is present in the liver in only trace quantities. Arginine and ornithine are capable of reversing the alcohol-induced effects or depression of albumin synthesis but are ineffective in either stimulating polysome reaggregation or albumin synthesis when the liver is derived from a fasted donor and this liver is exposed to ethanol. In this situation, the addition of spermine is needed to produce a reversal of the acute ethanol effects. It is as if arginine is the rate limiting amino acid and that adequate quantities of spermine are necessary to maintain an effective aggregated subcellular synthesizing system.

The role of acetaldehyde in producing alterations in protein synthesis is receiving more and more attention. Changes in cardiac muscle protein synthesis have been ascribed to this agent and not to ethanol. Acetaldehyde has also been shown to interfere with protein synthesis in liver slice studies (49) though the latter design is complicated by the fact that the integrity of the cells within the slice is much less than that of the cells near the surface. However acetaldehyde, in an amount far in excess of what is found in vivo, has only a minimal effect in decreasing albumin synthesis in the perfused liver from a fed donor, has no effect in decreasing albumin synthesis when

TABLE VII

ETHANOL VS. ACETALDEHYDE VS. FASTING

	ETHANOL	ACETALDEHYDE	FASTING
ALBUMIN SYNTHESIS	DECREASED IN LIVERS FROM FED OR FASTED DONORS BY 60-70%.	DECREASED IN LIVERS FROM FED DONORS BY 39%; NO CHANGE WHEN LIVER IS OBTAINED FROM FASTED DONORS.	DECREASED BY 40 - 50%
TOTAL RNA	NO CHANGE	NO CHANGE	DECREASED BY 30 - 40%
FREE POLYSOME	AGGREGATED	AGGREGATED	AGGREGATED
BOUND POLYSOME	DISAGGREGATED	AGGREGATED	PARTIALLY DISAGGREGATED
RIBOSOME EXCHANGE	DECREASED	UNCHANGED	UNCHANGED OR STIMULATED
FASTING PLUS	BOUND AND FREE POLYSOMES DISAGGREGATED. NO RESPONSE TO AMINO ACIDS	BOUND POLYSOME PARTIALLY DISAGGREGATED. GOOD RESPONSE TO AMINO ACIDS	

the liver is derived from a fasted donor, does not result in polysome disaggregation and does not interfere with the cycling of newly synthesized RNA on to the bound polysome. Thus, while acetaldehyde may interfere at some step following protein initiation, the mechanism of action of ethanol cannot be ascribed to acetaldehyde per se (Table VII). It is conceivable that the production of acetaldehyde by the liver may even be protective to this organ.

The first step in the metabolism of ethanol is a reversible oxidation to acetaldehyde catalyzed by alcohol dehydrogenase (ADH). ADH activity is influenced by diet (61). Livers from fed donors will have ADH activity greater than those derived from fasted donors, and it is conceivable that in livers from fed donors the presence of high levels of acetaldehyde will form ethanol through a reversal of the above reaction (44). Thus, the depressant effects of acetaldehyde in "fed" livers may be the consequence of ethanol formation. On the other hand, the livers from fasted donors with depressed ADH activity cannot convert acetaldehyde to an amount of ethanol that may be toxic.

If one continues on this line of reasoning one comes to the conclusion that the reason a liver from a fed donor can better withstand the effects of ethanol is because it is capable of converting ethanol to the less toxic acetaldehyde than a liver from a fasted donor with depressed ADH activity.

As indicated in the introduction, the mechanism responsible for protein synthesis is a highly complex one involving many steps. The results of these current studies only indicate that gross changes in the system may be produced, in particular, by exposure to or by the metabolism of ethanol. The exact steps whereby ethanol interferes in this system are clearly not known. In vivo measurements of protein production during ethanol exposure, do not appear to offer any chance of delineating the cause of the disruption of protein synthesis since the in vivo regulatory systems are as diverse as the protein synthesizing system itself. It will be necessary to utilize specific isolated systems and to ask of these systems very specific questions in order that adequate answers may be obtained.

SUMMARY

Utilizing the isolated perfused rabbit liver as the model, the effects of ethanol, acetaldehyde and fasting on albumin synthesis are described. A 24-48 hour fast decreases albumin synthesis by 50% associated with a 30% loss of hepatic RNA and disaggregation of the endoplasmic membrane bound polysome without any alteration in the degree of incorporation of newly synthesized RNA into this polysome species. Perfusion of the liver from a fed donor with ethanol decreases albumin synthesis by 67%, disaggregates the bound polysome, and inhibits the cycling of newly synthesized ribosomal RNA into this bound polysome, without any loss of RNA. The combination of stresses, namely fasting plus ethanol, is more toxic than either stress alone. Excess arginine and ornithine are capable of reversing the ethanol induced effects as long as the liver is obtained from a fed donor and spermine is effective in causing polysome reaggregation.

Acetaldehyde reduces albumin synthesis by 39% when the liver is derived from a fed donor but has no effect on the other parameters. Further, acetaldehyde at levels of 2 mg% does not influence albumin synthesis in the fasted state.

ACKNOWLEDGEMENTS

This work was supported in part by grants from the U.S. Public Health Service No. AA00959 and HL 09562; and the Louise and Bernard Palitz Fund.

REFERENCES

1. POST J, PATEK AJ, JR.: Serum proteins in cirrhosis of the liver. Arch Intern Med 69: 67-82, 83-89, 1942

2. BERSON SA, YALOW RS: The distribution of I^{131} labeled human serum albumin introduced into ascitic fluid: analysis of the kinetics of a three compartment catenary transfer system in man and speculations on possible sites of degradation. J Clin Invest 33: 377-387, 1954

3. HASCH E, JARNUM S, TYGSTRUP N: Albumin synthesis rate as a measure of liver function in patients with cirrhosis. Acta Med Scand 182: 83-92, 1967

4. DYKES PW: A study of the effects of albumin infusions in patients with cirrhosis of the liver. Q J Med 30: 297-327, 1961

5. WILKINSON P, MENDENHALL CL: Serum albumin turnover in normal subjects and patients with cirrhosis measured by ^{131}I-labeled human albumin. Clin Sci 25: 281-292, 1963

6. DYKES PW: The rates of distribution and catabolism of albumin in normal subjects and in patients with cirrhosis of the liver. Clin Sci 34: 161-183, 1968

7. CHERRICK GR, KERR DNS, READ AE, et al: Colloid osmotic pressure and hydrostatic pressure relationships in the formation of ascites in hepatic cirrhosis. Clin Sci 19: 361-375, 1960

8. ROTHSCHILD MA, ORATZ M, SCHREIBER SS: Changing concepts of albumin metabolism and distribution in cirrhosis of the liver. Scand J Gastroenterol 7: 17-23, 1970

9. ROTHSCHILD MA, ORATZ M, SCHREIBER SS: Albumin synthesis. N
    Engl J Med 286: 748-757; 816-821, 1972

10. MUNRO HN: A general survey of mechanisms regulating protein
    metabolism in mammals. In Mammalian Protein Metabolism, vol. 4.
    HN Munro (ed.). New York, Academic Press 1970. pp. 3-130

11. REDMAN CM: The synthesis of serum proteins on attached rather than
    free ribosomes of rat liver. Biochem & Biophys Res Commun 31:
    845-850, 1968

12. TAKAGI M, OGOTA K: Direct evidence for albumin biosynthesis by
    membrane bound polysomes in rat liver. Biochem & Biophys Res
    Commun 33: 55-60, 1968

13. QUINN PS, GAMBLE M, JUDAH JD: Biosynthesis of serum albumin in
    rat liver: isolation and probable structure of 'proalbumin' from rat
    liver. Biochem J 146: 389-393, 1975

14. URBAN J, INGLIS AS, EDWARDS K, SCHREIBER G: Chemical
    evidence for the difference between albumins from microsomes and
    serum and a possible precursor-product relationship. Biochem &
    Biophys Res Commun 61: 444-450, 1974

15. MECHLER B, VASSALLI P: Membrane-bound ribosomes of myeloma
    cells: III. The role of Messenger RNA and the nascent polypeptide
    chain in the binding of ribosomes to membranes. J Cell Biol 67:
    25-37, 1973

16. JUDAH JD, GAMBLE M, STEADMAN JH: Biosynthesis of serum
    albumin in rat liver: Evidence for the existence of 'proalbumin'.
    Biochem J 134: 1083-1091, 1973

17. RUSSELL JH, GELLER DM: Rat serum albumin biosynthesis: Evidence
    for a precursor. Biochem & Biophys Res Commun 55: 239-245,
    1973

18. BLOBEL G, DOBBERSTEIN B: Transfer of proteins across membranes:
    I. Presence of proteolytically processed and unprocessed nascent
    immunoglobin light chains on membrane-bound ribosomes of murine
    myeloma. J Cell Biol 67: 835-851, 1975

19. JACOBS-LORENA M, BAGLIONI C: A study of ribosomal subunits
    during cell free protein synthesis. Biochim Biophys Acta 224:
    165-173, 1970

20. HENSHAW EC, GUINEY DG, HIRSCH, CA: The ribosome cycle in
    mammalian protein synthesis. I. The place of monomeric
    ribosomes and ribosomal subunits in the cycle. J Biol Chem 248:
    4367-4376, 4377-4385, 1973

21. ADELMAN MR, SABATINI DD, BLOBEL G: Ribosome - membrane interaction. Non destructive disassembly of rat liver rough microsomes into ribosomal and membranous components. J Cell Biol 56: 206-229, 1973

22. HARRISON TM, BROWNLEE GG, MILSTEIN C: Studies on polysome - membrane interactions in mouse myeloma cells. Euro J Biochem 47: 613-620, 1974

23. SKOGERSON L, MOLDAVE K: Characterization of the interaction of aminoacyl transferase II with ribosomes; binding of transferase II and translocation of peptidyl transfer ribonucleic acid. J Biol Chem 243: 5354-5360, 1968

24. SKOGERSON L, MOLDAVE, K: Evidence for the role of aminoacyl-transferase II and translocation of peptidyl transfer ribonucleic acid. J Biol Chem 243: 5345-5360, 1968

25. SKOGERSON L, MOLDAVE K: Evidence for aminoacyl-tRNA binding, peptide bond synthesis, and translocase activities in the aminoacyl transfer reactions. Arch Biochem 125: 497-505, 1968

26. CULP W, McKEEHAN W, HARDESTY B: The mechanism of messenger RNA translocation through ribosomes. Proc Natl Acad Sci USA 64: 388-395, 1969

27. GAREN A: Sense and nonsense in the genetic code. Three exceptional triplets can serve as both chain terminating signals and amino acid codons. Science 160: 149-159, 1968

28. CASKEY CT: The universal RNA genetic code. Quart Rev Biophys 3: 295-326, 1970

29. GOLDSTEIN JL, BEAUDET AL, CASKEY CT: Peptide chain termination with mammalian release factor. Proc Natl Acad Sci USA 67: 99-106, 1970

30. VOGEL A, ZAMIR A, ELSON D: The possible involvement of peptidyl tranferase in the termination step of protein biosynthesis. Bioch 8: 5161-5168, 1969

31. CAPECCHI MR, KLEIN HA: Characterization of three proteins involved in polypeptide chain termination. Cold Spring Harbor Symp: Quart Biol 34: 469-477, 1969

32. BEAUDET AL, CASKEY CT: Mammalian peptide chain termination. II codon specificity and GTPase activity of release factor. Proc Natl Acad Sci USA 68: 619-624, 1971

33. GOLDSTEIN JL, CASKEY CT: Peptide chain termination effect of protein on ribosomal binding of release factors. Proc Natl Acad Sci USA 67: 537-543, 1970

34. ROTHSCHILD MA, ORATZ M, ZIMMON D, SCHREIBER SS, WEINER I, VAN CANEGHEM A: Albumin synthesis in cirrhotic subjects with ascites studied with carbonate-^{14}C.   J Clin Invest 48: 344-350, 1969

35. ROTHSCHILD MA, ORATZ M, MONGELLI J, SCHREIBER SS: Effect of a short-term fast on albumin synthesis studied in vivo, in the perfused liver, and on amino acid incorporation by hepatic microsomes. J Clin Invest 47: 2591-2599, 1968

36. KIRSCH R, FRITH L, BLACK E, HOFFENBERG R: Regulation of albumin synthesis and catabolism by alteration of dietary protein. Nature 217: 578-579, 1968

37. STAEHELIN T, VERNEY E, SIDRANSKY H: The influence of nutritional change on polyribosomes of the liver. Biochim Biophys Acta 145: 105-119, 1967

38. MARSH JB: Effects of fasting and alloxan diabetes on albumin synthesis by perfused rat liver. Am J Physiol 201: 55-57, 1961

39. ROTHSCHILD MA, ORATZ M, SCHREIBER SS: Alcohol, amino acids and albumin synthesis. Gastro 67: 1200-1213, 1974

40. HULSE JL, WETTSTEIN FO: Two separable pools of native ribosomal subunits in chick embryo tissue culture cells. Biochim Biophys Acta 269: 265-275, 1972

41. NORMAN M, GAMULIN S, CLARK K: The distribution of ribosomes between different functional states in livers of fed and starved mice. Biochem J 134: 387-398, 1973

42. ORATZ M, ROTHSCHILD MA, SCHREIBER SS: Alcohol, amino acids and albumin synthesis. II. Alcohol inhibition of albumin synthesis reversed by arginine. Gastro 71: 123-127, 1976

43. LINDROS KO: Acetaldehyde oxidation and its role in the overall metabolic effects of ethanol in the liver. In Alfred Benzon Symp. 6th, Regulation of hepatic metabolism. J Lindquist (ed.).   New York, London. Academic Press, 1974. pp. 417-432

44. LINDROS KO, VIHMA R, FORSANDER OA: Utilization and metabolic effects of acetaldehyde and ethanol in the perfused rat liver. Biochem J 126: 945-952, 1972

45. RAHWAN RG: Toxic effects of ethanol: Possible role of acetaldehyde tetrahydroisoquinolines, and tetrahydro-β-carbolines. Toxicol Appl Pharmacol 34: 3-27, 1975

46. KOIVULA T, LINDROS KO: Effects of long-term ethanol treatment on aldehyde and alcohol dehydrogenase activities in rat liver. Biochem Pharmacol 24: 1937-1942, 1975

47. KORSTEN MA, MATSUZAKI S, FEINMAN L, LIEBER CS: High blood acetaldehyde levels after ethanol administration: Difference between alcoholic and nonalcoholic subjects. N Engl J Med 292: 386-389, 1975

48. HASWMURA Y, TESCHKE R, LIEBER CS: Acetaldehyde oxidation by hepatic mitochondria: Decrease after chronic ethanol consumption. Science 189: 727-728, 1975

49. PERIN A, SCALABRINO G, SESSA A, ARNABOLDI A: In vitro inhibition of protein synthesis in rat liver as a consequence of ethanol metabolism. Biochim Biophys Acta 366: 101-108, 1974

50. RUBIN E, CEDERBAUM AI: Effects of ethanol and acetaldehyde on hepatic mitochondria. In Alcoholic Liver Pathology. Y Israel, H Kalant, (eds.). Ontario, Addiction Research Foundation 1975. pp. 305

51. SCHREIBER SS, BRIDEN K, ORATZ M, ROTHSCHILD MA: Ethanol, acetaldehyde and myocardial protein synthesis. J Clin Invest 51: 2820-2826, 1972

52. SCHREIBER SS: Stress and myocardial protein synthesis: The effect of alcohol and acetaldehyde. In Alcohol and Abnormal Protein Biosynthesis. MA Rothschild, M Oratz, SS Schreiber, (eds.). New York, Pergamon Press, 1975. pp. 273-291

53. ORATZ M, ROTHSCHILD MA, SCHREIBER SS: Differing effects of acetaldehyde and ethanol on hepatic albumin synthesis and cardiac muscle protein synthesis. Natl Council on Alcoholism. Wash DC. In Press, 1976

54. CLIFFORD AJ, RIUMALLO JA, BAGLIA BS, MUNRO HN, BROWN PR: Liver nucleotide metabolism in relation to amino acid supply. Biochim Biophys Acta 277: 443-448, 1972

55. GUYNN RW, PIEKLIK JR: Dependence on dose of the acute effects of ethanol on liver metabolism in vivo. J Clin Invest 56: 1411-1419, 1975

56. ISRAEL Y, VALENZUELA JE, SALAZAR I, UGARTE G: Alcohol and amino acid transport in the human small intestine. J Nutr 98: 222-224, 1969

57. CHEN T, GLAZKO AJ: Effect of ethanol on amino acid transport. In Alcohol and Abnormal Protein Biosynthesis: Biochemical and Clinical. MA Rothschild, M Oratz, SS Schreiber, (eds.). New York, Pergamon Press, 1975. pp. 95-110

58. ROTHSCHILD MA, ORATZ M, SCHREIBER SS: The hepatic protein synthesizing response to alcohol and fasting. In Plasma Protein Turnover. R Bianchi, G Mariani, AS McFarlane, (eds.). Baltimore, Md., 1976. In press

59. RUBIN E, LIEBER CS: Experimental alcohol hepatitis: A new primate model. Science 182: 712-713, 1973

60. RUBIN E, LIEBER CS: Fatty liver, alcohol hepatitis and cirrhosis produced by alcohol in subhuman primates. N Engl J Med 290: 128-135, 1974

61. BODE, JC: Factors influencing ethanol metabolism in man. In Alcohol and Aldehyde Metabolizing Systems. RG Thurman, JR Williamson, T Yonetani and B Chance, (eds.). New York, Academic Press, 1974. pp. 457-468

MECHANISM OF INDUCTION BY ETHANOL OF HEPATIC MICROSOMAL DRUG METABOLIZING ENZYMES

Jean-Gil Joly, Jean-Pierre Villeneuve, P. Mavier and C. Hétu

Clinical Research Center and Department of Medicine

Hôpital Saint-Luc and Université de Montréal, Québec

INTRODUCTION

It is widely accepted that alcoholics when sober are tolerant to a number of drugs. Although some effects of chronic ethanol administration are due to alterations of the sensitivity of the target organ to drugs (1), it has also been shown that ethanol accelerates the metabolism of xenobiotics (2). It is now accepted that microsomal hepatic drug biotransformation is stimulated by chronic ethanol administration (3,4).

When ethanol is chronically fed to rats, toxic and adaptive changes are observed in the liver (5). One adaptive change is the proliferation of the smooth endoplasmic reticulum first observed in the rat by Iseri et al. (6) and confirmed in the human by Lane et al. (7). These morphological alterations have been confirmed by biochemical methods when it was shown that the protein and phospholipid mass of the smooth microsomes was indeed increased following chronic ethanol administration (8). The essential microsomal mixed function oxidases components (9), cytochrome P-450 (10), NADPH-cytochrome P-450 reductase (11) and microsomal phospholipids (8), have all been shown to increase in content or in activity after chronic ethanol administration. Therefore, it is logical to observe that various drug metabolizing enzyme activities are enhanced by ethanol (3,4,11-13). An increase in hepatic drug biotransformation could explain, at least in part, why the clearance of drugs is more rapid in animals or in humans chronically fed with ethanol (2).

The mechanism(s) through which ethanol increases microsomal drug biotransformation is (are) as yet unclear. Studies with phenobarbital and methylcholanthrene have shown that microsomal phospholipid mass and composition were differently altered by the administration of these drugs, suggesting that microsomal phospholipid alterations could be related to the

TABLE I

EFFECT OF CHRONIC ALCOHOL FEEDING (36% OF CALORIES) WITH HIGH AND LOW FAT DIETS ON MICROSOMAL CYTOCHROME P-450 CONTENT, NADPH-CYTOCHROME P-450 REDUCTASE ACTIVITY, PHOSPHOLIPID CONTENT AND THE ACTIVITIES OF BENZPHETAMINE DEMETHYLASE AND ANILINE HYDROXYLASE (MEAN SE)

	35% cal. as fat (high fat diet)			2% cal. as fat (low fat diet)		
	n*	Control	Ethanol	n	Control	Ethanol
Cytochrome P-450						
(n moles/mg protein)	30	0.959±0.052	1.457±0.118 Ψ	22	0.819±0.032	1.030±0.044 Ψ
(n moles/g liver)	30	40.32±1.90	61.84±5.23 Ψ	22	35.35±1.95	39.89±2.51 §
NADPH-cytochrome P-450 reductase (ΔO.D. 465–450 sec^{-1} X 10^{-3})						
ΔO.D./mg protein	9	24.54±1.85	41.72±4.39 ¶	9	26.37±1.09	30.62±2.17
ΔO.D./100 g body weight	9	4679±427	9748±1600 ¶	9	4992±173	5443±516
Microsomal phospholipids						
(mg/mg protein)	29	0.421±0.022	0.447±0.095 Σ	22	0.420±0.020	0.460±0.020
(mg/100 g body weight)	29	70.58±5.69	89.43±83.93	22	73.69±5.31	73.50±6.02
Benzphetamine demethylase (n moles formaldehyde min^{-1})						
/mg protein	23	5.24±0.53	6.46±0.54 Ψ	21	4.68±0.47	6.32±0.73 Ψ
/100 g body weight	23	907±115	1178±135 Ψ	21	831±196	1023±142 ¶

TABLE I . . . Cont'd

	35% cal. as fat (high fat diet)			2% cal. as fat (low fat diet)		
	n*	Control	Ethanol	n	Control	Ethanol
Aniline hydroxylase (n moles p-aminophenol min^{-1})						
/mg protein	26	0.855±0.032	2.300±0.080$^{\Psi}$	22	0.810±0.106	1.830±0.080$^{\Psi}$
/100 g body weight	26	137±5	391±20	22	135±15	280±18

* number of pairs
Ψ p < 0.001
§ p < 0.05
Σ p < 0.02
¶ p < 0.01

(From: Joly J-G, Hétu C: Effect of chronic ethanol administration in the rat: relative dependency on dietary lipids. I. Induction of hepatic drug metabolizing enzymes in vitro. Biochemical Pharmacology 24: 1475–1480, 1975)

induction of microsomal enzymes (14). Other lines of evidence, however, tend to suggest that various inducers produce both an increase in cytochrome P-450 content and the induction of cytochrome P-450 species different in their substrate specificity (15). In the present work we will give experimental evidence showing that induction of microsomal drug metabolizing enzymes by ethanol is not related to microsomal phospholipid changes but to cytochrome P-450 alterations.

Chronic Ethanol Administration with High Fat Diets: Lack of relationship between qualitative microsomal phospholipid alterations and reconstituted microsomal benzphetamine demethylation activity.

Chronic administration of ethanol (36% of total calories) in the liquid diet rich in dietary lipids (35% of total calories) designed by De Carli and Lieber (16), increases cytochrome P-450 content, NADPH-cytochrome P-450 reductase activity and microsomal phospholipid content in the rat (Table I). Moreover, the composition of microsomal phospholipid, studied by thin layer chromatography, is found to be significantly altered if ethanol is given with high fat diets (Table II). Phosphatidylcholine is quantitatively the most important component accounting for about 60% of microsomal phospholipids. Phosphatidylethanolamine accounts for 20% and phosphatidylinositol and lysophosphatidylcholine together for 10% of total microsomal phospholipids. Sphingomyelin, phosphatidylserine and phosphatidic acid are present in smaller proportions. When the absolute amounts of phospholipids are calculated from these data, we observe that after ethanol, phosphatidylcholine increases 22% per mg of protein ($p < 0.001$) and 25% per gram of liver ($p < 0.005$); phosphatidylethanolamine does not change significantly and sphingomyelin decreases 22% per mg of protein ($p < 0.005$) and 21% per gram of liver ($p < 0.02$).

Because phosphatidylcholine has been shown to be the phospholipid of importance in microsomal drug biotransformation in vitro (17,18), its fatty acid composition has been studied by gas chromatography (Table III). Saturated fatty acids account for more than 50% of all fatty acids present in phosphatidylcholine, mainly in the form of stearic acid. The remaining fatty acids are unsaturated fatty acids, arachidonic acid being present in nearly twice the amount of oleic and linoleic acids together. After ethanol, saturated fatty acids decrease slightly ($p < 0.05$) mainly because of a change in palmitic acid. Unsaturated fatty acids increase 4% (p: N.S.) due to significant increases in oleic (28%, $p < 0.005$) and linoleic (18%, $p < 0.025$) acids. These increases are associated with a slight decrease in arachidonic acid ($p < 0.05$). Since the latter is quantitatively the most abundant, the net increase in absolute content of unsaturated fatty acids is therefore reduced to 4%.

The fatty acid composition of phosphatidylethanolamine, another quantitatively important microsomal phospholipid, was also studied. Saturated fatty acids and unsaturated fatty acids are present in almost the

TABLE II

EFFECT OF ETHANOL AND DIETARY FAT ON PERCENT COMPOSITION
OF HEPATIC MICROSOMAL PHOSPHOLIPIDS

(Values are presented as mean percent of total phospholipid phosphorus ± S.E.)

	35% cal. as fat (high fat diet)*			2% cal. as fat (low fat diet) Ψ		
	Control	Ethanol	Ethanol/Control	Control	Ethanol	Ethanol/Control
Origin	0.43±0.13	0.39±0.09	0.91	0.95±0.21	1.20±0.63	1.26
Phosphatidic acid	0.80±0.22	0.81±0.14	1.01	0.62±0.14	0.59±0.19	0.95
G#	0.26±0.11	0.21±0.07	0.81	0.25±0.08	0.23±0.09	0.92
Phosphatidylserine	3.64±0.39	3.09±0.18	0.85	2.93±0.21	2.73±0.16	0.93
Sphingomyelin	3.45±0.18	2.12±0.15¶	0.61	3.78±0.29	2.84±0.24Σ	0.75
Phosphatidylinositol and Lysophosphatidylcholine	10.20±1.76	10.82±0.30	1.06	10.30±0.36	10.48±0.29	1.02
Phosphatidylcholine	59.80±1.20	62.88±1.11§	1.05	59.03±0.74	59.52±0.40	1.01
Phosphatidylethanolamine	21.09±1.09	19.57±0.73	0.93	21.36±0.82	21.72±0.57	1.02

* 15 pairs   § $p < 0.01$
Ψ 13 pairs   Σ $p < 0.005$
unidentified spot   ¶ $p < 0.001$

(From: Joly J-G, Hétu C, Mavier P, Villeneuve J-P: Mechanism of induction of hepatic drug metabolizing enzymes by ethanol. I. Limited role of microsomal phospholipids. In Biochemical Pharmacology: in press.)

J.G. JOLY ET AL.

TABLE III

EFFECT OF ETHANOL AND DIETARY FAT ON FATTY ACID COMPOSITION OF HEPATIC MICROSOMAL PHOSPHATIDYLCHOLINE

(Values are presented as mean percent of total weight of fatty acids ± S.E.)

Fatty acid	35% cal. as fat (high fat diet)*			2% cal. as fat (low fat diet)$^\Psi$		
	Control	Ethanol	$\frac{\text{Ethanol}}{\text{Control}}$	Control	Ethanol	$\frac{\text{Ethanol}}{\text{Control}}$
14:0 (myristic)	1.16±0.17	1.25±0.18	1.08	1.59±0.16	1.17±0.11 #	0.74
16:0 (palmitic)	17.66±0.55	15.86±0.50 Σ	0.90	21.08±0.69	21.30±1.07	1.01
16:1 (palmitoleic)	0.57±0.12	0.77±0.09	1.35	1.24±0.42	1.38±0.39	1.11
18:0 (stearic)	34.64±0.87	33.97±0.91	0.98	31.37±1.19	29.69±1.32	0.95
18:1 (oleic)	6.65±0.51	8.49±0.45 ¶	1.28	11.05±0.78	12.02±0.63	1.09
18:2 (linoleic)	7.63±0.59	9.02±0.67 §	1.18	5.87±0.26	6.69±0.36	1.14
18:3 (linolenic)	–	–	–	0.43±0.07	0.65±0.08 #	1.51
20:4 (arachidonic)	26.11±0.64	25.11±0.62 #	0.96	22.19±0.87	21.27±1.02	0.96
22:6 (docosahexaenoic)	4.03±0.51	3.34±0.38	0.83	3.32±0.21	3.49±0.18	1.05

* 14 pairs
Ψ 13 pairs

# $p < 0.05$
§ $p < 0.025$
Σ $p < 0.01$
¶ $p < 0.005$

(From: Joly J-G, Hétu C, Mavier P, Villeneuve J-P: Mechanism of induction of hepatic drug metabolizing enzymes by ethanol. I. Limited role of microsomal phospholipids. In Biochemical Pharmacology: in press.)

same proportion in phosphatidylethanolamine. The saturated fatty acid composition of this phospholipid in control animals is similar to that of phosphatidylcholine. Unsaturated fatty acids, however, show a greater proportion of docosahexaenoic acid, the percentage of which is also greater than that of linoleic and oleic acids. When ethanol is administered with high fat diets, there is no significant change in phosphatidylethanolamine fatty acid composition.

Phosphatidylcholine is essential for in vitro drug metabolism (17). Phosphatidylcholines of different fatty acid composition stimulate differently in vitro drug metabolism by reconstituted systems of drug hydroxylation (18). Differences in microsomal phospholipid composition associated with dietary manipulations (19), induction by drugs (14) or related to sex (20), have been suggested to account for corresponding alterations in drug metabolism. Thus, we wondered whether the alterations of microsomal phospholipids observed with chronic ethanol administration with high fat diets could account for the observed increase in microsomal drug biotransformation. If differences in microsomal phospholipid composition were to explain the enhancement by ethanol of microsomal drug metabolizing enzymes, one would expect the microsomal lipid fraction of rats fed ethanol with high fat diets to have a greater stimulatory activity on the reconstituted system of benzphetamine demethylation than the microsomal lipid fraction of control animals. The benzphetamine demethylation stimulation observed by addition of microsomal lipids, obtained from solubilized microsomes of control and ethanol-fed rats, was compared in the presence of purified cytochrome P-450 and purified NADPH-cytochrome c reductase obtained from solubilized microsomes of ethanol-fed rats. It can be seen that the curves of activation of benzphetamine demethylation by either lipid fraction are identical (Fig. 1). This observation strongly suggests that significant alterations by ethanol of microsomal phospholipid composition do not explain the ethanol induction of microsomal benzphetamine demethylation activity.

Chronic Ethanol Administration in Presence of Low Fat Diets: Lack of effect on microsomal phospholipid content and composition and enhancement of in vitro and in vivo drug biotransformation.

The above conclusion was further verified by experiments in which similar amounts of ethanol were given but this time with low fat diets containing always 2% of total calories as linoleate as the only source of fat in order to prevent fatty acid deficiency (13). With such diets, ethanol does not increase the microsomal phospholipid mass even when expressed per 100 grams of body weight (Table I). Only minor changes in microsomal phospholipid composition are observed when ethanol is given with low fat diets (Table II). Sphingomyelin, accounting for less than 4% of the total microsomal phospholipids, decreases significantly but phosphatidylcholine and phosphatidylethanolamine, accounting respectively for 60% and 20% of total microsomal phospholipids, are not altered in their content.

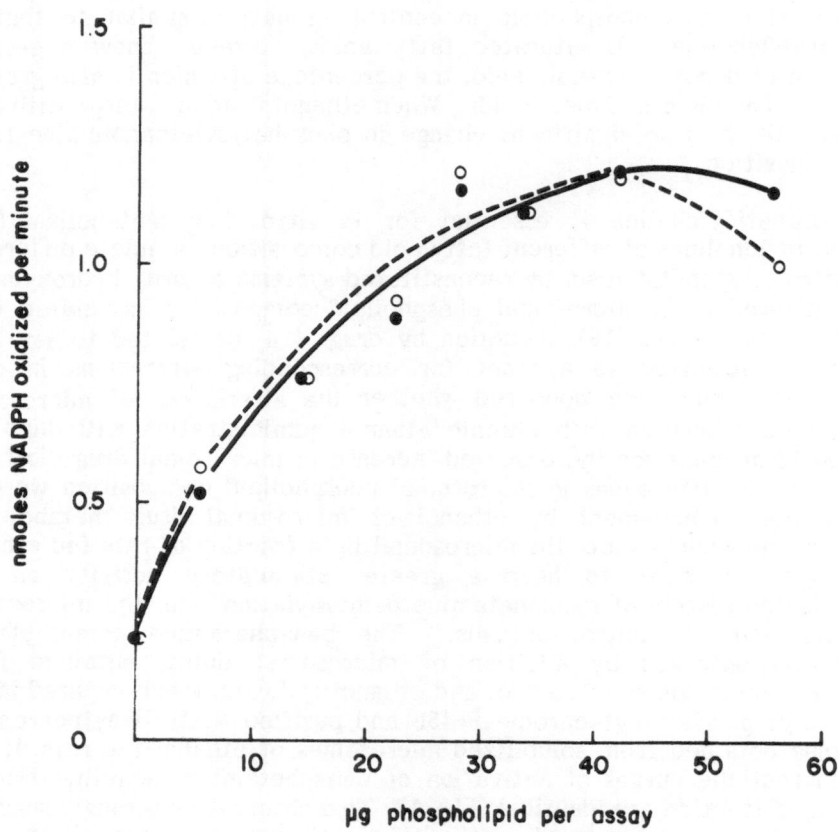

Fig. 1   Benzphetamine N-demethylation in presence of fixed amounts
           of cytochrome P-450 and NADPH-cytochrome c reductase; the
           amount of phospholipids varied from 0 to 56µg phospholipid per
           assay.   The reaction mixture contained potassium phosphate
           buffer 100µmoles (pH 7.4, 30°C), MgCl$_2$ 3µmoles, EDTA 0.05
           µmole, benzphetamine 1 µmole, NADPH 0.1 µmole, step III
           cytochrome P-450 (from microsomes of rats fed ethanol with
           the high fat diet) 0.198 nmole per assay, reductase (from
           microsomes of rats fed ethanol with the high fat diet) 165 units
           per assay, in a total volume of 1 ml. The activity was measured
           by following the rate of oxidation of NADPH (9).   Closed
           circles: lipid fractions from microsomes of control rats; open
           circles: lipid fractions from microsomes of ethanol-fed rats.
           (From: Joly J-G, Hétu C: Effect of chronic ethanol
           administration in the rat: relative dependency on dietary lipids.
           I. Induction of hepatic drug metabolizing enzymes in vitro.
           Biochemical Pharmacology 24: 1475-1480, 1975).

The fatty acid composition of microsomal phosphatidylcholine was also studied in this model (Table III). The proportion of saturated and unsaturated fatty acids was similar to that found with the high fat model with the slight difference that in the controls the saturated fatty acids contained less stearic acid and the unsaturated fatty acids contained slightly less arachidonic and linoleic acids and slightly more oleic acid than in the control rats given the high fat diets. Ethanol administration with the low fat diet only caused a slight (3.6%) but significant ($p < 0.02$) decrease in saturated fatty acids; myristic acid, accounting for less than 2% of total phosphatidylcholine fatty acids, decreased 26% and linolenic acid, accounting for less than 1% of total phosphatidylcholine fatty acids, increased 51%.

When phosphatidylethanolamine fatty acid composition was studied in this model, the only significant alteration observed after ethanol was a 22% decrease in oleic acid that accounts for less than 7% of total phosphatidylethanolamine fatty acids. Thus, when ethanol is administered with low fat diets, no change is observed in the microsomal phospholipid content and only minor alterations are observed in phospholipid composition. However ethanol, even when given with this model, enhances benzphetamine demethylation activity to an extent similar to that observed with the high fat diet model. It also increased aniline hydroxylation activity very significantly, (Table I). Moreover, hexobarbital total body clearance is accelerated after ethanol (Fig. 2), when studied in the same dietary model in which the microsomal phospholipid content per 100 grams of body weight is unchanged after ethanol. If ethanol increases in vitro benzphetamine demethylation and aniline hydroxylation and in vivo hexobarbital total body clearance without significantly altering either the content or the composition of hepatic microsomal phospholipid, we must search for other factors to explain the ethanol induction of microsomal drug metabolizing enzymes.

Partial Purification of Hepatic Microsomal Cytochrome P-450 of Control Rats, Ethanol-Fed Rats, Phenobarbital and Methylcholanthrene-Treated Rats: Evidence for an ethanol-induced species of cytochrome P-450.

As previously stated, the mixed function oxidase system is known to require at least three essential components: cytochrome P-450, NADPH-cytochrome c reductase and phospholipids (9). Studies using reconstituted systems of microsomal drug hydroxylation have shown that phenobarbital and methylcholanthrene induce species of cytochrome P-450 different in their substrate specificity (15). The hemoprotein induced by chronic feeding of ethanol was initially described as having spectral characteristics similar to those of the hemoprotein induced by phenobarbital when it was studied on whole microsomes (10). A cytochrome P-450 species showing high affinity for cyanide was later reported as preferentially induced by ethanol (21,22). More recently, Ullrich et al. reported that ethoxycoumarin O-dealkylation was more inhibited by tetrahydrofurane when using microsomes of ethanol-fed rats than when using microsomes of phenobarbital or benzpyrene-treated animals (23). We have also observed that ethanol induces microsomal aniline

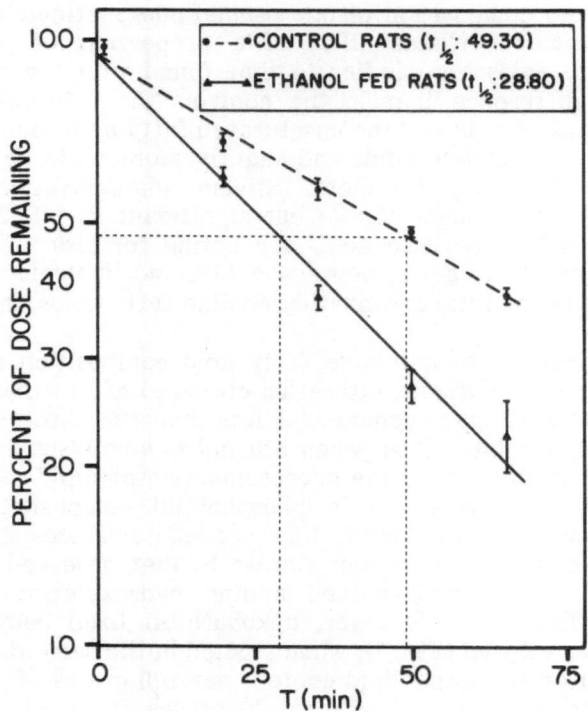

Fig. 2   *Hexobarbital total body clearance in rats fed ethanol with the low fat diet and their controls. The animals were given 100 mg/Kg of sodium hexobarbital-2-^{14}C (0.164 μCi/mg) intraperitoneally. Each point is the mean of 4 animals sacrificed at 1, 20, 35, 50 and 65 minutes after injection.*

hydroxylation more than phenobarbital or methylcholanthrene in Sprague-Dawley rats (Fig. 3) and that this reaction is also more strongly inhibited in microsomes of ethanol-fed rats than in microsomes of phenobarbital or methylcholanthrene-treated animals (Fig. 4). Tetrahydrofurane binds more avidly to microsomes of ethanol-fed rats than to those of controls or phenobarbital or methylcholanthrene-treated animals. The Ks value of tetrahydrofurane for microsomes of ethanol-fed rats is 0.25 mM whereas that of microsomes of control, phenobarbital and methylcholanthrene-treated rats is 10 mM. The existence of a substrate specific ethanol-induced cytochrome P-450 might explain these findings.

To verify this further, we have partially purified cytochrome P-450 of controls, ethanol-fed, phenobarbital-treated and methylcholanthrene-treated animals. Cytochrome P-450 was partially purified to step III according to

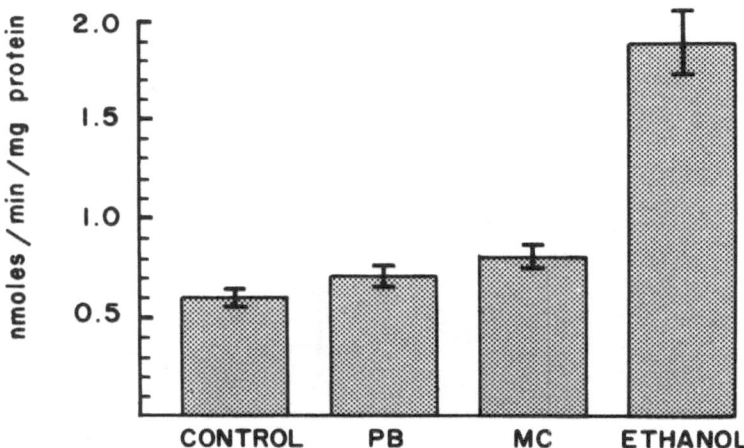

Fig. 3   *Microsomal aniline hydroxylation activity in control, pheno-*
barbital (PB)-treated (75 mg/kg i.p. X 3 days), methyl-
cholanthrene (MC)-treated (25 mg/Kg i.p. X 3 days) and
ethanol-fed (36% of total calories with high fat diets X 21 days)
rats. The reaction mixture contained MgCl₂ 25 μmoles, aniline
40 μmoles, NADP 5 μmoles, glucose-6-phosphate 25 μmoles,
glucose-6-phosphate dehydrogenase 2 units, potassium
phosphate buffer 625 μmoles (pH 7.4, 37°C), microsomal protein
7 mg in a final volume of 5.0 ml. The reaction was stopped with
2 ml of trichloro-acetic acid 23% (w/v) after 20 minutes of
incubation at 37°. The para-aminophenol formed was measured
spectrophotometrically (27).

Levin et al. (2). Spectral characteristics of the partially purified
hemoproteins are given in Table IV. NADPH-cytochrome c reductase and
lipid fractions were also partially purified from microsomes of ethanol-fed
rats according to the methods of Lu et al. (24) and Lu and Coon (25)
respectively. The cytochromes P-450 were then tested for their catalytic
activity in presence of each of three substrates: benzphetamine, benzpyrene
and aniline. In a reconstituted system of drug hydroxylation, it is possible to
compare the relative catalytic activity of cytochrome P-450 from various
sources by using fixed amounts of the same reductase and lipid, and
increasing amounts of each hemoprotein. If the hemoproteins are identical,
the rate of metabolism of a substrate should be the same, when equal
amounts of hemoproteins are used.

Phenobarbital-cytochrome P-450 was found to be much more active for
the N-demethylation of benzphetamine. Methylcholanthrene-cytochrome P-
450 activity is greatest in presence of benzpyrene. Ethanol- cytochrome P-
450 is the most active in the presence of aniline. Control cytochrome P-450

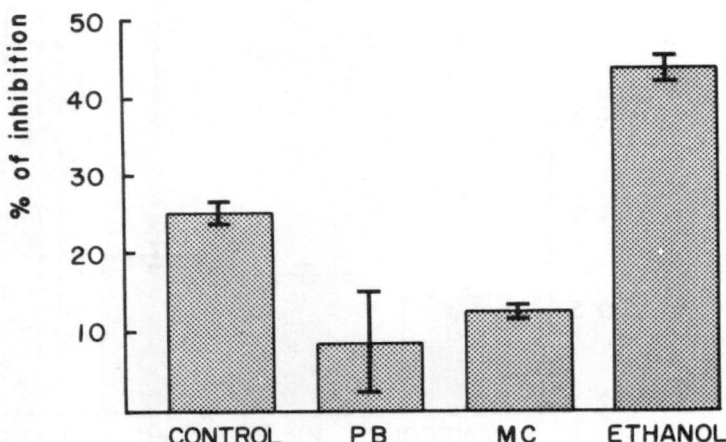

Fig. 4   *Percentage of inhibition by tetrahydrofurane of microsomal*
aniline hydroxylation in control, phenobarbital (PB)-treated (75
mg/Kg i.p. X 3 days), methylcholanthrene (MC)-treated (25
mg/Kg i.p. X 3 days) and ethanol-fed (36% of total calories
with high fat diets X 21 days) rats. The conditions of the
reactions are given in the legend to figure 3 except for the
addition of tetrahydrofurane at a final concentration of 50 mM.

has a low activity with all three substrates (Table V). Since in all assays the amounts of reductase and lipid were kept constant, we can therefore conclude that each of the hemoproteins studied has a different substrate specificity. Thus, chronic ethanol administration results in the appearance of a form of cytochrome P-450 spectrally and catalytically different from the corresponding hemoproteins of controls, phenobarbital and methyl-cholanthrene-treated animals.

From these studies we suggest that the reported increases in micro-somal benzphetamine demethylation (11,13) and benzpyrene hydroxylation (12) in ethanol-fed rats can be explained mainly by a proportional increase in cytochrome P-450 content since ethanol-induced cytochrome P-450 shows no substrate specificity for either substrate. By contrast the reported induction by ethanol of microsomal aniline hydroxylation activity (12,13) can be explained mainly by the appearance of a form of cytochrome P-450 showing substrate specificity for aniline.

The existence of a catalytically different species of cytochrome P-450 induced by chronic ethanol feeding may be of importance in the under-standing of some biological effects of ethanol.

TABLE IV

SPECTRAL CHARACTERISTICS OF PARTIALLY PURIFIED CYTOCHROME
P-450 OF CONTROL, ETHANOL-FED, PHENOBARBITAL-TREATED
AND METHYLCHOLANTHRENE-TREATED RATS

Parameter	C[*]	PB[*]	MC[*]	E[*]
1. CO-reduced difference spectra - A max. (nm)	449.5	450.0	448.0	450.5
2. Cyanide difference spectra - Ks (mM)				
Form I	0.77	0.50	1.08	1.68
Form II	5.60	3.10	9.64	7.00
Form III	30.00	20.40	60.50	19.10
3. Tetrahydrofurane difference spectra - Ks (mM)	>3.60	>3.60	>3.60	1.25
4. Aniline difference a)	0.75	-	-	0.46
spectra - Ks (mM) b)	1.19	-	-	1.06
5. Ethylisocyanide difference spectra				
a) absorbance maximum (nm)	455,430	455,430	452.430	455,430
b) ratio $\frac{455 \text{ nm peak}}{430 \text{ nm peak}}$	1.05	0.71	1.31	0.84
c) pH intercept	7.33	7.80	7.10	7.65

* C: control,   PB: phenobarbital,   MC: methylcholanthrene,   E: ethanol
cytochrome P-450

TABLE V

TURNOVER NUMBERS FOR EACH HEMOPROTEIN FOR THE ACTIVITIES
OF BENZPHETAMINE DEMETHYLATION (BD), BENZPYRENE
HYDROXYLATION (BH), AND ANILINE HYDROXYLATION (AH), ASSAYED
IN RECONSTITUTED SYSTEMS OF MICROSOMAL DRUG HYDROXYLATION

	BD[*]	BH[Ψ]	AH[§]
Phenobarbital-P-450	19.5	0.11	0.230
3-Methylcholanthrene-P-450	3.6	6.67	0.197
Ethanol-P-450	9.7	0.10	0.980
Control-P-450	7.9	0.06	0.260

[*]BD   The reaction mixture, in a final volume of 1.0 ml, contained potassium phosphate buffer 100 μmole (pH 7.4, 30°C), MgCl$_2$ 3 μmoles, benzphetamine 1 μmole, NADPH 0.1 μmole, reductase 150 units, lipid fraction 29μg phospholipids and increasing amounts (0.0 to 0.3 nmole) of each hemoprotein. The reaction was initiated by the addition of NADPH. The activity was measured by following the rate of NADPH oxidation (9).

[Ψ]BH   The reaction mixture, in a final volume of 1.0 ml, contained potassium phosphate buffer 100 μmoles (pH 7.0, 37°C), MgCl$_2$ 3 μmoles, { ^{3}H }-3,4-benzpyrene 10 nmoles (0.5 μCi), NADPH 0.4 μmoles, reductase 150 units, lipid fraction 29μg phospholipids, and increasing amounts (0.00 to 0.65 nmole) of each hemoprotein. The reaction was initiated by the addition of NADPH. The activity was determined by measuring the rate of formation of the radioactive products (26).

[§]AH   The reaction mixture, in a final volume of 1.0 ml, contained Tris-HCl buffer 50μmoles (pH 7.4, 37°C), glycerol 10% v/v, MgCl$_2$ 10 μmoles, aniline 8 μmoles, NADP 1 μmole, glucose-6-phosphate 5 μmoles, glucose-6-phosphate dehydrogenase 2 units, reductase 400 units, lipid fraction 29 μg phospholipids, and increasing amounts (1.0 to 3.0 nmoles) of each hemoprotein. The reaction was initiated by the addition of the NADPH-generating system. The activity was measured by determination of the rate of formation of para-aminophenol (27).

SUMMARY

The possibility that qualitative and/or quantitative alterations by ethanol of hepatic microsomal phospholipids in the rat explain increased microsomal drug biotransformation was studied. Ethanol, administered with high fat diets, increased microsomal phospholipid content and altered phospholipid composition. However, when such lipids were isolated from solubilized liver microsomes and used in a reconstituted system of drug hydroxylation using purified cytochrome P-450 and reductase fractions, the lipid fractions of both ethanol and control animals showed the same stimulatory effect on reconstituted benzphetamine demethylation activity. If ethanol was administered with low fat diets, it enhanced in vitro and in vivo hepatic drug metabolism without significantly altering the content or composition of hepatic microsomal phospholipids. Thus, the alterations by ethanol of microsomal phospholipids were not correlated with the induction by ethanol of mixed function oxidase activity. The possibility that ethanol might induce a new species of cytochrome P-450 was then studied. Cytochrome P-450, partially purified from solubilized microsomes of ethanol-fed rats, was found to be spectrally and catalytically different from the cytochromes P-450 partially purified from microsomes of control, phenobarbital-treated or methylcholanthrene-treated animals. It is concluded that the induction by chronic ethanol feeding of hepatic microsomal drug metabolizing enzymes may be explained by the appearance of a spectrally and catalytically characteristic species of cytochrome P-450.

ACKNOWLEDGEMENTS

We wish to thank Mr. P. Giroux, Mr. R. Duffy, Mr. D. Piché for their technical assistance, Miss M.J. Lachance for her medical art work, and Mr. J. Pruneau and Mr. J. Marchi for their photographic work. We also wish to thank Mrs. Y. Fréchette and Mrs. F. Duchesne for typing the manuscript.

REFERENCES

1. LeBLANC AE, KALANT H, GIBBINS RJ, BERMAN ND: Acquisition and loss of tolerance to ethanol by the rat. J Pharmac Exp Ther 168: 244-250, 1969

2. MISRA P, LEFÈVRE A, ISHII H, RUBIN E, LIEBER CS: Increase of ethanol, meprobamate and pentobarbital after chronic ethanol administration in man and in rats. Amer J Med 51: 346-351, 1971

3. KHANNA JM, KALANT H, YEE Y, CHUNG S, SIEMENS AJ: Effect of chronic ethanol treatment on metabolism of drugs in vitro and in vivo. Biochem Pharmac 25: 329-335, 1976

4. KALANT H, KHANNA JM, LIN GY, CHUNG S: Ethanol - A direct inducer of drug metabolism. Biochem Pharmac 25: 337-342, 1976

5. LIEBER CS, TESCHKE R, HASUMURA Y, DE CARLI LM: Differences in hepatic and metabolic changes after acute and chronic alcohol consumption. Fed Proc 34: 2060-2074, 1975

6. ISERI OA, LIEBER CS, GOTTLIEB LS: The ultrastructure of fatty liver induced by prolonged ethanol ingestion. Am J Pathol 48: 535-555, 1966

7. LANE BP, LIEBER CS: Ultrastructural alterations in human hepatocytes following ingestion of ethanol with adequate diets. Am J Pathol 49: 593-603, 1966

8. ISHII H, JOLY J-G, LIEBER CS: Effect of ethanol on the amount and enzyme activities of hepatic rough and smooth microsomal membranes. Biochim Biophys Acta 291: 411-420, 1973

9. LU AY, STROBEL HW, COON MJ: Properties of a solubilized form of the cytochrome P-450-containing mixed function oxidase of liver microsomes. Mol Pharmacol 6: 213-220, 1970

10. RUBIN E, LIEBER CS, ALVARES AP, LEVIN W, KUNTZMAN R: Ethanol binding to hepatic microsomes. Its increase by ethanol consumption. Biochem Pharmac 20: 229-231, 1971

11. JOLY J-G, ISHII H, TESCHKE R, HASUMURA Y, LIEBER CS: Effect of chronic ethanol feeding on the activities and sub-microsomal distribution of reduced nicotinamide adenine dinucleotide phosphate-cytochrome P-450 reductase and the demethylases for aminopyrine and ethylmorphine. Biochem Pharmac 22: 1532-1535, 1973

12. RUBIN E, LIEBER CS: Hepatic microsomal enzymes in man and rat: induction and inhibition by ethanol. Science 162: 690-691, 1968

13. JOLY J-G, HETU C: Effects of chronic ethanol administration in the rat: relative dependency on dietary lipids. I. Induction of hepatic drug metabolizing enzymes in vitro. Biochem Pharmac 24: 1475-1480, 1975

14. DAVIDSON SC, WILLS ED: Studies on the lipid composition of the rat liver endoplasmic reticulum after induction with phenobarbitone and 20-methyl-cholanthrene. Biochem J 140: 461-468, 1974

15. LEVIN W, LU AY, RYAN D, WEST S, KUNTZMAN R, CONNEY AH: Partial purification and properties of cytochrome P-450 and P-448 from rat liver microsomes. Arch Biochem Biophys 153: 543-553, 1972

16. DE CARLI LM, LIEBER CS: Fatty liver in the rat after prolonged intake of ethanol with a nutritionally adequate new liquid diet. J Nutr 91: 331-336, 1967

17. LU AY, STROBEL HW, COON MJ: Hydroxylation of benzphetamine and other drugs by a solubilized form of cytochrome P-450 from liver microsomes: lipid requirement for drug demethylation. Biochem Biophys Res Commun 36: 545-551, 1969

18. STROBEL HW, LU AY, HEIDEMA J, COON MJ: Phosphatidylcholine requirement in the enzymatic reduction of hemoprotein P-450 and in fatty acid, hydrocarbon and drug hydroxylation. J Biol Chem 245: 4851-4854, 1970

19. CENTURY B: A role of dietary lipid in the ability of phenobarbital to stimulate drug detoxification. J Pharmac Exp Ther 185: 185-194, 1973

20. BELINA H, COOPER SD, FARKAS R, FEUER G: Sex difference in the phospholipid composition of rat liver microsomes. Biochem Pharmac 24: 301-303, 1975

21. JOLY J-G, ISHII H, LIEBER CS: Microsomal cyanide-binding cytochrome: its role in hepatic ethanol oxidation. Gastroenterology 62: 174, 1972

22. COMAI K, GAYLOR JL: Existence and separation of three forms of cytochrome P-450 from rat liver microsomes. J Biol Chem 248: 4947-4955, 1973

23. ULLRICH V, WEBER P, WOLLENBERG P: Tetrahydrofurane - an inhibitor for ethanol-induced liver microsomal cytochrome P-450. Biochem Biophys Res Commun 64: 808-813, 1975

24. LU AY, WEST SB, VORE M, RYAN D, LEVIN W: Role of cytochrome b_5 in hydroxylation by a reconstituted cytochrome P-450-containing system. J Biol Chem 249: 6701-6709, 1974

25. LU AY, COON MJ: Role of hemoprotein P-450 in fatty acid ω-hydroxylation in a soluble enzyme system from liver microsomes. J Biol Chem 243: 1331-1332, 1968

26. DE PIERRE JW, MORON MS, JOHANNESEN KA, ERNSTER L: A reliable, sensitive and convenient radioactive assay for benzpyrene monooxygenase. Anal Biochem 63: 470-484, 1975

27. IMAI Y, ITO R, SATA J: Evidence for biochemically different types of vesicles in the hepatic microsomal fraction. J Biochem (Japan) 60: 417-428, 1966

ACCELERATION OF ETHANOL METABOLISM BY HIGH ETHANOL CONCENTRATIONS AND CHRONIC ETHANOL CONSUMPTION: ROLE OF THE MICROSOMAL ETHANOL OXIDIZING SYSTEM (MEOS)

Shohei Matsuzaki, R. Teschke, K. Ohnishi, and C.S. Lieber

Laboratory of Liver Disease, Nutrition and Alcoholism, Veterans Administration Hospital, Bronx, New York 10468 and Mount Sinai School of Medicine, City University of New York (CUNY)

A. INTRODUCTION

Chronic ethanol consumption has been shown to be associated with an acceleration of ethanol metabolism in man (1-3) and rats (4-6). This phenomenon could not be explained by the activity of alcohol dehydrogenase itself, as reviewed elsewhere (7). Some other possible mechanisms have been suggested, including the adaptive increase of the microsomal ethanol oxidizing system (MEOS) (5, 8, 9), increased mitochondrial reoxidation of NADH (10-12) and enhanced catalase-H_2O_2 mediated peroxidation (13, 14).

The respective roles of these mechanisms however, have been the subject of controversy in recent years. Moreover, acetaldehyde, the first metabolite of ethanol, was also found to be elevated in the blood of alcoholics (15), which further suggested an alteration of ethanol and acetaldehyde metabolism in the liver of alcoholics.

The present paper will focus on the respective roles of the enzyme pathways for ethanol oxidation in liver tissue, and the metabolic changes after chronic ethanol consumption.

B. PATHWAYS FOR ETHANOL OXIDATION

Three enzyme systems have been proposed for ethanol oxidation.

$$1) \quad CH_3CH_2OH + NAD^+ \xrightarrow{ADH} CH_3CHO + NADH + H^+$$

$$2) \quad CH_3CH_2OH + NADPH + H^+ + O_2 \xrightarrow{MEOS} CH_3CHO + NADP^+ + 2H_2O$$

3) $CH_3CH_2OH + H_2O_2 \xrightarrow{\text{catalase}} CH_3CHO + 2H_2O$

The first pathway mediated by alcohol dehydrogenase (ADH), is a well known enzyme system which plays a major role in the metabolism of alcohols including ethanol and other aliphatic alcohols (16) and endogenous substrates such as steroids (17). ADH is located in the cytosol, the soluble fraction of the hepatocyte, although low activity is also present in other tissues such as the gastric mucosa (18). ADH requires predominantly NAD as a cofactor, and reoxidation of this cofactor is generally accepted as the rate-limiting factor of this enzyme system rather than the activity of ADH itself. The optimum pH of ADH is 9.6 or more and its K_m for ethanol has been reported to be 0.5 - 2 mM (19-21) or even much lower (0.07 mM) in situ (22).

The second pathway, the NADPH-dependent microsomal ethanol oxidizing system (MEOS), is predominantly dependent upon NADPH and is relatively insensitive to azide and cyanide (8, 9). In addition, the activity of MEOS strikingly increases after chronic ethanol feeding in rats (8, 9). MEOS was demonstrated in human liver (9) and an increase of the NADPH-dependent ethanol oxidizing activity was also reported in the liver of alcoholics (23). The increase in MEOS activity is consistent with the morphologic change of the proliferation of the hepatic smooth endoplasmic reticulum (SER) after chronic ethanol intake in rats (24, 25) and in humans (26-28). The localization of the MEOS activity and its increase in the hepatic SER were confirmed by a biochemical study (29). The characteristics of MEOS differ from those of ADH not only by the subcellular localization but also by the neutral pH optimum in vitro (7-9), cofactor requirements (NADPH rather than NAD), K_m value for ethanol (8-10 mM) and the insensitivity to an ADH inhibitor, pyrazole (8, 9).

Alcohol oxidizing activity in hepatic microsomes was also described by Orme-Johnson and Ziegler (30), but the rate of ethanol oxidation in their system was only half that of methanol and one tenth of the rate of the system described by Lieber and DeCarli (8, 9). Furthermore, it could not oxidize long chain aliphatic alcohols such as butanol and was sensitive to catalase inhibitors, azide and cyanide. Therefore Ziegler concluded that this system is clearly different from the cytochrome P-450 dependent system and involves the H_2O_2 mediated ethanol peroxidation by catalase (31). More recently, indeed, the MEOS was differentiated from the system reported by Orme-Johnson and Ziegler (30) and from catalase by its ability to oxidize long chain aliphatic alcohols (32) which are not substrates for catalase (33).

The third pathway, catalase, is located primarily in peroxisomes, with some activity found in microsomal fractions, probably as a contaminant rather than a component of the microsomal membranes (34). It has been shown by Keilin and Hartree (35) that catalase is capable of oxidizing ethanol in vitro in the presence of H_2O_2 generating systems. It is generally accepted that the rate of H_2O_2 mediated peroxidation of ethanol by catalase is limited by the rate of H_2O_2 generation rather than the activity of catalase itself. The rate of H_2O_2 generation in the liver, however, has been reported to be very low: 3.6 μmoles/hour/g liver under physiological conditions (36). This rate represents only 2% of the rate of ethanol oxidation in vivo (178 μmoles/hour/g liver) (5). In perfused liver experiments a similar low rate of H_2O_2 generation (50-80 nmoles/min/g) has been reported by Oshino et al. (37). Furthermore, not all of the H_2O_2 generated in the liver could be utilized for the peroxidation of ethanol by catalase (38). Therefore ethanol peroxidation by catalase can theoretically account for less than 10% of the rate of ethanol oxidation by the nonADH pathway (which will be discussed subsequently). A significant role of catalase in ethanol oxidation has been rejected by many (39-41). The relationship of MEOS to catalase, however, has been a subject of controversy in recent years. MEOS has been attributed to NADPH-oxidase dependent H_2O_2 generation combined with the peroxidatic activity of catalase (13,14) or with catalase and ADH (42), and an unidentified enzyme (43).

C. DIFFERENTIATION OF MEOS FROM ADH AND CATALASE

Recently, MEOS has been separated from both ADH and catalase: microsomes were solubilized by ultrasonication and treatment with deoxycholate, and MEOS was separated from ADH and catalase by DEAE-cellulose column chromatography (44). The MEOS fraction contained three microsomal components, namely cytochrome P-450, NADPH cytochrome c reductase and phospholipid (Fig. 1). The activity of MEOS was different-iated from other alcohol oxidizing systems by its apparent K_m for ethanol (7.2 mM), by its insensitivity to the ADH inhibitor pyrazole and to catalase inhibitors such as azide and cyanide, and by the inability of a H_2O_2 generating system (glucose-glucose oxidase) to sustain ethanol oxidation (44). The capacity of the isolated MEOS fraction also to oxidize higher aliphatic alcohols such as propanol and butanol which are not substrates for catalase further differentiated MEOS from catalase (32).

More recently, the reconstitution of the ethanol oxidizing activity with the three microsomal components cytochrome P-450, NADPH cytochrome c reductase and lecithin was demonstrated (45). In these experiments cytochrome P-450 was partially purified by protease treatment and subsequently by column chromatography on DEAE-cellulose using a stepwise KCl gradient (46). NADPH cytochrome c reductase was partially purified essentially by the method of Levin et al. (47) with omission of the Emulgen 911 step. The activity of the reconstituted microsomal ethanol oxidizing system (reconstituted MEOS) showed a dependency upon the former two microsomal components and required synthetic phospholipids (such as lecithin) for its maximal activity. The K_m of the reconstituted MEOS for ethanol was 10 mM, which is similar to the K_m measured in crude microsomes and the MEOS fraction isolated by column chromatography (8, 9, 44). This reconstituted system required NADPH as a cofactor but did not react to a H_2O_2 generating system, and was insensitive to the catalase inhibitor azide. These characteristics were also similar to those observed in crude microsomes.

From all these data it is evident that MEOS can be clearly different-
iated from both alcohol dehydrogenase and catalase activity by a variety of
characteristics.

The importance of the physiological role of the MEOS, however, is still
the subject of controversy (48). To study this question, we used liver slices
and isolated hepatocytes.

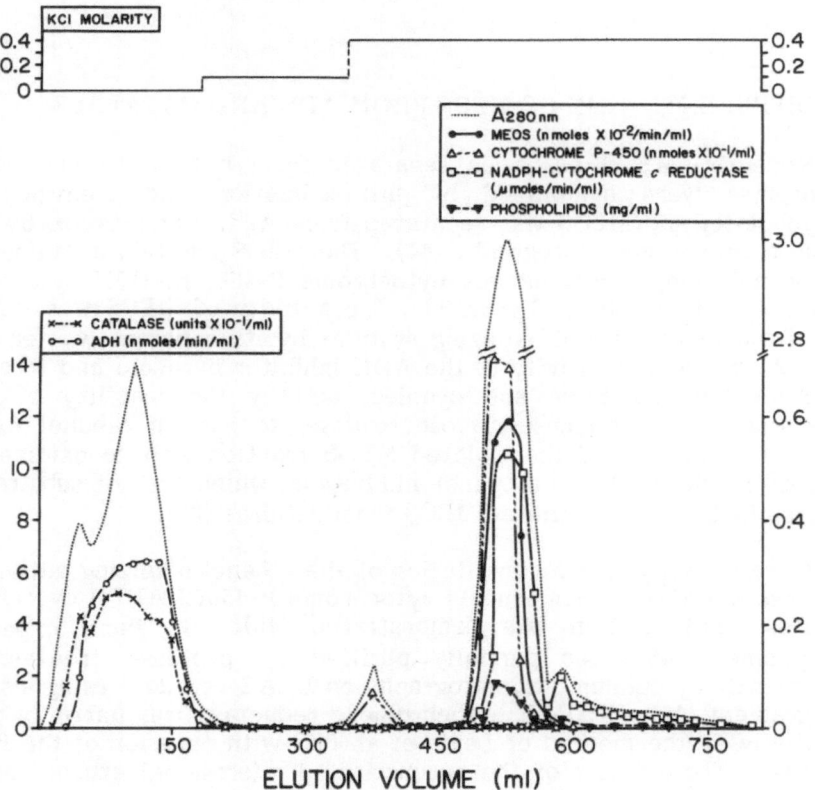

Fig. 1   *Separation of the MEOS from ADH and catalase activities by
          ion exchange column chromatography on DEAE-cellulose*
          *Sonicated microsomes from rats fed laboratory chow were
          further solubilized by treatment with sodium deoxycholate and
          put onto DEAE-cellulose column (2.5 x 45 cm). The separation
          of enzyme activities was achieved by stepwise elution with the
          salt gradient. From Teschke et al. (44).*

D. ETHANOL METABOLISM IN LIVER TISSUE

To avoid factors which complicate experiments in vivo, such as variable blood flow with varying ethanol concentration (49), we studied ethanol metabolism in isolated hepatocytes. Isolated rat hepatocytes are particularly suited for the study of the effects of various inhibitors. Their ethanol metabolism is higher than that in liver slices, although it is still lower than in vivo. Isolated hepatocytes were prepared enzymatically from female Sprague-Dawley rats fed Purina chow using the method of Berry and Friend (50), as modified by Jeejeebhoy et al. (51).

Activities of alcohol dehydrogenase (ADH) and catalase were examined photometrically in homogenates of isolated hepatocytes in six rats by the methods of Bonnicksen (52) and Lück (53) respectively. The ADH activity was 2.02 ± 0.21 μ moles NADH produced/min/g liver and the catalatic activity of catalase was 5,040 ± 530 units/g liver. These values were similar to those measured in total homogenates of rat liver. The results demonstrated that these enzymes remain unaffected throughout the isolation procedure of the hepatocytes.

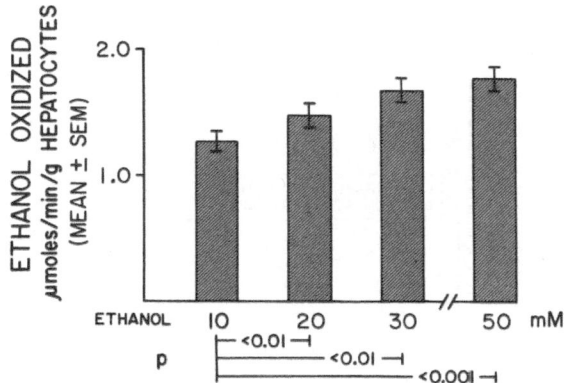

Fig. 2   *Effect of ethanol concentrations on the rates of ethanol oxidation by isolated hepatocytes*
100-150 mg of isolated hepatocytes were suspended in 3 ml of sodium bicarbonate buffer containing 1% bovine albumin and ethanol at final concentrations as indicated in the figure. The incubation was conducted in closed 25 ml flasks at 37ºC in a shaking water-bath (60 strokes/min) for 60-90 min. 0.2 ml of samples were collected every 30 min. The concentration of ethanol in the incubation medium was measured by gas liquid chromatography and ethanol oxidation was calculated by its disappearance. Samples were studied at least in duplicate. The study was conducted in 6 rats. p: comparison of the means calculated by the paired Student t-test.

The effects of an ADH inhibitor, pyrazole (2 mM), and a catalase inhibitor, azide (1 mM) were tested by incubating hepatocytes with the respective inhibitors for 30 min in the absence and presence of 50 mM ethanol. Hepatocytes were then sedimented by centrifugation (600 g) for 5 min and the pellets were resuspended in the buffer without the inhibitors. The resuspended hepatocytes were then sonicated. The activities of ADH and catalase were found to be completely inhibited both in the absence and presence of ethanol during this preincubation period.

1. Effect of Ethanol Concentrations on Ethanol Metabolism

When the concentration of ethanol in the incubation medium was increased progressively from 10 to 50 mM, the rates of ethanol oxidation were significantly accelerated (Fig. 2). This observation was similar to that of Grunnet et al. (54). The lowest concentration of 10 mM ethanol employed in this experiment is already fully saturating for ADH which has a K_m value lower than 2 mM as mentioned before. Therefore, the accelerated ethanol oxidation rates observed with increasing ethanol concentration indicate the presence of a nonADH pathway with a higher K_m than that of ADH. Then the effect of ADH inhibitor pyrazole (2 mM) on the concentration dependent ethanol oxidation was studied: 18-30% of the activities remained as indicated by the shaded parts of the bars (Fig. 3). Similar observations of a nonADH pathway have also been reported in experiments in liver slices (9, 55, 56), isolated hepatocytes (54) and in vivo (5). In the present experiment

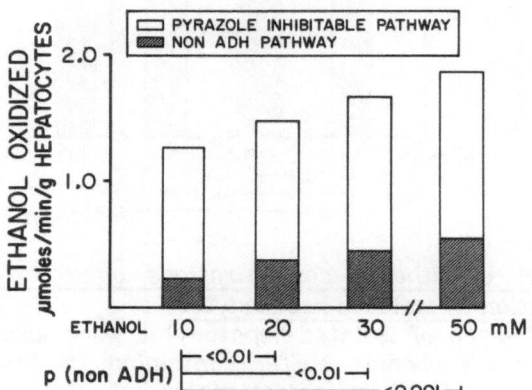

Fig. 3   *Effect of pyrazole (2 mM) on the concentration dependent ethanol oxidation in isolated hepatocytes*
To inhibit ADH activity, hepatocytes were preincubated with pyrazole for 30 min, thereafter the incubation was conducted as described in Fig. 2. Data represent means of experiments in 6 rats.

the remaining activity (the "nonADH pathway") was significantly accelerated with increasing ethanol concentrations. The increase in the activity of
the nonADH pathway represents at least half of the concentration dependent
part of ethanol metabolism in isolated hepatocytes. On the other hand, the
activity inhibitable by pyrazole (the "ADH pathway") was also slightly
enhanced by high ethanol levels (1.02 ± 0.07 µmoles/min/g liver at 10 mM vs.
1.23 ± 0.09 at 30 mM, $p < 0.05$).

The apparent K_m value of the nonADH pathway was determined by
replotting the activities remaining after ADH inhibition according to the
method of Lineweaver-Burk (Fig. 4). The value was 13 mM for ethanol,
which is comparable to the values measured in other in vitro systems (8-10
mM) (8,9,44,45). Actually, the apparent K_m of MEOS in crude microsomes
determined in the presence of 2 mM pyrazole was found to be slightly higher
compared to the value measured in its absence (Fig. 5).

To estimate the respective role of MEOS and catalase in the nonADH
pathway, the effect of 1 mM azide was tested as well as the effect of
increased H_2O_2 generation. When H_2O_2 generation was stimulated by
activating D-amino acid-oxidase in peroxisomes by 5 mM DL-alanine, the
rate of ethanol oxidation by the nonADH pathway was increased 40% (Fig.
6).

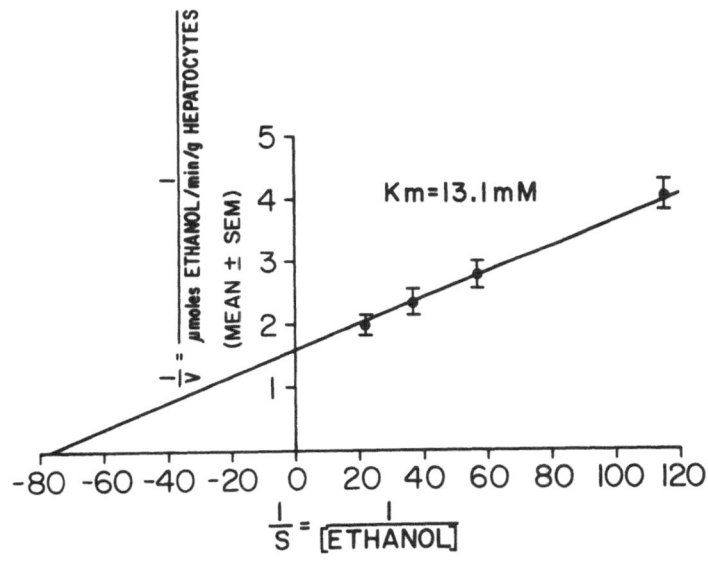

Fig. 4   Lineweaver-Burk plot of the concentration dependent rates of
           ethanol oxidation by the nonADH pathway in isolated hepato-
           cytes

These results confirm that in the presence of increased H_2O_2 generation, catalase is indeed capable of oxidizing ethanol. But these results also indicate that 1 mM azide does inhibit the peroxidatic activity of catalase in the liver. However, in the absence of unphysiologic H_2O_2 generating substrates, the rate of ethanol oxidation was only slightly lowered by 1 mM azide. These results were comparable to the findings reported by Teschke et al. in liver slices (55) and show that under physiologic conditions catalase plays no significant role in ethanol metabolism.

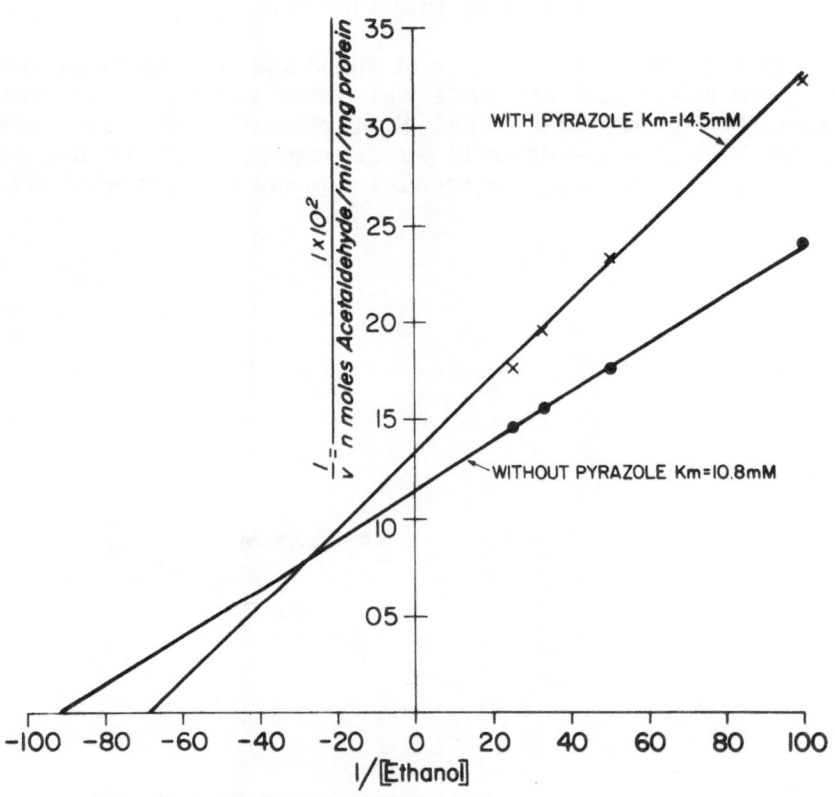

Fig. 5   *Effect of pyrazole (2 mM) on the apparent K_m of MEOS for ethanol*
Isolated hepatic microsomes from normal rats were incubated with 10 to 40 mM ethanol in the system reported (9). Rates of acetaldehyde production in the incubation medium were measured by gas-liquid chromatography. Data represent averages of experiments in 4 rats.

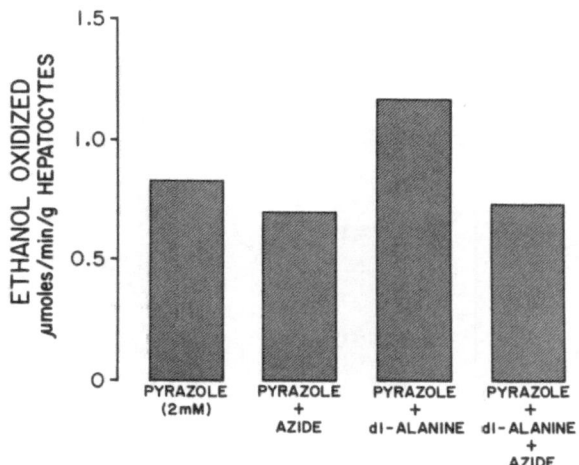

Fig. 6   *Inhibitory effect of azide on the peroxidatic activity of catalase
in isolated hepatocytes*
*100-150 mg of isolated hepatocytes were suspended in an
incubation medium containing 2 mM pyrazole plus azide. After
30 min preincubation, hepatocytes were incubated wtih 30 mM
ethanol with or without 5 mM DL-alanine for 90 min. Data
represent averages of rates of ethanol oxidation in experiments
with three rats.*

2. Effects of Chronic Ethanol Feeding on Ethanol Metabolism in Liver Tissue

Effects of chronic ethanol feeding were studied in rats fed ethanol chronically for 4-6 weeks as 36% of total calories in nutritionally adequate liquid diets. In pair-fed controls ethanol was substituted with carbohydrate as described elsewhere (57). Liver slices and isolated hepatocytes were prepared from rats fasted over-night. Liver slices of ethanol-fed rats oxidized ethanol at a significantly higher rate than those of controls (0.75 ± 0.03 μmoles/min/g liver in ethanol-fed vs. 0.58 ± 0.02 in the controls at 30 mM ethanol, $p < 0.01$) (58). Even after inhibition of ADH by 2 mM pyrazole, approximately 30% of the total ethanol oxidizing activities remained and a significantly higher rate in the nonADH pathway was found in ethanol-fed rats (0.31 ± 0.01 vs. 0.20 ± 0.02, $p < 0.001$). Inclusion of 1 mM azide in addition to the pyrazole affected only $6.6 \pm 2.0\%$ and $4.3 \pm 1.6\%$ of the ethanol oxidation rates by the nonADH pathway in ethanol-fed rats and the controls respectively, which again indicates a quantitatively minor role for catalase, even after chronic ethanol feeding (58).

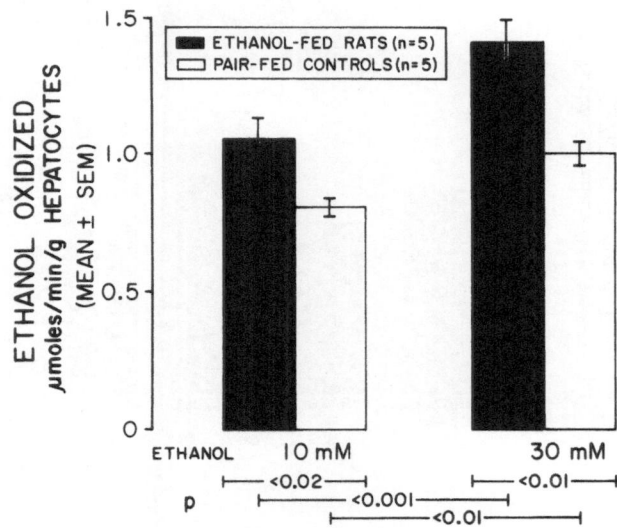

Fig. 7   *Effect of chronic ethanol feeding and ethanol concentrations on*
the rates of ethanol oxidation in isolated hepatocytes
Incubation of isolated hepatocytes was conducted as described
in Fig. 3.

     In isolated hepatocytes rates of ethanol oxidation were also accelerated
with increasing ethanol concentrations from 10 to 30 mM both in ethanol-fed
rats and in the pair-fed controls (Fig. 7). The rates were, however,
significantly greater in the ethanol-fed rats at both ethanol concentrations.
Furthermore, the magnitude of the acceleration by 30 mM ethanol was more
striking in ethanol-fed rats than in the controls. These results indicate that
the nonADH pathway (most likely MEOS as suggested by the preceding
studies) is subject to greater activation by the high ethanol concentrations in
ethanol-fed rats than in the controls.

     To test whether or not the MEOS is involved in the adaptive increase of
ethanol oxidation after chronic ethanol feeding, both ADH and catalase were
inhibited by 2 mM pyrazole and 1 mM azide. The activity of the nonADH and
non-catalase pathway was significantly higher in ethanol-fed rats and was
more strikingly activated by the increased ethanol concentration (Fig. 8).
The increase in the nonADH pathway in these fasted rats accounts for more
than 70% of the total increase in ethanol oxidation of ethanol-fed rats
measured in the absence of the inhibitors. Moreover, the activity of MEOS
is known to be inhibited by pyrazole to some extent in vitro using isolated
microsomes (9). When the inhibitory effect of the drug on the MEOS
activity is taken into account, the adaptive increase of ethanol metabolism
in ethanol fed rats could certainly be attributed to the increased activity of
the non-ADH pathway, most likely MEOS. Indeed, after 24 days of ethanol
feeding in rats, a striking increase of the MEOS activity has been reported
(5, 9).

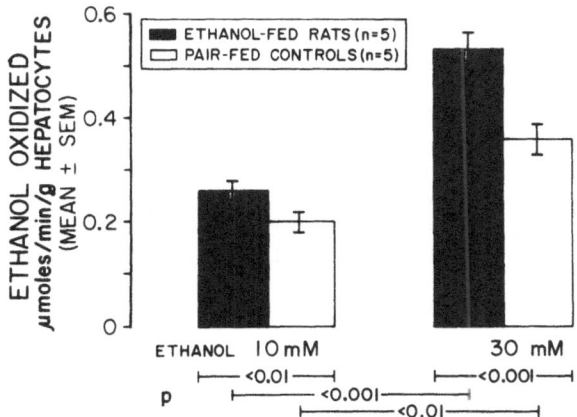

Fig. 8   *Effect of 2 mM pyrazole and 1 mM azide on ethanol oxidation in*
            isolated hepatocytes of ethanol-fed rats and controls
            Incubation of isolated hepatocytes with the inhibitors was
            conducted as described in Figs. 2 and 3.

       Thus, if MEOS were to function in vivo at rates comparable to (or even
half of) those in vitro, it could account for the total increase in ethanol
metabolism of isolated hepatocytes and to a large extent of that seen in vivo
after chronic ethanol feeding (5) (vide infra).

       However other investigators have considered an increase of the activity
of the ADH pathway after chronic ethanol consumption as a likely
mechanism.

       It is now generally accepted that the activity of ADH is not a rate
limiting factor for ethanol oxidation which depends upon the rate of NADH
reoxidation. Therefore, the question whether or not NADH reoxidation is
accelerated after chronic ethanol intake has to be examined. Two possible
mechanisms have been proposed for the increased reoxidation of NADH.
First, increased reoxidation of NADH by the mitochondrial respiratory chain
has been proposed by Bernstein et al. (11). This theory involves enhanced
(Na$^+$K$^+$)-stimulated ATPase activity and secondary stimulation of the
respiratory chain by increased availability of ADP, a situation similar to the
hypermetabolic state in hyperthyroidism (12). There are, however, some
discrepant observations. First, the hepatic mitochondria exhibit morphologic evidence of damage after chronic ethanol intake (24-28, 59-61). In
recent years functional signs of damage have also been reported: oxygen
consumption of hepatic mitochondria with NAD-dependent substrates was
decreased (62). Furthermore, for the reoxidation of NADH, mitochondrial
shuttles have to be involved to transport the H equivalents from the cytosol
into the mitochondria. The activities of mitochondrial shuttles in ethanol-
fed rats were found to be unchanged or slightly decreased (63). In our
present study, the rates of oxygen consumption in mitochondria of ethanol-

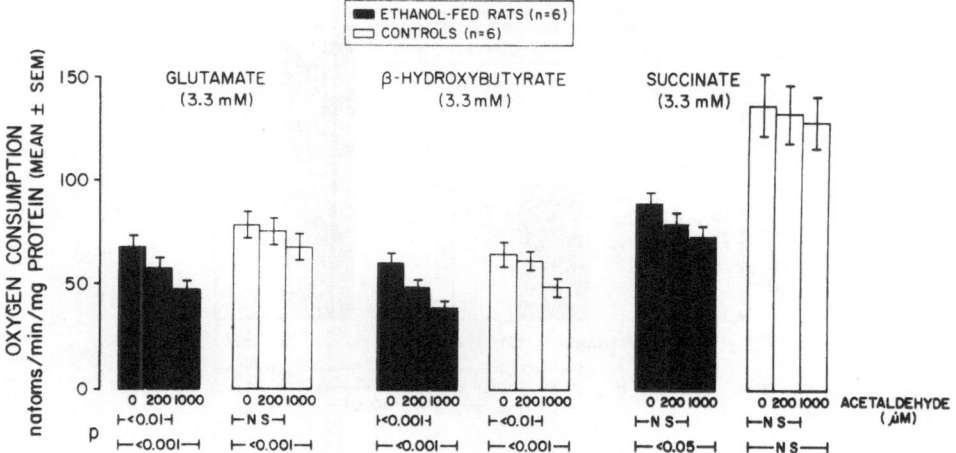

Fig. 9   *Effect of chronic ethanol feeding and the presence of acetalde-*
           hyde on the oxygen consumption at State 3 in hepatic
           mitochondria
           Isolated mitochondria (1.5 - 3 mg protein) were incubated in 3
           ml buffer containing 225 mM mannitol, 75 mM sucrose, 10 mM
           $MgCl_2$ *in 10 mM phosphate buffer (pH 7.4) at 26°C with the*
           NAD-dependent substrates. State 3 respiration was initiated by
           adding 600-900 nmoles of ADP. To examine the effect of
           acetaldehyde, acetaldehyde was added together with other
           NAD-dependent-substrates 3 min before adding ADP. Rates of
           oxygen consumption were measured polarographically with a
           Clark oxygen electrode. Samples were analyzed at least in
           duplicate.

fed rats were significantly depressed in the presence of 200 µM acetaldehyde
although this low concentration did not affect the respiration of controls
(Fig. 9). This concentration of acetaldehyde is known to occur in the liver
and in the hepatic vein blood during ethanol oxidation in vivo (64, 65).

Moreover, the oxidation of acetaldehyde itself in mitochondria was also
found to be decreased after chronic ethanol feeding (66, 67). A similar
result is shown in Fig. 10. These studies also revealed that the response of
mitochondria of ethanol-fed rats to the stimulatory effect of ADP was
decreased when acetaldehyde was used as a substrate. This decrease of
acetaldehyde oxidation is most probably due to its own toxicity to the
mitochondrial respiratory chain, as was found by the addition of 200 µM
acetaldehyde to other substrates (Fig. 9). These results indicated an
increased susceptibility of the mitochondrial respiratory chain to the
toxicity of acetaldehyde after chronic ethanol consumption. Acetaldehyde
exerts a similar toxicity on mitochondrial fatty acid oxidation (Fig. 11).

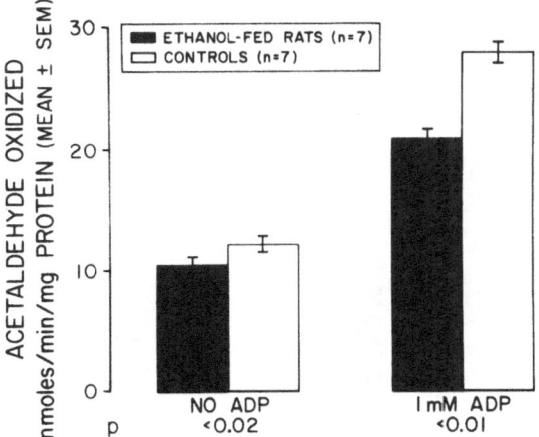

Fig. 10   *Effect of chronic ethanol feeding on acetaldehyde oxidation in*
              hepatic mitochondria
              Mitochondria (0.5 – 1 mg protein) were incubated in 0.7 ml
              buffer described in Fig. 8 with further addition of 1 mM
              pyrazole at 37°C. After 5 min preincubation, the reaction was
              started by adding acetaldehyde at a concentration of 200 μM
              and terminated at 0, 2, 4 and 6 min by 0.2 ml of 0.6 M
              perchloric acid containing 25 mM thiourea. The concentration
              of acetaldehyde in each flask was measured by gas-liquid
              chromatography and the rate of acetaldehyde oxidation was
              calculated from its disappearance rate.

Thus, in view of the evidence for widespread mitochondrial impairment, the
theory of the acceleration of the ADH pathway mediated by mitochondrial
NADH reoxidation raises serious questions, especially since other investigators failed to verify the increase in ATPase activity after chronic ethanol
feeding under conditions which still lead to accelerated ethanol metabolism
(68).

Another possible explanation for the enhanced reoxidation of NADH
may be given indirectly by the increased MEOS activity which is dependent
upon NADPH. After chronic ethanol intake the increased MEOS activity
accelerates NADPH utilization, and, to a lesser extent, NADH utilization
(44). Thus, the availability of NAD for the ADH pathway will increase by
the above mechanism since the hepatic NADPH-NADP couple is linked with
the NADH-NAD system (69). Increased ethanol metabolism (probably via
the ADH pathway) due to NADPH-mediated drug metabolism in microsomes
was also reported recently by Grundin (70). Furthermore, it is known that
ethanol oxidation by ADH can be mediated by NADP, albeit to a lesser
extent than by NAD (71). One could therefore expect increased availability
of the cofactors for both ADH and MEOS and activation of the ADH
pathway secondary to the increased activity of MEOS.

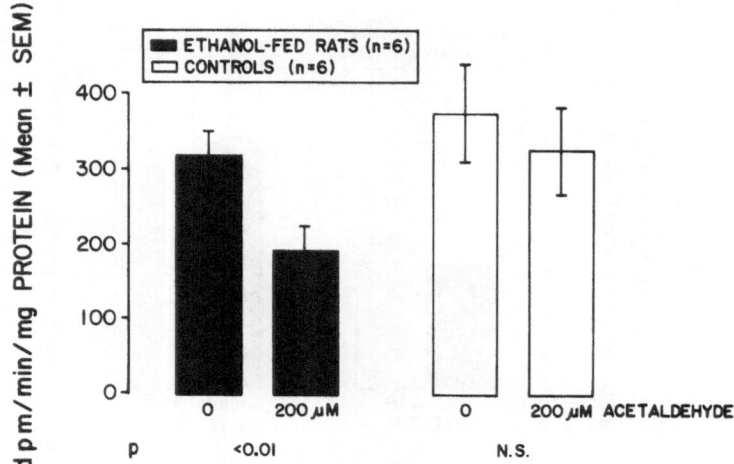

Fig. 11   *Effect of chronic ethanol feeding and the presence of acetal-*
dehyde on fatty acid oxidation in hepatic mitochondria
Palmitic acid oxidation was studied by measuring CO_2
production at $37°C$ using $1\text{-}^{14}C$-labelled palmitic acid, adjusted
to approximately 1250 dpm per nmole. The reaction system
consisted of 3 ml of the medium described in Fig. 8 without
EDTA, 0.2% defatted bovine albumin, 0.4 mM malate, 3 mM
carnitine, 3 mM ATP, 1.5 mM ADP, 3-5 mg of mitochondrial
protein and 100 µM of substrate. The incubation was conducted
for 30 min with or without acetaldehyde at an initial concentration of 200 µM. To replace the acetaldehyde oxidized in this
system, 300 nmoles were supplied at 10 and 20 min. The CO_2
produced was trapped by 0.3 ml of hyamine hydroxide in the
center-well and the radioactivity was determined in a liquid
scintillation counter.

Thus, increased MEOS activity after chronic ethanol intake seems to
represent a major mechanism for the acceleration of ethanol metabolism
either directly, or indirectly by activating the ADH pathway.

E.   FUNCTION OF MEOS IN VIVO

It has been reported that blood ethanol continues to disappear even
after the inhibition of ADH by pyrazole in rats in vivo (5, 48), (Fig. 12).
Similar observations were also reported in man (72, 73). In the rat study (5),
kinetic analysis of the blood ethanol clearance showed a K_m of 8 mM for
ethanol (Fig. 13) which is comparable to the K_m of MEOS in vitro (9, 25, 44).

Furthermore, significantly higher rates of ethanol clearance were
observed in ethanol fed rats after ADH inhibition in vivo (5, 48). Although

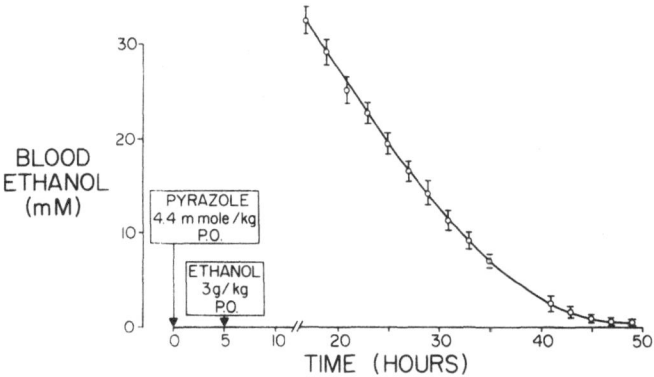

BLOOD
ETHANOL
(mM)

PYRAZOLE
4.4 m mole /kg
P.O.

ETHANOL
3g/ kg
P.O.

TIME (HOURS)

Fig. 12   *Blood ethanol clearance in rats pretreated with pyrazole*
The results represent the average of blood ethanol concentra-
tions obtained in nine rats fed Purina chow (± SEM) (5).

the results of these two studies (5, 48) in vivo in rats were comparable, the
functioning of MEOS in vivo was questioned by Kalant et al. (48). Since
Kalant et al. observed no blood ethanol clearance in pyrazole treated rats
during the first several hours, they attributed the disappearance of ethanol
after 7-8 hours to an incomplete inhibition of ADH due to a decrease of
pyrazole by its metabolism in the liver. It is more likely however that
ethanol disappearance from the blood could not be observed during the first
several hours because of continuous absorption of the relatively large dose
given. Early disappearance of the inhibitory effect of pyrazole, which was
administered in a large amount (4.4 mmoles/Kg b.w.), is also unlikely.
Pyrazole is a competitive inhibitor of ADH (74), with a half-life of 14 hours
in the absence of ethanol (39) and a significantly longer one in its presence
(75). Therefore, if the original residual ethanol metabolism after pyrazole
were due to incomplete ADH inhibition, the depression should be significantly reduced with time. Actually, as shown in figure 12, this was not the case
and rates of ethanol metabolism were virtually the same for instance 13 to
27 hours after pyrazole despite the 14 hour interval. Furthermore, in the
time period from 27 to 49 hours after pyrazole, there was progressive
deceleration of ethanol metabolism instead of the acceleration one would
have expected with progressively less complete inhibition. Moreover, the
rates of ethanol metabolism plotted according to Lineweaver–Burk yielded a
linear regression line (Fig. 13) which would not be expected if one were
dealing with incomplete inhibition by a competitive inhibitor with a half-life
much shorter than the duration of the test. In the case of complete
inhibition, the apparent K_m should have progressively decreased to approach
the K_m of noninhibited ADH, which is below 2 mM (20). Moreover, using a
pyrazole dose in vivo comparable to the one we employed and assessing
inhibition of liver ADH activity in vitro, Deitrich et al. (76) found that
pyrazole has an effective half-life for in vitro inhibition of about 76 hours
and, since there was a dilution factor of 300 from the whole liver to the

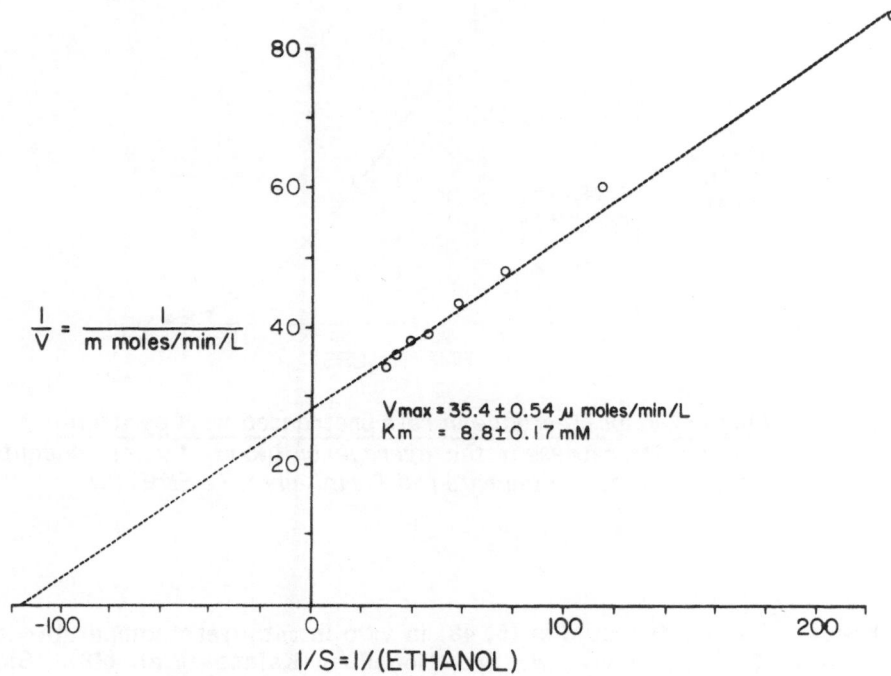

Fig. 13   *Lineweaver-Burk plot of blood ethanol clearance after pyrazole*
Rates of disappearance of ethanol from the blood were derived
from the curve shown in figure 12 for various blood ethanol
concentrations. V equals millimoles of ethanol oxidized per
minute per liter of blood. S equals molar concentrations of
ethanol (5).

assay cuvette, it was concluded that "smaller doses probably are completely inhibitory in vivo." For all these reasons, it is likely that most of the residual metabolism of ethanol after pyrazole administration in vivo (Figure 12) is due primarily to a nonADH pathway rather than to incomplete ADH inhibition.

Increased rates of blood ethanol disappearance in alcoholics have been reported by some (1-3). Furthermore, it has been observed by Salaspuro et al. (73) that higher rates of ethanol disappearance in alcoholics were sustained even after ADH inhibition by 4-methyl pyrazole and that the effect of ADH inhibition on ethanol metabolism was much less in alcoholics (particularly those with poor nutrition) than in controls. This finding indicates that the nonADH pathway is playing a more important role in alcoholics. This view is also supported by the fact that after chronic ethanol feeding, redox changes produced by an acute dose of ethanol are much less striking than in similarly treated control animals (77).

The effect of ethanol concentration on its metabolism in vivo has not been fully clarified yet.   However, the effect of the dose of ethanol administered has been reported in dogs (78).   Furthermore, additional, albeit indirect evidence in favor of the operation, in vivo, of a nonADH pathway for ethanol metabolism can be derived from a study of Guynn and Pieklik (79) who demonstrated dependence on dose of the acute effects of ethanol on liver metabolism in vivo. Ethanol was given to rats i.p. in doses of 0.69, 1.7, and 3.0 g/kg. The liver was freeze-clamped 120 min after injection. Each group showed a significantly different pattern of metabolites, redox states, and phosphorylation potentials although the rate of ethanol disappearance, at least between the two highest dose groups, was not significantly different.   The mitochondrial free $(NAD^+)/(NADH)$ ratio and the cytoplasmic free $(NADP^+)/(NADPH)$ ratio were paradoxically most reduced with the lowest dose of ethanol and became progressively more oxidized with increasing dose. In a somewhat different pattern, the phosphorylation potential (ATP / ADP Pi) remained at the control level in the low-dose group but was significantly elevated in the two higher-dose groups. Although these complex results may not be explained completely by any one hypothesis, the authors conclude that the increasing oxidation of the cytoplasmic free $(NADP^+)/(NADPH)$ ratio and the mitochondrial free $(NAD^+)/(NADH)$ ratio from the lowest to highest doses in the current study is compatible with a significant in vivo contribution by the microsomal ethanol oxidizing system, and that "even though the important factors operative in vivo are yet to be resolved, it can at least be concluded from the differential effects of dose of the current study that the rate of NADH production alone cannot explain the findings." Thus the evidence which has accumulated over the last few years clearly indicates that the ADH pathway alone cannot explain all the effects of ethanol.

Interpretation of changes of ethanol metabolism in vivo may be difficult because of complicating factors encountered in vivo at high ethanol concentrations. In addition to changes in hepatic blood flow (49) alluded to before, high ethanol concentrations inhibit ADH activity (substrate inhibition) (80, 81). In our rat experiments, the activity of cytosolic ADH of rat liver measured by NAD-NADH change at pH 9.6 was found inhibited by 16.4 and 31.1% at 30 and 60 mM ethanol respectively compared to the activity at 10 mM ethanol. Furthermore, at high ethanol levels we found high concentrations of blood acetaldehyde particularly in alcoholics (15). The NADH reoxidation in mitochondria could be depressed by the toxicity of acetaldehyde, and consequently the function of the ADH pathway could be decreased.   Moreover, it is known that ADH can reduce acetaldehyde to ethanol in the presence of NADH. This "back" reaction (and possibly also product inhibition) may occur when acetaldehyde concentrations and NADH/NAD ratios are increased in the liver by the decreased acetaldehyde oxidation and NADH reoxidation in the mitochondria, conditions favored by the impairment of hepatic mitochondrial function after chronic ethanol intake as described before. Actually, the slowing of ethanol oxidation by the increased acetaldehyde level in vivo in rats (82) lends credence to such a mechanism.

For these as well as other reasons, assessment of pathways of hepatic ethanol metabolism from interpretations of blood ethanol clearance curves in vivo is complicated. However, enough results are presently available to indicate that the ADH pathway alone cannot explain all observed results and that a nonADH pathway must be invoked, particularly at high ethanol concentrations and after chronic ethanol consumption. The original claim that catalase accounts for MEOS activity (13) has now been retracted (83) and as discussed before, the studies conducted in vivo and in isolated hepatocytes and liver slices indicate that MEOS accounts for the bulk of the activity of the nonADH pathway of hepatic ethanol metabolism.

SUMMARY

The rate of ethanol oxidation adaptively increases during chronic ethanol intake in man and in experimental animals. Each of the three hepatic ethanol oxidizing enzyme systems namely, alcohol dehydrogenase (ADH), the microsomal ethanol oxidizing system (MEOS) and catalase has been incriminated but their respective roles have not been fully clarified.

In rat liver tissues (isolated hepatocytes and liver slices) rates of ethanol oxidation were accelerated by increasing ethanol concentration well beyond ADH saturation. This concentration dependent increase was maintained even after ADH inhibition by 2 mM pyrazole and was for the most part insensitive to a catalase inhibitor, azide (1 mM). Furthermore, the K_m of the nonADH pathway (13 mM for ethanol) was comparable to that of MEOS measured in the presence of pyrazole. It was calculated that a major part of the nonADH pathway can be attributed to the function of MEOS in the liver.

After chronic ethanol feeding, the activity of MEOS measured in isolated hepatic microsomes strikingly increased, but the activity of ADH and catalase in the liver did not. A rate limiting factor for ethanol oxidation by ADH, the rate of NADH reoxidation in mitochondria, was probably not increased in ethanol-fed rats, since various mitochondrial functions were significantly decreased particularly in the presence of concentrations of acetaldehyde known to occur in vivo. Nevertheless, rates of ethanol oxidation in isolated hepatocytes of ethanol-fed rats were significantly greater than those in controls and the differences were more striking at 30 mM ethanol than at 10 mM. The significantly higher ethanol oxidation was maintained even in the presence of pyrazole and azide. The increase in the nonADH and non-catalase pathway (most likely MEOS) can account for the bulk of the adaptive increase in ethanol oxidation. Thus, the acceleration of ethanol oxidation at high ethanol concentrations and a major part of the adaptive increase in ethanol metabolism after chronic ethanol intake can be attributed to the increase in MEOS activity.

REFERENCES

1. MISRA PS, LEFEVERE A, ISHII H, RUBIN E, LIEBER CS: Increase in ethanol, meprobamate and pentobarbital metabolism after chronic ethanol administration in man and in rats. Am J Med 51: 346-351, 1971

2. KATER RM, CARULLI N, IBER FL: Differences in the rate of ethanol metabolism in recently drinking alcoholic and nondrinking subjects. Am J Clin Nutr 22: 1608-1617, 1969

3. MEZEY E, TOBON F: Rates of ethanol clearance and activities of the ethanol-oxidizing enzymes in chronic alcoholic patients. Gastroenterology 61: 707-715, 1971

4. HAWKINS RD, KALANT H, KHANNA JM: Effect of chronic intake of ethanol on rate of ethanol metabolism. Canad J Physiol Pharmacol 44: 241-257, 1966

5. LIEBER CS, DE CARLI LM: The role of the microsomal ethanol oxidizing system (MEOS) for ethanol metabolism in vivo. J Pharmacol Exp Ther 181: 279-287, 1972

6. VIDELA L, BERNSTEIN J, ISRAEL Y: Metabolic alterations produced in the liver by chronic ethanol administration. Increased oxidative capacity. Biochem J 134: 507-514, 1973

7. LIEBER CS: Hepatic and metabolic effects of alcohol (1966-1973). Gastroenterology 65: 821-846, 1973

8. LIEBER CS, DE CARLI LM: Ethanol oxidation by hepatic microsomes: Adaptive increase after ethanol feeding. Science 162: 917-918, 1968

9. LIEBER CS, DECARLI LM: Hepatic microsomal ethanol oxidizing system: In vitro characteristics and adaptive properties in vivo. J Biol Chem 245: 2505-2512, 1970

10. VIDELA L, ISRAEL Y: Factors that modify the metabolism of ethanol in rat liver and adaptive changes produced by its chronic administration. Biochem J 118: 275-281, 1970

11. BERNSTEIN J, VIDELA L, ISRAEL Y: Metabolic alterations produced in the liver by chronic ethanol administration. II. Changes related to energetic parameters of the cell. Biochem J 134: 515-521, 1973

12. ISRAEL Y, VIDELA L, VIDELA VF, BERNSTEIN J: Effects of chronic ethanol treatment and thyroxine administration on ethanol metabolism and liver oxidative capacity. J Pharmacol Exp Ther 192: 565-574, 1975

13. THURMAN RG, LEY HG, SCHOLZ R: Hepatic microsomal ethanol oxidation. Hydrogen peroxide formation and the role of catalase. Eur J Biochem 25: 420-430, 1972

14. THURMAN RG: Induction of hepatic microsomal reduced nicotinamide adenine dinucleotide phosphate-dependent production of hydrogen peroxide by chronic prior treatment with ethanol. Molec Pharmacol 9: 670-675, 1973

15. KORSTEN MA, MATSUZAKI S, FEINMAN L, LIEBER CS: High blood acetaldehyde levels after ethanol administration in alcoholics. New Eng J Med 292: 386-389, 1975

16. ARSLANIAN MJ, PASCOE E, REINHOLD JG: Rat liver alcohol dehydrogenase. Purification and properties. Biochem J 125: 1039-1047, 1971

17. OKUDA K, TAKIGAWA N: Rat liver 5 β-cholestane-3α,7α,12α, 26-tetrol dehydrogenase as a liver alcohol dehydrogenase. Biochim Biophys Acta 220: 141-148, 1970

18. MISTILIS SP, GARSKE A: Induction of alcohol dehydrogenase in liver and gastrointestinal tract. Aust Ann Med 18: 227-231, 1969

19. LUNDQUIST F, WOLTHERS H: The kinetics of alcohol elimination in man. Acta Pharmacol 14: 265-289, 1958

20. MAKAR AB, MANNERING GJ: Pyrazole inhibition and kinetics of ethanol metabolism in the intact rat and monkey. Biochem Pharmacol 19: 2017-2022, 1970

21. REYNIER M: Pyrazole inhibition and kinetic studies of ethanol and retinol oxidation catalyzed by rat liver alcohol dehydrogenase. Acta Chem Scand 23: 1119-1129, 1969

22. LINDROS KO, OSHINO N, PARRILLA R, WILLIAMSON J: Characteristics of ethanol oxidation on flavin and pyridine nucleotide fluorescence changes in perfused rat liver. J Biol Chem 249: 7956-7963, 1974

23. MEZEY E, TOBON F: Rates of ethanol clearance and activities of the ethanol-oxidizing enzymes in chronic alcoholic patients. Gastroenterology 61: 707-715, 1971

24. ISERI OA, LIEBER CS, GOTTLIEB LS: The ultrastructure of fatty liver induced by prolonged ethanol ingestion. Am J Pathol 48: 535-555, 1966

25. RUBIN E, HUTTERER F, LIEBER CS: Ethanol increases hepatic smooth endoplasmic reticulum and drug-metabolizing enzymes. Science 159: 1469-1470, 1968

26. LANE BP, LIEBER CS: Ultrastructural alterations in human hepatocytes following ingestion of ethanol with adequate diets. Am J Pathol 49: 593-603, 1966

27. RUBIN E, LIEBER CS: Early fine structural changes in the human liver induced by alcohol. Gastroenterology 52: 1-13, 1967

28. RUBIN E, LIEBER CS: Alcohol-induced hepatic injury in non-alcoholic volunteers. N Eng J Med 278: 869-876, 1968

29. ISHII H, JOLY J-G, LIEBER CS: Effect of ethanol on the amount and enzyme activities of hepatic rough and smooth microsomal membranes. Biochem Biophys Acta 291: 411-420, 1973

30. ORME-JOHNSON WH, ZIEGLER DM: Alcohol mixed function oxidase activity of mammalian liver microsomes. Biochem Biophys Res Commun 21: 78-82, 1965

31. ZIEGLER DM: Discussion in Microsomes and Drug Oxidation. RW Estabrook, JR Gillette and KC Liebman (eds.). Baltimore, Williams and Wilkins, 1972, pp. 458

32. TESCHKE R, HASUMURA Y, LIEBER CS: Hepatic microsomal alcohol oxidizing system. Affinity for methanol, ethanol and propanol. J Biol Chem 250: 7397-7404, 1975

33. CHANCE B, OSHINO N: Kinetics and mechanisms of catalase in peroxisomes of the mitochondrial fraction. Biochem J 122: 225-233, 1971

34. REDMAN CM, GRAB DJ, IRUKULLA R: The intracellular pathway of newly formed rat liver catalase. Arch Biochem Biophys 152: 496-501, 1972

35. KEILIN D, HARTREE EF: Properties of catalase. Catalysis of compiled oxidation of alcohols. Biochem J 39: 293-301, 1945

36. BOVERIS A, OSHINO N, CHANCE B: The cellular production of hydrogen peroxide. Biochem J 128: 617-630, 1972

37. OSHINO N, CHANCE B, SIES H, BUCHER T: The role of H_2O_2 generation in perfused rat liver and the reaction of catalase compound I and hydrogen donors. Arch Biochem Biophys 154: 117-131, 1973

38. OSHINO N, JAMIESON D, CHANCE B: The properties of hydrogen peroxide production under hyperoxic and hypoxic conditions of perfused rat liver. Biochem J 146: 53-65, 1975

39. LESTER B, BENSON GD: Alcohol oxidation in rats inhibited by pyrazole oximes and amides. Science 169: 282-284, 1970

40. PAPENBERG J, von WARTBURG JP, AEBI H: Metabolism of ethanol and fructose in the perfused rat liver. Enzym Biol Clin 11: 237-250, 1970

41. FEYTMANS E, LEIGHTON F: Effects of pyrazole and 3-amino-1, 2, 4-triazole on methanol and ethanol metabolism by the rat. Biochem Pharmacol 22: 349-360, 1973

42. ISSELBACHER KJ, CARTER EA: Ethanol oxidation by liver microsomes: Evidence against a separate and distinct enzyme system. Biochem Biophys Res Commun 39: 530-537, 1970

43. ROACH MK, REESE WN, CREAVEN PJ: Ethanol oxidation in the microsomal fraction of rat liver. Biochem Biophys Res Commun 36: 596-602, 1969

44. TESCHKE R, HASUMURA Y, LIEBER CS: Hepatic microsomal ethanol oxidizing system: Solubilization, isolation and characterization. Arch Biochem Biophys 163: 404-415, 1974

45. OHNISHI K, LIEBER CS: Reconstitution of the hepatic microsomal ethanol oxidizing system. Fed Proc 35: 706, 1976

46. COMAI K, GAYLOR JL: Existence and separation of three forms of cytochrome P-450 from rat liver microsomes. J Biol Chem 248: 4949-4955, 1973

47. LEVIN W, RYAN D, WEST S, LU AY: Preparation of partially purified lipid-depleted cytochrome P-450 and reduced nicotinamide adenine dinucleotide phosphate-cytochrome c reductase from rat liver microsomes. J Biol Chem 249: 1747-1754, 1974

48. KALANT H, KHANNA JM, ENDRENYI I: Effect of pyrazole on ethanol metabolism in ethanol treated rats. Canad J Physiol Pharmacol 53: 416-422, 1975

49. STEIN WS, LIEBER CS, LEEVY CM, CHERRICK GR, ABELMANN WH: The effect of ethanol upon systemic and hepatic blood flow in man. Am J Clin Nutr 13: 68-74, 1963

50. BERRY MN, FRIEND DS: High yield preparation of isolated rat liver parenchymal cells. A biochemical and fine structural study. J Cell Biol 43: 506-520, 1969

51. JEEJEEBHOY KN, HO J, GREENBERG R, PHILLIPS MJ, BRUCE-
     ROBERTSON A, SODTKE U: Albumin fibrinogen and transferrin
     synthesis in isolated rat hepatocyte suspension. Biochem J 146:
     141-155, 1975

52. BONNICHSEN R, BRINK NG: Liver alcohol dehydrogenase. In Methods
     of Enzymology, vol 1. SP Colowick and NO Kaplan (eds.). New
     York, Academic Press, 1965. pp. 495-503

53. LUCK H: Catalase.   In Methods of Enzymatic Analysis.   HU
     Bergmeyer, (ed.). New York, Academic Press, 1963. pp. 885-894

54. GRUNNET N, QUISTORFF B, THIEDEN HI: Rate limiting factors in
     ethanol oxidation by isolated rat liver parenchymal cells. Eur J
     Biochem 40: 275-282, 1973

55. TESCHKE R, HASUMURA Y, LIEBER CS: Hepatic ethanol metabolism:
     Respective roles of alcohol dehydrogenase, the microsomal ethanol
     oxidizing system and catalase. Arch Biochem Biophys 175: 635-
     643, 1976

56. THIEDEN HI: The effect of ethanol concentration on ethanol oxidation
     rate in rat liver slices. Acta Chem Scand 25: 3421-3427, 1971

57. DE CARLI LM, LIEBER CS: Fatty liver in the rat after prolonged
     intake of ethanol with a nutritionally adequate liquid diet. J Nutr
     91: 331-336, 1967

58. MATSUZAKI S, LIEBER CS: ADH independent ethanol oxidation in the
     liver and its increase by chronic ethanol consumption. Gastro-
     enterology 69: A45/845, 1975

59. SVOBODA DJ, MANNING RT: Chronic alcoholism with fatty meta-
     morphosis of the liver. Mitochondrial alterations in hepatic cells.
     Am J Pathol 44: 645-662, 1964

60. KIESSLING K-H, PILSTROM L: Ethanol and the human liver.
     Structural and metabolic changes in liver mitochondria. Cyto-
     biologie 4: 339-348, 1971

61. FRENCH SW: Fragility of liver mitochondria in ethanol-fed rats.
     Gastroenterology 54: 1106-1114, 1968

62. CEDERBAUM AI, LIEBER CS, RUBIN E: Effect of chronic ethanol
     treatment on mitochondrial functions damage to coupling site I.
     Arch Biochem Biophys 165: 560-569, 1974

63. CEDERBAUM AI, LIEBER CS, TOTH A, BEATTIE DS, RUBIN E:
     Effects of ethanol and fat on the transport of reducing equivalents
     into rat liver mitochondria. J Biol Chem 248: 4977-4986, 1973

64. ERIKSSON CJ: Ethanol and acetaldehyde metabolism in rat strains genetically selected for their ethanol preference.   Biochem Pharmacol 22: 2283-2292, 1973

65. TOTTMAR O, MARCHNER H: Characteristics of the acetaldehyde oxidation in rat liver, and the effects of antabuse, 4-methyl-pyrazole and unknown dietary factors on the hepatic output of acetaldehyde.   In The Role of Acetaldehyde in the Actions of Ethanol, vol 23.   KO Lindros and CJP Ericksson, (eds.).   The Finnish Foundation for Alcohol Studies, Helsinki, 1975.   pp. 47-66

66. HASUMURA Y, TESCHKE R, LIEBER CS: Acetaldehyde oxidation by hepatic mitochondria.   Decrease after chronic ethanol consumption.   Science 189: 727-729, 1975

67. HASUMURA Y, TESCHKE R, LIEBER CS: Characteristics of acetaldehyde oxidation in rat liver mitochondria.   J Biol Chem, in press, 1976

68. GORDON E: ATP metabolism in an ethanol-induced fatty liver.   Alcoholism: Clinical and Experimental Research, in press, 1977

69. VEECH RL, EGGLESTON LV, KREBS HA: The redox state of free nicotinamide-adenine dinucleotide phosphate in the cytoplasm of rat liver.   Biochem J 115: 609-619, 1969

70. GRUNDIN R: Metabolic interaction of ethanol and alprenolol in isolated liver cells.   Acta Pharmacol Toxicol 37: 185-200, 1975

71. DALZIEL K, DICKINSON FM: The activity of liver alcohol dehydrogenase with nicotinamide-adenine dinucleotide phosphate as coenzyme.   Biochem J 95: 311-320, 1965

72. BLOMSTRAND R, THEORELL H: Inhibitory effect on ethanol oxidation in man after administration of 4-methylpyrazole.   Life Sci 9: 631-640, 1970

73. SALASPURO MP, LINDROS KO, PIKKARAINEN P: Ethanol and galactose metabolism as influenced by 4-methylpyrazole in alcoholics with and without nutritional deficiency.   Ann Clin Res 7: 269-272, 1975

74. THEORELL H, YONETANI T: On the effects of some heterocyclic compounds on the enzymic activity of liver alcohol dehydrogenase.   Acta Chem Scand 5: 1105-1126, 1951

75. RYDBERG U, BUIJTEN J, NERI A: Kinetics of some pyrazole derivatives in the rat.   J Pharm Pharmacol 24: 651-652, 1972

76. DEITRICH RA, COLLINS AC, ERWIN VG: Effect of pyrazole in vivo on aldehyde metabolism in rat liver and brain. Biochem Pharmacol 20: 2663-2669, 1971

77. DOMSCHKE S, DOMSCHKE W, LIEBER CS: Hepatic redox state: Attenuation of the acute effects of ethanol induced by chronic ethanol consumption. Life Sci 15: 1327-1334, 1974

78. NEWMAN HW, LEBMAN AJ, CUTTING WC: Effect of dosage on rate of disappearance of alcohol from its blood stream. J Pharmacol 61: 58-61, 1937

79. GUYNN RW, PIEKLIK JR: Dependence on dose of the acute effects of ethanol on liver metabolism in vivo. J Clin Invest 56: 1411-1419, 1975

80. THEORELL H, NYGAARD AP, BONNICHSEN R: Studies on liver alcohol dehydrogenase. III. The influence of pH and some anions on the reaction velocity constants. Acta Chem Scand 9: 1148-1165, 1955

81. von WARTBURG J-P, BETHUNE JL, VALLEE BL: Human liver alcohol dehydrogenase. Kinetic and physiochemical properties. Biochem 3: 1775-1782, 1964

82. GERSHMAN H: Acetaldehyde-ethanol change in vivo during ethanol oxidation. Arch Biochem Biophys 168: 327-330, 1975

83. THURMAN RG, BRENTZEL HJ: The role of alcohol dehydrogenase in microsomal ethanol oxidation and the adaptive increase in ethanol metabolism due to chronic treatment with ethanol. Alcoholism: Clinical and Experimental Research 1: in press, 1977

DISCUSSION

CHAIRMAN: H. KALANT

GORDON: What type of ethanol did you use in your experiments on the isotope exchange reactions? Was it labelled specifically or uniformly labelled?

LUNDQUIST: It was R-1-^{3}H-ethanol.

KISILEVSKY: If ethanol is a source of ATP, why does the AMP level increase during ethanol metabolism?

LUNDQUIST: It is not known with certainty but probably it is due to activation of acetate. Acetate is formed and some of it, depending on the species and state of nutrition of the experimental animal, is activated to acetyl CoA. In this process AMP is formed. I must admit that there are problems.

LIEBER: Can you estimate the effect of the specific dynamic action of alcohol on the consumption of a mixed diet?

LUNDQUIST: It should be possible to calculate oxygen uptake from the amount of alcohol consumed. Stoke and Stuart found that alcohol induced a 13% increase in the total oxygen uptake and this may be quite a reasonable figure. I believe it would depend on quite a number of conditions and I can't really say anything very definite.

LIEBER: One of the reasons for interest in this is the inconsistency in the weight gain of pair fed animals on alcohol containing diets and on diets in which the alcohol has been replaced by the theoretical caloric equivalent of either carbohydrate or fat. One would predict that the alcohol animals should regularly lose weight relative to the controls, and in many studies this is the case. But in many other studies it isn't the case and there doesn't seem to be any consistent information on this point. Let me just add that there is no question in my mind that the isocaloric substitution for alcohol involves a deficit in terms of caloric balance that cannot be explained except perhaps on the basis of this specific dynamic action of ethanol related to a lack of coupling with AMP formation.

KHANNA: We have been involved in the study of animals chronically treated with ethanol and pair fed and I would disagree with what Dr. Lieber has said. We find that the weight gains are equal in the two groups especially if one gives a high protein diet, about 20% of the calories, along with the ethanol. In fact we find a bit more weight gain in the ethanol treated animals compared to the controls. On the high fat diet my impression is that if you start the animals around 150 g then they gain just about the same weight. If you start the animals younger, around 90 g, then there is less of a weight gain in the ethanol treated animals. It really depends on when you start and what type of diet you give along with ethanol.

JOLY: How do you explain the triglyceride accumulation secondary to lipid peroxidation?

DI LUZIO: We are looking at the possibility that the sites of peroxidation and loss of anti-oxidants are mitochondrial. It is the mitochondria which show increased peroxidation and decreased anti-oxidant levels after alcohol. We can tie in the work showing a failure of fatty acid oxidation by the mitochondria to explain the production of the fatty liver.

RUBIN: We actually agree with most of the data that Dr. Gordon presented. But we have measured adenine translocase activity in our model and have been unable to determine any difference in the ethanol treated and control animals. I think it's important to note that the adenine translocase system is linear up to 15 seconds and if one goes much longer than this one is not in the linear range. I wonder if this might not explain some of the differences which we found.

GORDON: We are quite aware of this problem and have only reported data involving linearity. However there is another very important point. I get no change in the adenine nucleotide translocase system unless I get an increase in the long chain coA derivatives of fatty acids, and if I remove those long chain coA derivatives of fatty acids then I remove the effect. Sometimes this takes different periods of time.

LIEBER: You have demonstrated that acetaldehyde has an effect on protein metabolism which is different from that of ethanol and have implied that the effect of ethanol on protein metabolism may not be by acetaldehyde. We should keep in mind alternate explanations because when we give acetaldehyde under these conditions it differs from the acetaldehyde generated by ethanol in at least three ways: (1) the concentration of acetaldehyde achieved in the blood is obviously different; (2) the site of acetaldehyde production from ethanol in the liver does not necessarily correspond to the site of penetration of acetaldehyde when it comes into the liver from the blood stream; and (3) acetaldehyde given in the absence of ethanol has a different effect on the ADH mediated pathway than does acetaldehyde given in the presence of ethanol. For these and other reasons I think we should keep in mind the possibility that these experiments do not necessarily indicate that the effect of ethanol is not mediated by acetaldehyde.

ROTHSCHILD: I couldn't agree with you more. The concentrations we haven't measured. The site of acetaldehyde formation is also compartmentalized and I'm really not certain how we can get around this. The use of pyrazole or 4-methylpyrazole while impeding the enzyme system nearly 95% will still allow significant ethanol metabolism and so far our studies with 4-methylpyrazole have shown absolutely no alteration in the reduction of albumin sythesis with ethanol perfusion. In two studies 4-methylpyrazole has reversed the acetaldehyde inhibition of albumin synthesis in the rat liver but this may not be the case in vivo when the acetaldehyde is produced from ethanol. Since acetaldehyde is rapidly diffusable caution must be taken in interpreting that the effects of ethanol metabolism are related to acetaldehyde.

LIEBER: Would the opposite approach, the use of a small dose of Disulfiram or calcium carbonimide shed any light?

ROTHSCHILD: That's a very good idea.

FISHER: We will be hearing a lot more about hypoxia later on, but I just wondered if either the ethanol or acetaldehyde concentrations you use are associated with haemolysis in your perfusion system?

ROTHSCHILD: There is some haemolysis that takes place regardless of what you do. We end up usually with a potassium level of 7.5 mEq/L whereas we may start with 4.5 or 5 mEq/L. Haemolysis with alcohol is a little bit more than with other substances but not significantly so and not routinely.

LIEBER: In support of the thesis that ethanol administration induces a specific type of P-450, I would like to mention two additional pieces of information. We have succeeded in reconstituting the microsomal ethanol oxidizing system using P-450 as a reducer of phospholipids. In preliminary experiments we have found that the activity of the system is significantly increased when the P-450 of alcohol fed animals is used. The second point is that we have some preliminary results indicating that the electrophoretic bands that appear in the P-

450 region after alcohol feeding are different than the P-450 induced by phenobarbital and methylcholanthrene.

JOLY: We have not used ethanol as a substrate because our preparation is contaminated with catalase. However ethanol may be a good substrate because in binding studies we found that the association constant of our ethanol P-450 is much lower than that obtained with control P-450.

LIEBER: I wonder if these marked differences in the curves relating activity to the amount of added P-450 after induction by different inducers will enable you to predict the differences in the effect on the in vivo metabolism of different types of binding substrates?

JOLY: This question is very important indeed because all we are doing really is trying to explain what happens in vivo. We are currently trying to find out if aniline given in vivo can be used as a marker of induction by ethanol.

ISRAEL: At what oxygen tension do you study the cells?

MATSUZAKI: I studied 95% oxygen and atmospheric air and could not find a significant difference. Initially these experiments were done in 95% oxygen but later experiments were done in atmospheric air.

ISRAEL: I wonder whether you are in fact inhibiting all the catalase in your system. Have you done formate controls in order to show that you still do not have some catalase activity?

MATSUZAKI: Our studies suggest that the intracellular inhibition is maintained until the reaction is started.

LIEBER: Formate is not a specific substrate for catalase. Formate can be metabolized by a variety of other pathways, including the microsomal hydroxylation pathway.

KHANNA: Are you studying one time period?

MATSUZAKI: I use a time curve.

KHANNA: What sort of time curve do you use?

MATSUZAKI: These hepatocytes can oxidize ethanol in a linear manner for 90 minutes or more.

KHANNA: Have you been doing all these studies with a time curve?

MATSUZAKI: Yes. In order to get such a small difference, especially in the presence of pyrazole, we have to take two or three more points.

LUNDQUIST: In our laboratory we found even higher non-ADH activity in isolated hepatocytes, as much as 2.4 micromoles/gram at 80 millimoles of ethanol.

KALANT: You showed a linear increase in the rate of alcohol oxidization and the non-ADH component or pyrazole resistant component as you increased the ethanol concentration from 10 to 30 millimoles. Other investigators finding such an increase have usually been working at a much higher concentration, something in the order of 100-200 millimolar. Is there something significantly different about isolated hepatocytes that alters their sensitivity to relatively small increases in the concentration of the alcohol?

MATSUZAKI: Such high concentrations are very unphysiological and I have never tried more than 15 millimolar. Such high concentrations may involve cellular toxicity. Furthermore it is difficult to measure ethanol disappearance with accuracy at concentrations more than 60 or 80 millimolar.

METABOLISM OF ETHANOL AND THE EFFECTS OF ETHANOL ON

METABOLISM: GENERAL DISCUSSION

CHAIRMAN: M.M. FISHER

FISHER: At least some of the controversies in this field are related to the many variations in technique. We are looking at ethanol metabolism in vivo and by a variety of in vitro models including isolated cell organelles, isolated liver cells and isolated perfused livers. And we are looking at animals that have been fed or fasted and of different strains and sexes. Surely some of the controversies merely reflect this variation in the experimental model being used. Furthermore there is unnecessary variety in our terminology. We have been comparing millimoles of ethanol and milligrams of acetaldehyde. Should we not use a molar approach in talking about blood and tissue levels of ethanol and its metabolites?

ROTHSCHILD: Yes. I think we should adopt a standardized chemical terminology. Whether we want to use mg% or molar doesn't matter but I think the terminology should be uniform.

LIEBER: If there is a hypermetabolic state during the chronic ingestion of ethanol does this account for the increased rate of ethanol oxidization? And if there is a hypermetabolic state why do we have a reduced state in the mitochondria?

ISRAEL: There are two groups that have found a hypermetabolic state, our group working with liver slices incubated within 3 minutes of killing the animal and in close to physiological conditions, and Dr. Thurman working with the perfused liver. Up to 50% more oxygen is consumed if the liver comes from alcohol treated animals. Dr. Gordon working with hepatocytes did not find this effect.

GORDON: I found the effect depending on the control I used. The effect you are looking at is the availability of substrate.

151

ISRAEL: We have reported this effect in fed animals as well. The feeding factor is not the reason for the discrepancy.

GORDON: But your rates of ethanol oxidation are those of a starved animal not a fed animal!

ISRAEL: Well, perhaps you would like to take Dr. Thurman's studies on the perfused livers of fed animals.

GORDON: No. Dr. Thurman's rates of ethanol consumption are those of starved animals.

ISRAEL: It is very difficult to compare cells with slices. The important thing here is that the two groups finding this effect have used cells that have not been much tampered with - the whole tissue is placed in an incubator as fast as possible. In your conditions, where you don't see this effect, you take the liver, and perfuse it with collagenase, perfuse it with proteolytic enzymes, smash it, centrifuge it and wash it several times before ending up with cells in the incubator after $1\frac{1}{2}$ or 2 hours! There is another factor of importance. Have you demonstrated that the rate limiting step of ethanol metabolism in your cell preparations is the same as that in vivo?

FISHER: I think we are off to a good start. The original question was - is there a hypermetabolic state? I think the answer is yes depending on the circumstances under which one looks for it. Is it too much to ask that we look for these metabolic effects under conditions that are uniform? Since most of us take our alcohol in the fed state, is there not something to be said for doing our experiments in the fed animal?

LIEBER: Before I comment on that particular point, I want to come back to the statement about the condition of the tissue used for experimentation. Dr. Israel pointed out some of the problems with isolated hepatocytes. But there are also major problems with other systems, tissue slices and perfused livers in particular. All these in vitro techniques have problems and we have to define the extent to which they mimic the in vivo conditions. This brings me back to the standardization of technique. I was very honoured to see the Toronto group modify our liquid diet. In Montreal another modification of the diet has been used and again we were very flattered. But I wonder what is the necessity for all these modifications. Wouldn't it be simpler if we could all agree on the technique? The reason we originated this liquid diet was to overcome the natural aversion of the rat for alcohol. If you put alcohol in its drinking water the rat will not take enough alcohol to produce liver lesions if the diet is adequate. The animals given our liquid alcohol diets have no choice but to take the alcohol and a good diet, and the model has reproduced at least some of the lesions seen in man. Certain individuals have used low fat alcohol diets. These do not result in the production of a fatty liver. What is the point of giving alcohol liquid diets if you are not going to produce lesions which mimic those you are interested in studying. I urge you therefore, if you do modify the diet, at least to give us a rationale in terms of producing a better lesion or producing a more severe lesion.

KHANNA: I don't believe in using one standardized diet for doing experiments. It depends on what the aim of the experiment is. Since we know the effects of ethanol are not just simply dependent on the amount of ethanol but are also dependent on the amount of protein, fat and carbohydrate in the diet, then we must do experiments under different dietary conditions. Perhaps some of the effects Dr. Lieber is getting are simply because of the particular diet he is using. For example, in one of my experiments I studied ethanol metabolism during its chronic administration. I used two types of diet – one the standard liquid alcohol diet and the other a high protein (28%) and a low fat (10%) diet. With the latter diet there was an increase in ethanol metabolism without any increase in MEOS activity. We must study ethanol metabolism under different dietary conditions.

LIEBER: All I meant was that if we study the pathogenesis of alcohol fatty liver, we ought to use a model which reproduces the lesion. Obviously if we are studying the effect of dietary protein, fat or carbohydrate we have to change these factors in the diet. And this we did. But there are studies in the literature which pertain to the pathogenesis of alcohol liver injury using a model which does not produce alcohol liver injury. These studies may be irrelevant.

LUNDQUIST: I want to underline the species differences involved in alcohol metabolism. As you may know in the rat the total capacity of ADH is actually used up in the fatty liver stage. No matter what you do, whether you use uncouplers or fructose or anything, you cannot make the rate of the ADH reaction go any faster at the same alcohol concentration. However in other species such as the pig or human there is a reserve of ADH activity and you may be able to boost the ADH activity under these conditions. I think it is quite important to realize that there are species differences.

ROTHSCHILD: I think that we are dwelling on an important point. If we cannot standardize the model system, perhaps we can standardize the criteria by which we evaluate the experimental models we are using. Perhaps we can standardize the measurement of certain parameters of hepatic cell function and viability so that different studies can be better compared.

JOLY: Although I agree with Dr. Khanna that the use of different diets may be helpful, the last two papers from his group actually contradict one another really just because the source of carbohydrate in the diets was changed. This change cancelled out the effects of ethanol on drug metabolism in vitro. Therefore it is important to have an experimental diet which is uniform quantitatively and qualitatively.

The second point is that the diet designed by Dr. Lieber's group reflects the diet consumed by North Americans. Therefore these two points have to be kept in mind: 1) we should try to use an experimental diet that approximates the diet consumed by man, and 2) whenever we start to modify this diet we might cancel out an effect that we want to study.

FISHER: Do we now all accept the conclusion that the rate-limiting step in ethanol metabolism is the mitochondrial re-oxidation of NADH?

LUNDQUIST: This is not quite right because the rate-limiting step of the NADH pathway is in fact the dissociation of NADH from the enzymes.   What determines the overall rate is then the rate of removal of the NADH.   Whether this is primarily by means of the respiratory chain or the shuttle processes depends upon the situation in the cell and whether the animal has been fed or not. I think it may be a simplification to put it the way you do.

GORDON: We should not forget that in addition to the mitochondrial mechanisms there are other ways in which the re-oxidation of NADH can occur.   For example there is coupling of the NADH and NADPH systems.   Therefore it is probably an over-simplification to consider the re-oxidation of NADH as the one great limiting factor. But the capacity of the mitochondria to re-oxidize NADH is obviously a very important over-riding consideration under many circumstances.

ROTHSCHILD: We also have to consider whether the ethanol feeding is acute or chronic because alteration of metabolic behaviour under the latter conditions ultimately depends on the ability of the cells to synthesize the proteins required for the various steps. At some point we must go back to altered RNA metabolism. Eventually we are going to have to go back one step if not many steps.

ISRAEL: I would like to add to what Dr. Lundquist said. It really depends on the state of the animal. Recent studies have shown that in the fed animal the re-oxidation of NADH is the rate-limiting step but in the fasting animal the rate of transfer of reducing substances to the shuttle system is the rate-limiting step.   Therefore it is an over-simplification to say that the rate-limiting step is the re-oxidation of NADH.

FISHER: Many of us have had problems coming to grips with the concept of the empty calorie. Dr. Lieber, what is an empty calorie?

LIEBER: Well, it is perhaps a dangerous word. We observed that the weight gain of rats fed isocaloric amounts of alcohol instead of carbohydrate was not as great as that of the control animals even though they had no greater loss of calories in the stool and urine. We then went to man and did a number of studies under metabolic ward conditions. We gave to volunteers diets that maintained their weight and then introduced alcohol as an isocaloric substitution. We observed a small but consistent drop in weight. Again we found no increased loss of calories. When you do isocaloric substitution of carbohydrate with ethanol you decrease the dietary carbohydrate and some people wondered whether the low intake of carbohydrate had something to do with our observations. So instead of an isocaloric substitution of ethanol for carbohydrate, we merely added ethanol to a normal diet. In the control period, during which weight was maintained, the volunteers received 2,200 calories. We then doubled the caloric intake by adding 2,200 calories of ethanol. Usually there was a slight increase of weight but then it petered out and after 3 weeks of 4,400 calories, the individual was back to his original weight. Again there was no increased loss of calories and no increased activity. These volunteers were perfectly capable of gaining weight. When we added 2,200 calories of chocolate to the diet, weight gain was rapid. So alcohol calories do not fully count, at least if one gives a large dose of alcohol. Now we don't have a good explanation for this, except from an energy point of view. There is actually an energy cost in the MEOS pathway. Instead of producing hydrogenic compounds we use hydrogenic compounds. All that is produced actually is heat and to the extent that this generation of heat exceeds body requirements it can be equated with a wastage of energy. This may explain some of the energy loss with alcohol and other drugs which induce the microsomal system.

JOLY: If we give the same amount of ethanol to two populations of rats, one fed a high fat diet and one fed a low fat diet, we find a lack of weight gain only in the former group. Yet both groups have MEOS activity in vitro and a MEOS activity which is increased by chronic ethanol feeding. I have trouble understanding these data.

LIEBER: Have you studied calorie losses in the stools of your two groups of animals?

JOLY: No.

LIEBER: I am afraid that they may be different.

LUNDQUIST: To my mind an empty calorie is simply one which doesn't give rise to ATP formation. If one gives a substance like ethanol which gives a lower yield of ATP one would expect that oxygen uptake from other sources would increase to keep ATP production maintained. So I think there is a real problem here. It may have something to do with futile cycles activated in the presence of alcohol. I think that is where you might look for a solution to this problem.

LIEBER: I think the concept is broader than just ethanol as a substrate for the microsomes. The induction of microsomal function pertains not only to exogenous substrates. It also pertains to endogenous substrates.   There are numerous endogenous substrates which get degraded on the microsomes even in the absence of ethanol. How is their metabolism influenced by induction of the microsomal system by alcohol?

KHANNA: When I first started in the alcohol field I decided to use Dr. Lieber's diet because the weight gain was very similar in the alcohol and control groups. Since he introduced the concept of MEOS and has had to account for this wastage of calories, he now is getting less weight gain in his animals chronically treated with ethanol. We started using his diet very precisely and we got equal weight gain in the ethanol treated and control animals after chronic ethanol treatment. In a paper published this year I showed very clearly that it also depends on the percentage of fat in the diet. With a low fat diet there is, if anything, more body weight gain in the ethanol treated animals. With our high protein diet we also found a somewhat higher weight gain in the ethanol treated animals compared to controls.

LIEBER: We have published in detail our experiments with two types of diets, an amino acid diet and a casein diet. We point out that there is not equal weight gain. I want you to verify this and then retract your statement that we have published equal weight gain.

ISRAEL: We have confirmed Dr. Khanna's observations and we have confirmed Dr. Lieber's observations. It all depends on the type of animal you use. If we use an animal that isn't hyperexcitable, we usually get the ethanol animals to grow the same or with a high protein diet even a little better than the controls. They are sleeping all day, they are not exercising. This is another problem; you have to consider the energy spent by the animals. Now we have another strain of animals that develops hypertension because of stress. These animals lose weight fantastically on the ethanol diets. So it may be a matter of the stress to which you subject the animals with the diet and how much the animals exercise.

FISHER: I think we had better move on. This is obviously one of those issues that is better raised but not discussed.

LIEBER: Let me point out that all the studies I have discussed were done in man, in order to avoid all these problems you are alluding to. I suggest that the rat presents problems in extrapolation and that we should go back to clinical investigation.

FISHER: Do we all agree that the liver injury caused by alcohol is caused by both the direct toxic effects of alcohol and by malnutrition?

LIEBER: Direct hepatotoxicity is a dangerous concept and hard to define. We would define a hepatotoxin as anything that interferes with the structure or function of the liver. Under many conditions we can show that alcohol in man as well as in experimental animals does produce functional and structural abnormalities of the liver. So we can call it a hepatotoxin. Now whether we call it direct, I am not sure what we mean by this. In our own experiments we have never tried to ascertain to what extent ethanol without being metabolized is toxic to the liver. In the intestines it seems to have a direct toxic effect by virtue of its high concentration. We have as yet not ascertained whether a high hepatocytic concentration of ethanol is damaging to the liver. But there have been experiments in both Toronto and New Orleans concerning the damage that alcohol can produce when its metabolism is stopped and maybe we should have the debate thrown to these two groups.

ISRAEL: We did carry out some studies to determine whether it is the ethanol or its metabolism which is hepatotoxic. The answer is very difficult. The one thing I can say is that if you increase the blood levels of ethanol you may increase the liver damage. For example, we did one study with pyrazole. This compound inhibits alcohol dehydrogenase and increases blood ethanol levels. After about one month of treatment we found that the triglyceride levels in the pyrazole/ethanol groups were five times higher than those seen in the ethanol group. Similar studies have also been done by Dr. Di Luzio and he reported the production of hepatic damage in the animals given pyrazole plus ethanol. An objection has been raised to the use of pyrazole but I must emphasize that the amount of pyrazole used in our studies was very small, about 37 mg/kilogram every 2 days. Dr. Rubin and Dr. Lieber used pyrazole every day in twice the dose for a month. So this is one type of evidence which we have which shows that if you increase the blood levels you can increase the liver damage.

DI LUZIO: This is a bit controversial in the sense that if you block ethanol metabolism with pyrazole you see no liver pathology in acute experiments.

Now I agree with Dr. Lieber than we have to design experimental models equivalent to those which we see in man but we have looked at vaporization studies where we maintained animals in isolated chambers, and exposed them constantly to alcohol vapour over a period of 28 days. Although they had very elevated blood alcohol levels initially, there was a fantastic tolerance induced and no liver pathology occurred. So the model becomes really important. Not only the blood alcohol level produced but how the animal is exposed to the alcohol is important. We suspect that it is not alcohol per se but really alcohol metabolism which contributes to the lesions.

FISHER: Unfortunately the programme is not as well balanced as it should have been. The catalase school has not been fairly represented. A recent copy of Federation Proceedings featured a symposium in which many members at this table took part. The Federation Proceedings Symposium indicates that there are still investigators who believe that catalase is important. Perhaps Dr. Lieber might address himself to this.

LIEBER: We all know that catalase does exist in the hepatocyte and we all know, if you furnish catalase with a hydrogen regenerating system and ethanol, that it will oxidize the ethanol. But what is the importance of this catalase mediated oxidation in vivo? Now it is generally accepted that the rate limiting step for catalase mediated ethanol oxidation is the rate of H_2O_2 generation in the liver. The best data available for H_2O_2 generation are those published by Chance and his colleagues in Philadelphia. Their reports assess the rate of H_2O_2 generation at a level so low that it could not conceivably contribute a major fraction of the ethanol oxidation.

There is another approach to the problem of the role of catalase. Catalase was first considered as a main pathway for ethanol metabolism many years ago. It was rejected on the basis that Aminotriazole, a good catalase inhibitor, does not affect ethanol metabolism in vivo. Thurman was the first to report that Aminotriazole inhibits ethanol metabolism in the perfused liver and in vivo. But to my knowledge nobody else has found this. And I would like to refer you to a paper that Dr. Thurman has published in Molecular Pharmacology early this year where he now himself reports a number of experiments in which he could not reproduce the inhibition of ethanol metabolism by Aminotriazole. I suggest that at the present time there is no good evidence indicating that the catalase pathway plays a major role in vivo under normal conditions. I would agree that if we stimulate H_2O_2 generation, then catalase could conceivably participate in ethanol oxidation.

FISHER: Many of us went through a phase where catalase was considered to be an experimental artifact. Do you consider it such?

LIEBER: No. Catalase exists in the hepatocyte and it can oxidize ethanol. I only point out that the evidence indicates that the contribution of catalase to ethanol metabolism in vivo is negligible quantitatively. But it certainly does exist and it can be increased under certain circumstances.

ISRAEL: Well, for once I would like to agree with Dr. Lieber. We worked with formate oxidation in vivo. The key word here is in vivo. There is no doubt that there can be metabolism of ethanol through catalase in vitro if you produce enough hydrogen peroxide. But there isn't enough H_2O_2 production in vivo to support a good catalase mediated ethanol metabolism.

KHANNA: I think that the only positive studies against catalase playing a major role in ethanol metabolism in vivo, either in acutely or chronically treated animals are the studies of Dr. Israel's group. The studies with Aminotriazole are less desirable because Aminotriazole is very non-specific and hinders many other systems. I think there is general agreement here.

FISHER: We have had some preliminary advertising for the role that acetaldehyde may be playing in the pathogenesis of liver injury. Dr. Lindros has worked actively in this field and I would like to ask him to initiate the discussion.

LINDROS: In a recent study at the Department of Medical Chemistry at the University of Helsinki we compared the metabolism of acetaldehyde in rats fed different kinds of diet. It had been reported previously that a low protein diet causes decreased ethanol metabolism and also causes a decrease in the alcohol dehydrogenase activity in the liver concomitant with a decreased protein content in the liver. We extended these studies to acetaldehyde and studied the effects of a low protein diet on acetaldehyde levels in the blood after the acute administration of ethanol. In the low protein diet group we saw a significant increase in the level of acetaldehyde in the blood. At the same time the rate of ethanol metabolism was significantly slower as compared to the rate in the other groups and normally we always see a decrease in blood acetaldehyde if the rate of ethanol metabolism is slower. We also found a significant decrease in the acetaldehyde dehydrogenase activity in the liver and in all of the subcellular fractions, the mitochondria, the microsomes and the cytosol. What relevance these results have in terms of a possible role of acetaldehyde or of malnutrition in alcohol induced liver damage we don't know. But we think that these results may be used as a basis for further studies.

ROTHSCHILD: Again the model system is seen to be important. The model based on a low protein diet is totally different from the model based on a zero protein diet.

As far as the cardiovascular system is concerned we have shown that acetaldehyde inhibits protein synthesis in vitro. We used subcellular systems and found no effect whatsoever with ethanol itself. In terms of cardiac muscle protein synthesis, it appears to be acetaldehyde which is the offending agent and not ethanol. In this system acetaldehyde does not disaggregate muscle polysomes and does not impede the ability of these isolated polysomes to synthesize nascent peptides.   Whatever effect acetaldehyde has on cardiovascular protein synthesis it is a much more subtle step than simple polysome disaggregation and alteration of the total mechanism of protein synthesis within the liver.

LINDROS: I think that methylpyrazole can distinguish between ethanol and acetaldehyde induced effects.   In vivo and in the isolated perfused liver a very low level of methylpyrazole will have a very slight effect on ethanol metabolism, but will produce a very marked reduction in acetaldehyde levels. I think this could be a very useful tool in the attempt to differentiate between the effects of ethanol and those of ethanol together with acetaldehyde.

LIEBER: I agree that this is a nice tool but you are just looking at the blood and this only reflects a very small overflow of acetaldehyde. Most of the ethanol and acetaldehyde metabolism takes place in sites which you do not consider in these studies.

Dr. Rothschild pointed out that he had acetaldehyde toxicity in the heart but not so much in the liver. We have shown that acetaldehyde has some effect on hepatic mitochondrial function. One of the problems was that we used relatively high concentrations of acet-aldehyde. But Dr. Matsuzaki's studies have demonstrated that the mitochondria of alcohol fed animals are much more susceptible to the effects of acetaldehyde, even in concentrations which are normally found in the liver and which do not affect normal mitochondrial function. Therefore its lack of action in a normal rat does not mean that acetaldehyde does not have a toxic effect in an alcohol fed rat.

FISHER: Does ethanol itself alter the activity of acetaldehyde dehydrogenase?

LINDROS: We studied this giving ethanol either in the liquid diet or by intubation. When we gave ethanol in the liquid diet we did not see any decrease in acetaldehyde dehydrogenase activity in the liver. However if we gave it by intubation in amounts sufficient to cause loss of body weight and poor food intake, then we did see a decrease in acetaldehyde dehydrogenase activity, especially of mitochondrial enzyme. Concomitantly with this we saw increased acetaldehyde levels. Again it depends on the model!

LIEBER: We measured acetaldehyde dehydrogenase activity in liver homogenates and mitochondria in the presence of different concentrations of ethanol. Ethanol did not inhibit the activity of the acetaldehyde dehydrogenase. But chronic ethanol feeding may affect acetaldehyde dehydrogenase activity in the liver. We studied the rate of acetaldehyde oxidation by intact mitochondria in vitro. Acetaldehyde dehydrogenase activity was found to be slightly but significantly increased in ethanol fed rats. In spite of this increased activity of acetaldehyde dehydrogenase the oxidation of acetaldehyde by the mitochondria was lower in the ethanol fed rats. Therefore after chronic ethanol feeding the amount of enzyme is increased or unchanged but its function in the mitochondria is decreased. Therefore after chronic ethanol feeding the amount of enzyme is increased or unchanged but its function in the mitochondria is decreased. Therefore we have to think of mitochondrial function as well as enzyme activity.

ISRAEL: But the important thing is the phosphorylation potential inside the cell of the alcohol treated animal as compared to the control. We cannot simply take the mitochondria out and forget about the in vivo controls of mitochondrial function. Dr. French, Dr. Gordon and I all agree that there is a reduction in the phosphorylation potential of the cell after chronic alcohol treatment. Perhaps the rate at which acetaldehyde is metabolized in the mitochondria is not decreased after chronic alcohol treatment but is actually increased.

LINDROS: How do you explain the discrepancy between the decreased acetaldehyde uptake and the increased rate of ethanol metabolism in the livers of your chronically treated animals?

You have impaired acetaldehyde utilization in the mitochondria isolated from chronically treated animals. Yet in the livers of such animals you find an increased rate of ethanol metabolism and therefore an increased rate of acetaldehyde oxidation. Do you find a huge amount of acetaldehyde leaving the liver?

LIEBER: You are perfectly logical! We do see an increased blood acetaldehyde level after alcohol consumption.

FISHER: Are the mitochondrial abnormalities that we see in this condition the cause or the effect?

LIEBER: We think that they are both the cause and the effect. We found during alcohol infusion studies that alcoholics have a higher blood acetaldehyde level than controls with the same dose of ethanol and at the same blood ethanol level. This increased acetaldehyde level could result in mitochondrial impairment. Since the mitochondria are the site of acetaldehyde metabolism and since there can be decreased acetaldehyde metabolism in the injured mitochondria, this mitochondria injury may result in a further increase in the acetaldehyde level and further liver toxicity.

FISHER: Then you claim that the mitochondria are actually injured in the first instance?

LIEBER: In this particular instance, they are.

FISHER: May we now leave the mitochondria but still have Dr. Lieber at the microphone. If ethanol metabolism in vivo follows zero order kinetics, that is does not bear any relationship to its concentration, does the apparent increase in MEOS activity in alcohol treated animals have any significance?

LIEBER: The question of blood alcohol disappearance curves in vivo, in man and in animals, has been highly controversial. In the literature one can find linear disappearance and not-so-linear disappearance. One can find papers with an accelerated rate at high concentrations and papers without this. The problem is that practically all papers have ignored a key factor, namely blood flow through the liver. And it has been well documented that hepatic blood flow is affected differently at different alcohol concentrations. By the way, we should be aware of this fact when we try to extrapolate from in vitro enzyme activities to in vivo enzyme activities. I have been quite amused to see two sets of standards applied to MEOS and to ADH. I have seen publications stating that the MEOS increases or decreases don't correlate perfectly well with the rates of alcohol metabolism measured in vivo, and therefore MEOS isn't really involved in vivo. But if we applied the same reasoning to ADH we would have to say that ADH plays no role in vivo. After chronic alcohol feeding ADH doesn't go up, it decreases. But the rate of ethanol metabolism goes up. Nobody would say, because there is no correlation, that ADH doesn't play a role. So we must be careful.

Now to come back to your question. I challenge the zero order concept because it isn't definitely established in the literature, because blood flow measurements have not been given and because ADH activity is inhibited by high ethanol concentrations. Furthermore there may be product inhibition which doesn't exist with MEOS. Acetaldehyde has a feedback inhibitory effect on the ADH pathway which it doesn't have in the MEOS system.

LINDROS: How can you say that ADH is not a rate limiting step and yet is subject to substrate inhibition? The latter implies that ADH is a rate limiting step.

LIEBER: It is not a rate limiting step under normal circumstances. But as you have shown, if you decrease ADH activity then it becomes rate limiting. Why is there a reduction with a low protein diet or with pyrazole? Because when you reduce its activity ADH may become rate limiting.

LINDROS: I agree on that point. But this means that you would really have very substantial substrate inhibition at higher ethanol levels. Has anybody shown that this is possible with the rat liver?

RUBIN: We published such data last year.

KHANNA: Dr. Lieber has asked why people expect a beautiful correlation between changes in MEOS and ethanol metabolism. The simple reason is that Dr. Lieber has said that there is such a correlation; a 20% increase in MEOS activity is associated with a 20% increased in ethanol metabolism!

LIEBER: The fact remains that there is a rough correlation between MEOS activity and the rate of ethanol metabolism and there is no correlation between ADH activity and the rate of ethanol metabolism. Now your group has published several papers indicating an increase of ADH activity after alcohol feeding. You make a major point out of these findings. Yet we have never been able to verify them. Now I understand that there have been changes in some of the results. What is the present status of your laboratory with ADH.

KHANNA: It does not really matter any more whether the ADH is increased or not. Originally we did find an increase in ADH activity and a number of investigators did likewise. On the other hand, other investigators did not find such an increase in ADH activity. We now know that ADH is not the rate limiting step. We also know that the atypical enzyme has a much higher activity in some humans that do not metabolize ethanol much faster than normals. So the question is immaterial.

LIEBER: Immaterial or not, does it increase or not in your hands?

KHANNA: Well, it depends. Sometimes we find an increase and sometimes we don't. I think that the inconsistency may be explained on the basis of changes in the diet and in the strain of animal. But I don't think it is an important question anymore.

FISHER: Could we have three minutes of your data that are presumably publishable and then we'll get on to a clinical theme before coffee.

KHANNA: The important question about liver fat and ethanol concentration is what happens in vivo and Dr. Lindros and I have been studying this for the last few months. We gave 4 groups of 8 animals 4 different doses of ethanol: 0.5 g/kilogram, 1 g/Kg, 2 g/Kg and 4 g/Kg. We found no differences in ethanol metabolism regardless of the dose given to the animal.

GORDON: Were your animals starved before you did the experiment?

KHANNA: No, these studies were done with fed animals.

Now if the MEOS system is responsible for increased ethanol metabolism in vivo, then one should get increased ethanol metabolism at the higher doses. Animals chronically treated with ethanol and pair fed were given a challenge dose of 0.5 g/Kg to saturate ADH or a dose of 2.5 g/Kg to saturate the MEOS system. Regardless of the dose, the percentage increase in ethanol metabolism was just about the same, approximately 20%. Previously we reported a 40% increase but since then we have been using a different strain of animal from a different supplier.

We also studied the effect of methylpyrazole. It produced 87-90% inhibition of ethanol metabolism. If you account for some loss by kidney and lungs most of the metabolism of ethanol must occur via the ADH route.

LIEBER: Dr. Khanna did not do blood flow estimations and therefore we really cannot make any conclusion from these studies in vivo. It is well known that alcohol at different concentrations will affect hepatic blood flow differently.

KHANNA: Please tell us how changes in blood flow are going to explain this situation.

LIEBER: I refer you to my review article in the Annals of Medicine, 1967.

FISHER: I will use the chairman's prerogative here. The hepatic world is still waiting for good measurements of hepatic blood flow.

RAISFELD: We are hearing a lot of discussion about ethanol metabolism but I am just seeing data relating to the plasma disappearance of ethanol. Is it fair to equate plasma disappearance with metabolism? I think we should clarify these terms before going any further.

LUNDQUIST: This is a very good question. Where you have absorption going on from the intestinal tract you cannot rely on the rate of the disappearance from the blood. You have to be absolutely sure that everything given is absorbed and distributed in the body before you can use any measurements of plasma disappearance. And even then, it might be quite difficult to measure small changes accurately.

KHANNA: We measure the blood ethanol level at various time intervals and get a linear curve of disappearance. Extrapolation of this line to zero ethanol concentration gives you the time in which the ethanol dose is eliminated. So there is really no problem of absorption in this case.

FISHER: There has been a suggestion over the years that some of us are more immune to the ravages of alcohol than are others. However, with further studies of the problem, we are beginning to wonder if this isn't just a dose-response phenomenon. If so, won't we all get alcohol-induced liver disease if we try.

LIEBER: Within a given population of patients not all heavy drinkers develop cirrhosis at a given time. Even in our baboons only one of three did. The reason for these different susceptibilities is not always clear but it seems to pertain to any pathogen. We don't all react the same to toxic compounds. This is why we talk of LD-50's. The same probably pertains to ethanol. There appear to be factors other than ethanol metabolism which determine our response to the toxin. But the overriding factor seems to be the dose because some effects are always observed when we give enough alcohol.

FISHER: Dr. Di Luzio, does the antioxidant have any role to play in protecting our society?

DI LUZIO: We have not yet studied this possibility in man and the answer
to your question is really unknown.

ORGANELLE PATHOLOGY OF ALCOHOL-INDUCED HEPATIC INJURY

Emanuel Rubin and Arthur I. Cederbaum

Department of Pathology, Mount Sinai School of Medicine

University of New York, New York, N.Y. 10029

Chronic ethanol ingestion has been shown to affect most cytoplasmic organelles of the hepatocyte, both morphologically and functionally. Some of these changes appear to be injurious i.e., they result in decreased function, while others are probably adaptive and lead to enhanced function.

Adaptive Changes

Smooth Endoplasmic Reticulum

Hypertrophy of the smooth endoplasmic reticulum, with a concomitant increase in drug metabolizing enzymes occurs after the administration of phenobarbital and a wide varity of drugs metabolized by hepatic microsomes (1). Chronic administration of ethanol to rats (2), baboons (3) and man (4,5,6) also results in hypertrophy of this organelle, which is responsible for the metabolism of xenobiotics. In these species, chronic ethanol administration leads to enhanced activities of microsomal drug metabolizing enzymes (7) and enhanced clearance of drugs from the blood. Together with these changes, the activity of the microsomal ethanol oxidizing system (MEOS) is enhanced (8) and the blood clearance of ethanol itself is accelerated (9,10).

Golgi Complex

The Golgi apparatus of the liver plays a part in the synthesis and release of lipoproteins (11). Chronic ethanol administration to man results in prominence of the hepatic Golgi apparatus and the accumulation of particles (assumed to be lipoproteins) (12) within the cisternae. In addition, after chronic ethanol ingestion, rats showed increased secretion of lipoproteins (13). Plasma lipoproteins are thought to be glycolipoproteins (14); the attachment of the carbohydrate moieties is mediated by the action of glycosyl transferases (14), enzymes which are located exclusively in the Golgi apparatus (15). We therefore investigated the effects of acute and chronic administration of ethanol on the activity of a glycosyl transferase in preparations of the Golgi apparatus isolated from rat liver (16).

In rats killed 16 hours after a single dose of ethanol, uridine diphosphogalactosyl transferase (UDPGT) activity was significantly increased, whether expressed per mg protein per g of liver, or total liver per 100 g of body weight (Table I).

To determine whether the increase in UDPGT activity was demonstrable with an acceptor other than a protein, and whether a qualitative change in Golgi membranes had occurred, we measured the activity of UDP galactose: N-acetylglucosamine galactosyl transferase in partially purified Golgi fractions, according to the method of Fleischer et al (17), with the addition of 0.5% "Triton X" (18) in a final volume of 0.4 ml. The ratio of hydrolysis to transferase activity was about 0.3. The Golgi apparatus was isolated using a modification of the method of Leelavathi et al (18).

TABLE I

EFFECT OF ETHANOL INGESTION ON UDPGT ACTIVITY (MEAN   S.E.M.) IN GOLGI APPARATUS OF RAT LIVER

	Units mg^{-1} Proteins	Units Per Total Protein Per g Liver	Units Per Total Liver Per 100 g Body Weight
Acute ethanol (16 h) Acceptor-ovalbumin			
Control (15)	18.0 ± 0.9	397 ± 26	$1,362 \pm 97$
Ethanol treated (14)	24.9 ± 1.1	494 ± 25	$1,871 \pm 115$
p	< 0.001	< 0.01	< 0.005
Acceptor-N-acetylgluco-samine			
Control (5)	12.4 ± 1.5	219 ± 31	$1,001 \pm 131$
Ethanol treated (5)	22.3 ± 2.4	368 ± 38	$1,759 \pm 208$
p	< 0.01	< 0.02	< 0.02
Chronic ethanol Acceptor-N-acetylgluco-samine			
Control (5)	14.1 ± 2.2	264 ± 42	780 ± 106
Ethanol treated (5)	29.6 ± 2.7	510 ± 62	$1,915 \pm 281$
p	< 0.005	< 0.01	< 0.005

Total UDPGT activity, measured as the sum of all fractions, was almost doubled when calculated as units per mg of total protein (Table I). The increase was about 75% when activity was referred either to total protein per g of liver or to total liver per 100 g of body weight. In rats killed 90 minutes after a single dose of ethanol, no significant change in UDPGT activity, using either acceptor, was observed, compared with controls. To determine whether the increase in UDPGT activity is affected by chronic ethanol administration, rats of initial weight 150 g were fed a nutritionally adequate liquid diet for 24 days (19). Pair-fed litter mates were given the same diet, except that ethanol isocalorically replaced carbohydrate, to the extent of 36% of the total number of calories. Using N-acetylglucosamine as the acceptor, the increase in UDPGT activity in chronically treated animals was comparable to that in rats given a single large dose of ethanol (Table I). The enhanced secretion of lipoproteins which follows ethanol ingestion may theoretically be considered an adaptive escape mechanism, by which the liver disposes of some of the excess lipids which accumulate in the cytoplasm.

In view of the need for lipoproteins to be transformed into glycolipo-proteins before being secreted, the induction of glycosyl transferase activity suggests that alterations of the Golgi apparatus should be included among adaptive responses to ethanol. This is the first demonstration of the induction of enzyme activity of the Golgi apparatus using either a hexosamine or a protein as an acceptor for the transferase.

Injurious Changes

Rough Endoplasmic Reticulum

In electronmicrographs of liver after chronic ethanol ingestion, the rough endoplasmic reticulum, i.e., the portion with attached polyribosomes, is decreased (4,5). Rothschild and colleagues have shown in the perfused liver that a 24 hour fast leads to disaggregation of polysomes bound to endoplasmic reticulum, together with a severe decrease in albumin synthesis (20). This process is reversed by tryptophan, lysine, arginine, ornithine and isoleucine. Exposure to ethanol in the perfusate also disaggregates bound polysomes and results in a low rate of albumin production. After exposure of the liver to ethanol in fed animals, the response to amino acids is similar to that in fasted animals not exposed to ethanol.

Mitochondria

The most dramatic injurious effect of chronic ethanol ingestion appears to be located in the mitochondria.

Chronic ethanol consumption in animals (21-24) and man (5,6) leads to fatty liver, in the absence of nutritional deficiencies. Several mechanisms have been suggested for the ethanol-induced steatosis, including decreased fatty acid oxidation by mitochondria (25). The lipids deposited in the liver after chronic ethanol intoxication are principally of dietary origin (26), suggesting reduced hepatic oxidation of fatty acids. Ethanol metabolism has been reported to decrease $^{14}CO_2$ production from labelled palmitate and acetate in liver slices (25), which points to decreased β-oxidation or reduced activity of the citric acid cycle (25) or both. The production of reducing equivalents by the oxidation of ethanol results in a lowering of the mitochondrial oxidation-reducing state, which causes reduction of oxalacetate to malate, thus decreasing activity of the citric acid cycle.

In contrast to acute ethanol intoxication, chronic ethanol ingestion is associated with striking ultrastructural changes in the mitochondria (2,27,28) and increased membrane fragility (29). In addition, oxygen consumption with a variety of substrates is impaired by chronic ethanol consumption (30). These findings suggested that chronically compromised integrity of the mitochondria, independent of the biochemical events associated with ethanol metabolism, might interfere with fatty acid oxidation. In this study we continued our investigations into the pathogenesis of fatty liver by determining the effect of chronic ethanol ingestion on the metabolism of fatty acids by isolated hepatic mitochondria.

Oxidation of ethanol by liver cells produces acetaldehyde, which is primarily oxidized within the mitochondria (31,32,33). Acetaldehyde is a toxic compound with numerous effects on mitochrondrial functions (34-36). We have reported that acetaldehyde inhibits the oxidation of NAD^+-dependent substrates (37). Thus, there are similarities between the effects of acetaldehyde and those of chronic ethanol feeding on mitochondrial functions (30,37,38). We, therefore, investigated the effects of acetaldehyde on fatty acid oxidation by isolated mitochondria to determine if this metabolite of ethanol oxidation may play a role in the ethanol-induced steatosis.

Preparations

Male Sprague-Dawley rats, weighing about 150 g, were fed for 24 days a nutritionally adequate liquid diet (19), in which carbohydrate provided 47% of total calories, protein 18%, and fat 35%. Pair-fed littermates consumed the same diet except that ethanol isocalorically replaced carbohydrate, accounting for 36% of total calories. The hepatic triglyceride content increased about 6-fold after ethanol feeding (19). For the experiments with acetaldehyde, rats maintained on a Purina Chow diet were used. Rat liver mitochondria were prepared in 0.25 M sucrose-0.01 M Tris-HC1, pH 7.4-0.001 M EDTA. In this report total oxidation of fatty acids refers to oxidation to CO_2 and H_2O, whereas β-oxidation refers to the classical Knoop oxidation pathway to the level of acetyl-CoA.

Oxygen consumption, CO_2 production with labelled fatty acids and citric acid cycle intermediates, ketone body production, oxidation of fatty acids in the presence of artificial electron acceptors and the activities of palmitoyl CoA synthetase and carnitine palmitoyltransferase were assayed as previously described (39-41).

Chronic ethanol consumption did not cause biochemical disruption of the mitochondrial membranes; mitochondria from ethanol-fed rats were impermeable to NADH and showed comparable ATPase activity as controls. Permeability to anions and susceptibility to anion inhibitors were not altered, and P:O or respiratory control ratios with succinate or ascorbate were similar to those found with pair-fed controls (30,42). Various inhibitors of mitochondrial functions (oligomycin, atractyloside, rotenone, cyanide, etc.) were as effective in mitochondria from ethanol-fed rats as in controls. The content of mitochondrial protein (milligrams per g wet weight) and the percentage yield of mitochondria were the same for mitochondria from ethanol-fed rats as controls (42).

Effect of Chronic Ethanol Consumption on Oxygen Uptake

In State 4, the rate of oxygen consumption associated with the oxidation of palmitoyl-1-carnitine, palmitoyl-CoA and palmitate was depressed 10 to 15% in mitochondria from ethanol-fed rats (Table II). The addition of ADP (State 3) increased the rate of oxygen consumption with all substrates. However, in mitochondria from ethanol-fed rats, the oxidation of fatty acids in State 3 was about 30% less than controls (Table II). The oxidation of other fatty acids of different chain length and extent of saturation (oleate, octanoate, linoleate and myristate) was also depressed after ethanol treatment. The reduction in palmitate or oleate oxidation after ethanol feeding was also found in the absence of carnitine or ATP and in the presence of 0.1 mM CoASH. The addition in vitro of up to 100 mM ethanol to mitochondria from chow-fed control rats had no effect on fatty acid oxidation. In view of the greater reduction in ADP-stimulated oxygen uptake (State 3) after ethanol feeding, compared to that in State 4, the respiratory control ratio was depressed in mitochondria from ethanol-fed animals oxidizing fatty acids as substrates (Table II). This reduction (18 to 23%) was somewhat less than that previously observed with α-ketoglutarate, glutamate or β-hydroxybutyrate (about 30%), but more than that observed with succinate (9%). This intermediate value for the decrease in the respiratory control ratio with fatty acids as substrates (between that of NAD^+-dependent substrates and flavin-linked substrates) may reflect the fact that reducing equivalents from the β-oxidation of fatty acids enter the respiratory chain both at the level of NADH-dehydrogenase and at the cytochrome b-ubiquinone level (via the electron transfer flavoprotein).

Effect of Chronic Ethanol Consumption on CO_2 Production from Fatty Acids and Citric Acid Cycle Intermediates

To confirm the oxygen uptake data, we studied the effect of ethanol feeding on CO_2 production from ^{14}C-labelled palmitate and octanoate. As shown in Table III, CO_2 production from palmitate was reduced 37% in mitochondria from ethanol-fed rats, a value comparable to the 32% decrease in State 3 oxygen consumption. CO_2 production from octanoate was reduced 20% by ethanol feeding, similar to the 17% decrease in State 3

TABLE II

EFFECT OF CHRONIC ETHANOL CONSUMPTION ON OXYGEN UPTAKE
ASSOCIATED WITH FATTY ACIDS AS SUBSTRATES

Substrate	Reaction	Activity		Effect %	p
		Control	Ethanol		
Palmitoyl-l-carnitine	State 4-oxygen uptake	20.93±1.40	18.0 ±1.46	-14	<0.05
	State 3-oxygen uptake	75.80±5.40	54.2 ±4.7	-29	<0.01
	Respiratory control	3.84±0.41	3.01±0.27	-22	<0.01
Palmitoyl-CoA	State 4	19.6 ±1.6	16.46±2.10	-16	<0.01
	State 3	76.83±1.8	52.0 ±6.80	-32	<0.01
	Respiratory Control	3.99±0.37	3.17±0.24	-21	<0.02
Palmitate	State 4	29.65±2.30	25.50±3.10	-14	<0.02
	State 3	81.50±5.70	55.2 ±6.0	-32	<0.01
	Respiratory Control	2.75±0.22	2.09±0.14	-24	<0.05

Activity refers to natoms oxygen consumed per min per mg mitochondrial protein. Respiratory control is the state 3 (+ ADP) rate of respiration divided by the rate in state 4 (– ADP).

TABLE III

EFFECT OF CHRONIC ETHANOL CONSUMPTION ON CO_2 PRODUCTION
FROM FATTY ACIDS AND CITRIC ACID CYCLE INTERMEDIATES

Substrate	Activity		Effect	p
	Control	Ethanol		
	(nmoles/min/mg protein)		(%)	
A. Palmitate-1-^{14}C	1.63±0.37	1.03±0.28	-37	<0.001
Octanoate-1-^{14}C	1.65±0.34	1.32±0.25	-20	<0.01
Acetate-1-^{14}C	15.3 ±1.2	12.4 ±1.4	-19	<0.01
Citrate-6- ^{14}C	13.7 ±1.4	10.7 ±1.3	-22	<0.05
α-Ketoglutarate-1-^{14}C	17.1 ±1.7	13.8 ±1.7	-19	<0.05
Succinate-1,4-^{14}C	14.6 ±2.6	12.1 ±3.1	-17	0.10>p>0.05
B. Citrate-6-^{14}C	9.6 ±1.1	7.1 ±1.0	-26	
Citrate-6-^{14}C plus 1 mM malate	12.7 ±1.7	9.6 ±0.9	-24	
Citrate-6-^{14}C plus 3.3 mM malate	11.8 ±1.2	8.1 ±1.1	-31	
α-Ketoglutarate-1-^{14}C	11.6 ±1.0	8.5 ±2.3	-27	
α-Ketoglutarate-1-^{14}C plus 1 mM malate	16.2 ±13.4	12.1 ±2.8	-25	
α-Ketoglutarate-1-^{14}C plus 3.3 mM malate	14.7 ±2.1	12.0 2.5	-18	

oxygen consumption. The decrease in CO_2 production from fatty acids may reflect impairment of the activity of the citric acid cycle by chronic consumption of ethanol, or impairment of the β-oxidation of fatty acids to the level of acetyl CoASH. Therefore the effects of ethanol feeding on CO_2 production from several citric acid cycle intermediates were tested.

CO_2, liberated in the isocitric dehydrogenase step of the citric acid cycle, is derived from the 6-C of citric acid, whereas CO_2 liberated in the α-ketoglutarate dehydrogenase reaction is derived from the 1-C of α-ketoglutarate (43). Therefore CO_2 production from citrate-6-^{14}C is a measure of the span citrate to isocitrate to α-ketoglutarate while CO_2 production from α-ketoglutarate-1-^{14}C or glutamate-1-^{14}C measures the span α-ketoglutarate to succinyl CoA (44). The use of succinate-1,4-^{14}C, or uniformly-labelled malate, coupled with the information derived from experiments with citrate-6-^{14}C and α-ketoglutarate-1-^{14}C, provides information concerning the spans succinate to citrate, or malate to citrate, respectively. The use of acetate-1-^{14}C allows assay of the complete citric acid cycle, since neither of the CO_2 molecules produced is derived from the acetate on the first turn of the cycle (43). Upon subsequent revolutions, labelled acetyl carbon is eliminated as radioactive CO_2. CO_2 production associated with the oxidation of acetate, citrate, α-ketoglutarate and succinate was depressed 20% in mitochondria from ethanol-fed rats (Table III). It has been established that with substrate-depleted mitochondria, the presence of malate is required for entry of exogenous α-ketoglutarate or citrate into mitochondria (45,46). Although substrate-depleted mitochondria were not used, it is possible that penetration of citrate or α-ketoglutarate into the mitochondria may have been rate-limiting under these experimental conditions. Therefore CO_2 production from citrate and α-ketoglutarate was assayed in the presence and absence of malate. The addition of malate increased the rate of CO_2 production from both citrate and α-ketoglutarate with both mitochondrial preparations. Under all conditions, CO_2 production from citrate and α-ketoglutarate was depressed in mitochondria from ethanol-fed rats (Table III).

Effect of Chronic Ethanol Consumption on Palmitoyl-CoA Synthetase and Carnitine Palmitoyltransferase

Factors which might play a role in the inhibition of fatty acids include the fatty acid synthetase of the outer membrane, which activates long chain fatty acids (47,48), and carnitine palmitoyltransferase, which transports long chain fatty acids into the mitochondria (49,50). We, therefore, investigated the effects of chronic ethanol feeding on the activities of these two enzymes. Palmitoyl-CoA synthetase activity was not affected by ethanol feeding (specific activity (micromoles of hydroxamate formed per hour per mg of protein) of 3.7 ± 0.4 for control mitochondria and 3.5 ± 0.5 for mitochondria from ethanol-fed rats). By contrast carnitine palmitoyl-transferase activity was stimulated 30% (specific activity (nanomoles of CoA released per min per mg of protein) of 27 ± 1.4 for control mitochondria and 35 ± 4 for mitochondria from ethanol-fed rats, $p < 0.05$). Thus, the depression of total fatty acid oxidation by ethanol feeding cannot be explained by an effect on the activities of these enzymes.

Effect of Chronic Ethanol Consumption on Ketogenesis

It seemed possible that chronic ethanol consumption might favor a flow of acetyl-CoA, derived from β-oxidation, into ketogenesis rather than to total oxidation to CO_2. Such a shift would cause CO_2 production and O_2 uptake to be reduced, but β-oxidation of fatty acids would not necessarily be depressed. We therefore investigated the effects of chronic ethanol feeding on ketone body production by hepatic mitochondria. Ethanol feeding had no effect on the endogenous rate of ketone body production (40.88 ± 5.4 nmol of β-hydroxybutyrate and acetoacetate formed per 30 min per mg of protein for control mitochondria and 42.5 ± 3.5 for mitochondria from ethanol-fed rats). The addition of palmitoyl-1-carnitine or palmitate increased ketone body production about 4-fold. There was a slight increase in ketone body production in mitochondria from ethanol-fed rats (+9 to +15%), but this did not reach statistical significance. Similar results were obtained with lower concentrations of fatty acids, e.g. with 30 μM palmitoyl-1-carnitine, there was an 11% increase in ketogenesis after ethanol feeding.

Pande (51) has suggested that ketone body production in liver may be enhanced by the suppression of the citric acid cycle. We therefore investigated ketogenesis after inhibiting the activity of the citric acid cycle with fluorocitrate. With labelled palmitate and octanoate, 25 μM fluoro-citrate inhibited CO_2 production 70 to 80% in mitochondria from ethanol-fed rats and 80 to 90% in controls. In the presence of fluorocitrate, there was no difference in the endogenous rate of ketone body production between control mitochondria and those from ethanol-fed rats (Fig. 1). However, compared to the rates in the absence of fluorocitrate, this endogenous rate

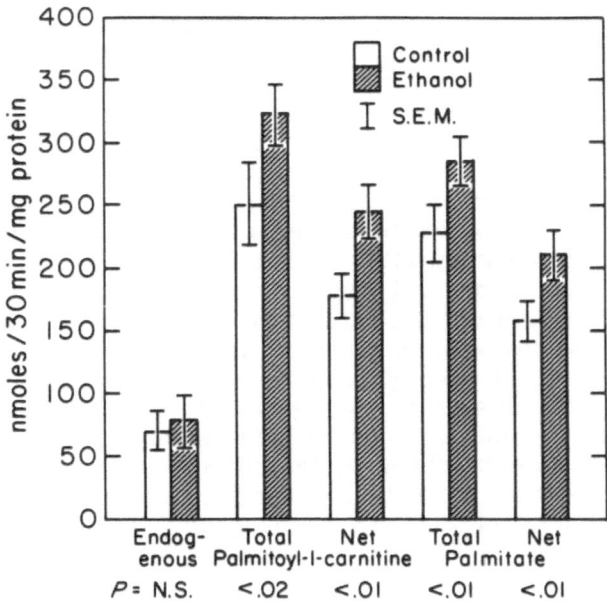

Fig. 1   *Effect of chronic ethanol consumption on ketone body production in the presence of fluorocitrate.*
The endogenous rate refers to the rate in the absence of added fatty acid. The net rate is the total rate minus the endogenous rate.

increased 70% in control mitochondria and 79% in those from animals given ethanol, suggesting diversion of acetyl-CoA into ketogenesis, a more accessible pathway.   Upon adding palmitoyl-l-carnitine or palmitate, ketogenesis was increased about 3-fold in control mitochondria, and about 4-fold in mitochondria from ethanol-fed rats (Fig. 1).   The total rates of ketogenesis were greater in the presence of fluorocitrate than in its absence, with both mitochondrial preparations. Both the total and net rates of ketone body production were greater in mitochondria from ethanol-fed rats than controls, with either substrate.   Thus, in the presence of fluorocitrate, ketogenesis was stimulated after ethanol feeding. This may explain, in part, the increase of serum ketone bodies which occurs after chronic ethanol feeding (52). The increase in ketone body production after ethanol ingestion may be due to increased activities of enzymes which participate in the formation of ketones or increased formation of acetyl-CoA via β-oxidation (or both). The increase in ketone body production (and formazan formation, see below) suggests that ethanol feeding does not impair β-oxidation of fatty acids to the level of acetyl-CoA.

Oxidation of Fatty Acids in Presence of Artificial Electron Acceptors

The ethanol-induced decrease in fatty acid oxidation under State 4 conditions or in the presence of an uncoupler points to some impairment of the respiratory chain.   The additional reduction in ADP-stimulated fatty acid oxidation suggests impairment of coupled phosphorylation (30). Others have suggested that ADP entry into the mitochondria may be compromised (53). To verify the results described above, and to eliminate the influence of changes in the respiratory chain, we studied fatty acid oxidation under anaerobic conditions with the use of artificial electron acceptors to reoxidize NADH. Mitochondria isolated from rats fed ethanol for 24 days displayed a slightly higher rate of endogenous formazan production than their pair-fed controls (Table IV). Upon the addition of palmitate the total rate, as well as the net rate of formazan production, was higher in mitochondria from ethanol-fed rats. Comparable results were obtained in mitochondria from two pairs of rats, with the use of octanoate or oleate as substrates. By contrast, there were no changes in formazan production after acute administration of ethanol (6 g/kg; 34.65 nmol of formazan/hour/mg for controls oxidizing palmitate, 34.98 for acute ethanol). Thus, in the absence of a functional respiratory chain, mitochondria from ethanol-fed rats show a higher rate of formazan production, either because of increased β-oxidation, or increased activity of the citric acid cycle.   To dissociate these two possibilities, we studied formazan production in the presence of fluoro-citrate, which inhibits the metabolism of two carbon fragments via the citric acid cycle.   Under anaerobic conditions in the presence of fluoro-citrate, formazan production upon the addition of palmitate presumably is a measure of β-oxidation. Fluorocitrate depressed the endogenous rate in the controls by 41%, but only by 23% in mitochondria from ethanol-fed rats (Table IV).   With palmitate as the substrate, the total rate of formazan production was increased 39% by ethanol ingestion, compared to pair-fed controls.   The net rate was also 28% greater in mitochondria from ethanol-

TABLE   IV

EFFECT OF CHRONIC ETHANOL CONSUMPTION ON FORMAZAN
PRODUCTION IN PRESENCE AND ABSENCE OF FLUOROCITRATE

Fluorocitrate	Addition	Formazan Production		Effect	p
		Control	Ethanol		
		(nmol/hr/mg protein)		(%)	
-(12)	None	24.42 ± 3.3	29.70 ± 4.62	+21	<0.05
	Palmitate	45.21 ± 5.94	54.12 ± 5.94	+20	<0.05
	(Net)	20.79 ± 3.63	24.42 ± 3.30	+17	<0.05
+ (3)	None	14.52 ± 3.63	22.77 ± 4.29	+57	
	Palmitate	35.31 ± 3.96	49.17 ± 5.61	+39	
	(Net)	20.78 ± 3.63	26.74 ± 4.29	+28	

treated animals (Table IV).   Therefore, β-oxidation does not appear to be
decreased by chronic ethanol feeding, since formazan production and
ketogenesis were actually increased by ethanol feeding.

Effect of Chronic Ethanol Consumption on Oxygen Consumption with other Substrates

β-oxidation of fatty acids to the level of acetyl CoASH is not impaired
by chronic ethanol consumption, whereas oxygen uptake and CO_2 production
are depressed. This impairment may involve, in part, inhibitory effects on
the activity of the citric acid cycle (Table II), but may also reflect
impairment of the activity of the mitochondrial respiratory chain. Indeed
the decrease in CO_2 production from the citric acid cycle intermediates
may be due to effects on the respiratory chain. Consequently oxygen uptake
with substrates supplying electrons to different segments of the respiratory
chain was studied. Under state 4 conditions, mitochondria from ethanol-fed
rats showed a 10 to 20% decrease in oxygen consumption associated with the
oxidation of NAD^+-dependent substrates, succinate and ascorbate (Table V).
In the presence of ADP (state 3) oxygen uptake associated with the oxidation
of NAD^+-dependent substrates was depressed 30 to 40% in mitochondria
from ethanol-fed rats (Table V). The impairment of oxygen uptake with
these substrates may reflect decreased activity of enzymatic components of
the respiratory chain or decreased content of respiratory components.
Indeed the activities of cytochrome oxidase and succinic dehydrogenase (42)
as well as the contents of cytochromes b, a, and a_3 (28) were decreased in
mitochondria from ethanol-fed rats.

TABLE V

EFFECT OF CHRONIC ETHANOL CONSUMPTION ON OXYGEN UPTAKE

| | State 4 Oxygen Uptake | | Effect | p | State 3 Oxygen Uptake | | Effect | p |
	Control	Ethanol	(%)		Control	Ethanol	(%)	
	(natoms O_2/min/mg protein)				(natoms O_2/min/mg/protein)			
Glutamate (9)	23.03±2.34	19.20±1.93	-17	<0.01	73.1 ± 7.8	46.3 ± 4.66	-37	<0.001
α-Ketoglutarate (8)	17.10±1.20	15.29 ±1.12	-11	<0.05	64.5 ± 3.71	45.1 ± 4.56	-30	<0.01
β-Hydroxybutyrate (6)	17.80±2.54	15.70±1.90	-12	<0.05	61.2 ± 8.3	38.3 ± 7.9	-38	<0.01
Succinate (9)	26.55±2.37	22.58±2.37	-15	<0.05	87.53±4.1	69.15±3.8	-21	<0.01
Ascorbate (9)	65.62±8.92	52.76±7.17	-20	<0.01	102.3±13.7	85.5±12.1	-17	<0.01

TABLE VI

EFFECT OF ACETALDEHYDE ON OXYGEN CONSUMPTION ASSOCIATED WITH THE OXIDATION OF PALMITOYL-1-CARNITINE AND PALMITOYL-CoA

Substrate	Concn. of Acetaldehyde (mM)	Oxygen Consumption		Percentage Change		Respiratory Control Ratio	Percentage Change
		State 4	State 3	State 4	State 3		
		(natoms oxygen/min/mg protein)		(%)			(%)
Palmitoyl-1-carnitine	---	15.1	69.8	---	---	4.62	---
	0.6	15.4	62.3	+2	-11	4.05	-12
	1.0	14.1	55.8	-6	-20	3.96	-14
	2.0	14.4	49.5	-5	-29	3.44	-26
	3.0	12.9	42.3	-14	-39	3.28	-29
	12.0	11.5	24.5	-24	-65	2.13	-52
Palmitoyl-CoA	---	17.9	63.0	---	---	3.52	---
	0.6	16.1	56.0	-10	-11	3.47	-2
	1.0	17.5	54.0	-2	-14	3.09	-12
	2.0	16.5	44.5	-8	-29	2.70	-23
	3.0	16.2	42.5	-9	-33	2.61	-26
	12.0	11.0	27.0	-38	-57	2.45	-30

Effect of Acetaldehyde on Oxygen Uptake

Acetaldehyde, at concentrations up to 3 mM, had little effect on state 4 oxidation of palmitoyl-l-carnitine or palmitoyl-CoA; inhibition was observed at higher concentrations (12 mM). By contrast, state 3 oxygen consumption was inhibited at concentrations of acetaldehyde which had little effect on state 4 oxygen uptake (Table VI). The extent of inhibition of fatty acid oxidation observed here is similar to that of NAD^+-dependent substrate oxidation (α-ketoglutarate, glutamate, β-hydroxybutyrate) observed previously (compare Table I, Ref. 37). On the other hand, the state 3 oxidation of a flavin-linked substrate (succinate) or ascorbate, which reduces cytochrome c, was not affected by 1-3 mM acetaldehyde (37).

The greater sensitivity of coupled (state 3) than resting (state 4) respiration to inhibition by acetaldehyde is evidenced by the decrease in the respiratory control ratio associated with the oxidation of palmitoyl-l-carnitine and palmitoyl CoA (Table VI). Acetaldehyde also decreased oxygen uptake in the presence of dinitrophenol. The state 3 rate of oxidation of the albumin-bound free fatty acids, palmitate and oleate, was inhibited by acetaldehyde to a similar extent as the activated fatty acids (Table VI).

Effect of Acetaldehyde on CO_2 Production from Fatty Acids

Since acetaldehyde is itself metabolized and gives rise to oxygen consumption, we studied the effects of acetaldehyde on CO_2 production from labelled palmitate and octanoate. Acetaldehyde is oxidized to acetate by the mitochondrial aldehyde dehydrogenase (32,33). The activation of acetate to acetyl CoA, with subsequent oxidation to CO_2, would be expected to cause a dilution of labelled CO_2 produced from the β-oxidation of labelled fatty acids. Formation of $^{14}CO_2$ produced from $\{1-^{14}C-\}$ palmitate and $\{1-^{14}C-\}$ octanoate was strikingly reduced by acetaldehyde (Fig. 2). Dilution effects may account for part of the inhibition, since labelled CO_2 production was more sensitive to inhibition by acetaldehyde than was oxygen consumption. For example, 1 mM acetaldehyde inhibited oxygen uptake 20% whereas labelled CO_2 production was depressed about 50%. However, dilution effects cannot explain all the effects of acetaldehyde on fatty acid oxidation because total oxygen consumption was depressed in the presence of acetaldehyde. In addition, comparable concentrations of acetate caused less depression of labelled CO_2 formation than did acetaldehyde (Fig. 3). In fact CO_2 production from labelled octanoate is relatively insensitive to dilution by acetate (Fig. 3). Therefore, factors other than dilution itself participate in the inhibition of CO_2 production by acetaldehyde.

Acetaldehyde, in concentrations as high as 12 mM did not affect the activity of enzymes involved in activating and translocating fatty acids into the mitochondria, i.e., palmitoyl CoA synthetase and carnitine palmitoyl-transferase activities.

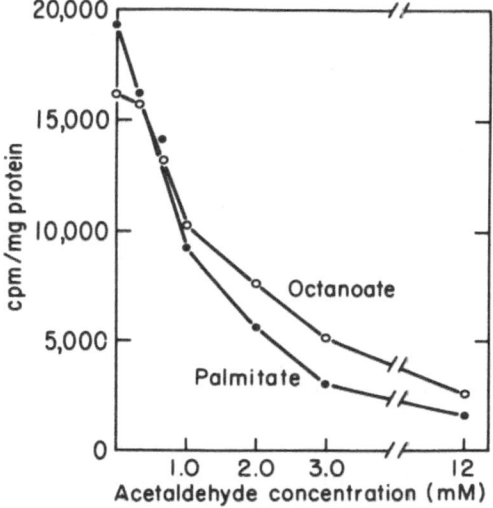

Fig. 2   Effect of acetaldehyde on $^{14}CO_2$ production from 1-^{14}C-palmitate and 1-^{14}C-octanoate.

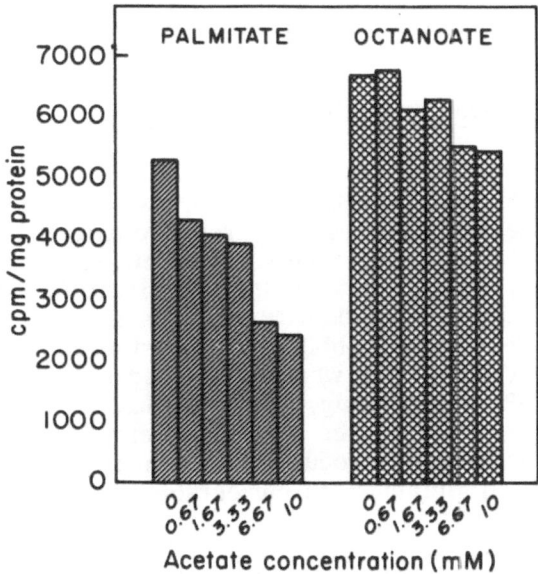

Fig. 3   Effect of acetate on $^{14}CO_2$ production from 1-^{14}C-palmitate and 1-^{14}C-octanoate.

Effect of Acetaldehyde on Ketone Body Formation

It seemed possible that acetaldehyde might cause a shift of acetyl CoA to ketogenesis rather than to total oxidation to CO_2. Such a redistribution of acetyl CoA was suggested to explain the inhibition of palmitate oxidation to CO_2 by acetate (39). If this were so, CO_2 production and O_2 uptake would be inhibited, but β-oxidation of fatty acids might not be depressed. We, therefore, investigated the effects of acetaldehyde on ketogenesis. In the absence of palmitoyl-l-carnitine, acetaldehyde slightly stimulated the endogenous rate of ketone body production (Table VII). This may reflect the participation of acetyl CoA derived from the oxidation of acetaldehyde in ketogenesis, an explanation in keeping with the report of Grunnet (33) that half of the acetate formed from acetaldehyde is incorporated into ketone bodies. Acetate did not affect endogenous ketogenesis (39), suggesting that the slight activation of ketogenesis by acetaldehyde may involve the step which converts acetaldehyde to acetate, a process which forms NADH. The lowering of the redox state by the oxidation of acetaldehyde inhibits the activity of the citric acid cycle; therefore, acetyl CoA is diverted to ketogenesis. This is supported by the observation that the endogenous content of acetoacetate is slightly reduced, whereas the β-hydroxybutyrate-acetoacetate ratio is increased, suggesting an acetaldehyde-induced lowering of the mitochondrial redox state. The addition of palmitoyl-l-carnitine increased ketone body production 3-fold (Table VII). Acetaldehyde decreased ketone body production from palmitoyl-l-carnitine. Whereas 0.6-3 mM acetaldehyde had little effect on β-hydroxybutyrate formation, the formation of acetoacetate was decreased, a finding which probably reflects the production of NADH during acetaldehyde oxidation.

Effect of Acetaldehyde on CO_2 Production from Citric Acid Cycle Intermediates

The oxidation of acetate to CO_2 was depressed by acetaldehyde (Table VIII). This may reflect dilution resulting from the oxidation of acetaldehyde to acetate, as well as possible effects on the citric acid cycle and/or the respiratory-phosphorylation chain. Palmitate oxidation to CO_2 was more sensitive to inhibition by acetaldehyde than was acetate oxidation to CO_2 e.g., 1 and 3 mM acetaldehyde inhibited labelled acetate oxidation 34 and 58%, respectively (Table VIII), whereas labelled palmitate oxidation was inhibited 52 and 73%, respectively (Fig. 2). Thus, acetaldehyde may have additional inhibitory effects on the β-oxidation of palmitate to acetyl CoA. Acetaldehyde depressed CO_2 production associated with the oxidation of malate, succinate and glutamate to comparable extents (Table VIII). CO_2 production from citrate-6-^{14}C was not affected by 0.6 or 1.25 mM acetaldehyde; inhibition was observed only at the higher level of 3 mM, and the extent of inhibition was less than that observed with the other citric acid cycle intermediates. However the addition of malate increased CO_2 production from citrate (Table VIII), probably by promoting increased transport of citrate into the mitochondria. In the presence of malate, acetaldehyde decreased CO_2 production from citrate to almost the same

TABLE VII

EFFECT OF ACETALDEHYDE ON KETONE BODY FORMATION [a]

Palmitoyl-1-Carnitine Concn.	Concn. of Acetaldehyde	Ketone Body Formation				Percentage Change	
		β-Hydroxy-butyrate	Aceto-Acetate	Total	Net	Total	Net
(mM)	(mM)					(%)	
0	--	8.1	42.8	50.9	--	--	--
	0.6	9.5	41.2	50.7	--	0	--
	1.0	14.2	41.4	55.6	--	+9	--
	2.0	22.0	40.0	62.0	--	+22	--
	3.0	20.0	36.0	56.0	--	+10	--
	12.0	21.0	35.5	56.5	--	+11	--
0.1	--	69.8	70.2	140.0	89.1	--	--
	0.6	73.7	57.6	131.3	80.6	-6	-10
	1.0	75.0	47.2	122.2	66.6	-13	-25
	2.0	66.9	46.2	113.1	51.1	-19	-43
	3.0	69.2	42.2	111.4	55.4	-20	-38
	12.0	31.5	41.2	72.7	16.2	-48	-82

[a]The endogenous rate refers to the rate in the absence of palmitoyl-l-carnitine. The net rate refers to the total rate minus the endogenous rate.

TABLE VIII

EFFECT OF ACETALDEHYDE ON $^{14}CO_2$ PRODUCTION
FROM CITRIC ACID CYCLE INTERMEDIATES

Substrate	Concn. of Acetaldehyde	Activity	Effect	p
	(mM)	(nmoles/min/mg)	(%)	
{u-^{14}C} Malate	---	11.89 ± 1.02	---	---
	0.6	9.35 ± 0.55	-21	< 0.05
	1.25	8.06 ± 0.58	-32	< 0.01
	3.0	5.46 ± 0.71	-54	< 0.001
{1,4-^{14}C} Succinate	---	14.74 ± 1.71	---	---
	0.6	11.29 ± 2.13	-23	N.S.
	1.25	9.49 ± 1.99	-36	< 0.05
	3.0	6.86 ± 1.55	-53	< 0.02
{1-^{14}C} Glutamate	---	17.87 ± 2.42	---	---
	0.6	13.63 ± 2.15	-24	N.S.
	1.25	11.79 ± 1.96	-34	< 0.02
	3.0	5.89 ± 2.16	-67	< 0.01
{1-^{14}C} Glutamate plus malate	---	21.56 ± 2.02	---	---
	0.6	17.92 ± 2.45	-17	N.S.
	1.25	13.40 ± 2.26	-38	< 0.02
	3.0	9.09 ± 2.46	-58	< 0.002
{6-^{14}C} Citrate	---	18.71 ± 1.45	---	---
	0.6	17.40 ± 1.20	- 7	N.S.
	1.25	16.18 ± 1.60	-14	N.S.
	3.0	12.72 ± 1.02	-32	< 0.02
{6-^{14}C} Citrate plus malate	---	24.03 ± 3.46	---	---
	0.6	21.86 ± 2.87	- 9	N.S.
	1.25	18.51 ± 2.80	-23	0.10>p>0.05
	3.0	10.66 ± 4.99	-56	< 0.05
{1-^{14}C} Acetate	---	16.19	---	
	0.6	11.86	-27	
	1.0	10.69	-34	
	3.0	6.79	-58	

extent as it decreased CO_2 production from the other substrates (Table VIII). Acetate (0.5 and 1.0 mM) had no effect on CO_2 production from any of these labelled substrates. At 3 mM acetate, some inhibition (dilution) of labelled CO_2 production was observed (10-15%). Thus acetaldehyde depressed CO_2 production from citric acid cycle intermediates at concentrations in which acetate had no effect, suggesting that the inhibition by acetaldehyde does not appear to be mediated by acetate.

Fatty acid oxidation by isolated hepatic mitochondria was depressed after chronic ethanol feeding, suggesting that persistent changes in mitochondrial functions, in addition to the effects produced by metabolism of ethanol, may play a role in the production of fatty liver. The decreases in oxygen uptake and CO_2 production from fatty acids do not by themselves prove that fatty acid utilization is impaired, because acetyl-CoA derived from β-oxidation may be diverted to other pathways, e.g. ketogenesis or fatty acid elongation, rather than to oxidation via the citric acid cycle. We, therefore, examined some of the factors which may participate in the depression of fatty acid oxidation after ethanol feeding, including activation and translocation of fatty acids, β-oxidation, ketone body production, and the activities of the citric acid cycle and the respiratory phosphorylating system. Chronic ethanol consumption did not inhibit the enzymes responsible for activating or transporting fatty acids into the mitochondria. Ethanol feeding induced a slight increase in ketone body production and formazan formation, which was augmented considerably in the presence of fluorocitrate. These data suggest that mitochondrial β-oxidation to the level of acetyl-CoA is increased, rather than decreased by chronic ethanol ingestion. This is consistent with the increased blood levels of ketone bodies and increased acetoacetate formation by liver slices from rats chronically fed ethanol (52). In view of the fact that formazan production and ketogenesis are increased rather than decreased in mitochondria from ethanol-fed rats, the decrease in CO_2 production from fatty acids may be caused either by depression of citric acid cycle activity or by impaired mitochondrial respiratory chain. The decreased rate of fatty acid oxidation cannot be attributed to the presence of ethanol in the tissue, since the washing procedures would have removed any contaminated ethanol. Furthermore, addition of ethanol in vitro had no effect on fatty acid oxidation. The addition of ATP, CoA, or NAD^+ did not prevent the reduction in fatty acid oxidation after ethanol feeding suggesting that nucleotide or cofactor depletion is not a factor.

The fact that formazan production and ketogenesis are stimulated, but total oxidation of fatty acids is depressed, suggests that acetyl-CoA is diverted from the citric acid cycle to other pathways, e.g. ketogenesis. The decrease in CO_2 production from labelled palmitate or octanoate suggests the possibility of an inhibitory effect of chronic ethanol feeding on the activity of the citric cycle. CO_2 production from several labelled intermediates of the citric acid cycle was depressed after chronic consumption of ethanol. The well-known inhibitory effects of ethanol on the activity of the citric acid cycle in studies with perfused livers (54) and isolated hepatocytes (44) are presumably due to the metabolism of ethanol, which lowers the mitochondrial redox state. However, similar effects of CO_2 production from citric acid cycle intermediates in the absence of ethanol metabolism can be produced by persistent damage to the mitochondria. Since oxygen uptake with all substrates was depressed after chronic ethanol consumption, it is probable that impairment of the respiratory chain after chronic ethanol consumption is responsible, at least in part, for the decrease in CO_2 production by mitochondria from ethanol-fed rats. Impairment of the activities of the respiratory chain in the citric acid cycle, or both, may contribute to the impairment of fatty acid oxidation found in mitochondria from ethanol-fed rats.

Acetaldehyde (0.6 to 3.0 mM) inhibited the oxidation of fatty acids by rat liver mitochondria, as assayed by oxygen consumption and CO_2 production. The mechanism behind the inhibition of fatty acid oxidation by acetaldehyde apparently does not involve activation of palmitate to palmitoyl CoA or transfer of palmitate into the mitochondria as the carnitine ester. Acetaldehyde, in concentrations which inhibited fatty acid oxidation, had no effect on the activities of palmitoyl CoA synthetase or carnitine palmitoyltransferase. Moreover, acetaldehyde inhibited octanoate oxidation; octanoate is activated in the mitochondria and does not require carnitine for transport into the mitochondria (47). The fact that ketogenesis and CO_2 production are both depressed suggests that acetaldehyde does not shift the end products of fatty acid oxidation from the citric acid cycle into ketogenesis. Since acetaldehyde inhibits CO_2 production from palmitate to a greater extent than that from acetate, an acetaldehyde-sensitive site may be in the β-oxidation pathway.

The decrease in CO_2 production from fatty acids also points to an inhibitory effect on the citric acid cycle. Acetaldehyde decreases CO_2 production from citric acid cycle intermediates at concentrations in which acetate has no effect, a finding which suggests that the inhibition by acetaldehyde is direct, and not due to acetate. NADH production in the oxidation of acetaldehyde by mitochondrial aldehyde dehydrogenase might be involved in the inhibition of CO_2 production from malate and succinate by acetaldehyde; oxalacetate could be reduced to malate in the presence of NADH, thereby decreasing the rate of the citrate synthase reaction (55). In addition, the activity of α-ketoglutarate dehydrogenase has been reported to be inhibited by NADH (56), and isocitric dehydrogenase is a regulatory enzyme which is inhibited by NADH (57). However, NADH produced from the oxidation of acetaldehyde cannot be entirely responsible for the inhibition of CO_2 production by acetaldehyde. Acetaldehyde is oxidized by a mitochondrial enzyme with a very high affinity for acetaldehyde (Km less than $10\,\mu M$, (33,58-60). An increase in the concentration of acetaldehyde from 0.08 to 1.0 mM did not result in an increase in the rate of acetaldehyde oxidation by liver mitochondria (61). Therefore, the greater extent of inhibition of CO_2 production produced by 1.25 or 3 mM acetaldehyde, compared to that produced at 0.6 mM, cannot be due only to NADH generated during the metabolism of acetaldehyde. However, acetaldehyde inhibits the respiratory chain in a concentration-dependent manner, thereby reducing the regeneration of NAD^+. Pande (51) has suggested that fatty acid oxidation in liver mitochondria is limited by the capacity of the electron transport–oxidative phosphorylation system. Acetaldehyde inhibits NAD^+-dependent state 3 oxygen consumption with fatty acids as the substrate. In view of the fact that acetaldehyde inhibits the state 3 oxidation of other NAD^+-dependent substrates (37), it is probable that effects on the respiratory-phosphorylation chain are also involved in the inhibition of fatty acid oxidation by acetaldehyde.

The major mechanisms mediating control of the citric acid cycle reactions may include allosteric control by adenine and pyridine nucleotides, control by the redox state, and control of the transport of intermediates across the mitochondrial membrane (for discussion see ref. 62,63). Feedback from the electron transport chain to the citric acid cycle is mediated by factors including the phosphorylation state of adenine and guanine nucleotides and the redox state of the pyridine nucleotides (62,63). It is therefore likely that the inhibition of CO_2 production from citric acid cycle intermediates by acetaldehyde represents several factors which interfere with the control of the citric acid cycle, including competition between acetaldehyde and the various substrates for NAD^+, relative feedback inhibition of citric acid cycle enzymes by NADH and inhibitory effects on the respiratory chain. Since the concentrations of acetaldehyde employed in this study (0.6 mM and greater) are higher than the maximum blood levels of acetaldehyde, the physiological significance and the role that acetaldehyde may play in the development of the ethanol-induced fatty liver must await further studies concerning the concentration of acetaldehyde in the liver cells after acute or chronic ethanol ingestion, or the effect of chronic exposure to lower concentrations of acetaldehyde (e.g. during chronic ethanol consumption) on fatty acid oxidation. In contrast to acetaldehyde, ethanol in vitro had no effect on fatty acid oxidation by isolated mitochondria. Concentrations of acetaldehyde which do inhibit fatty acid oxidation in vitro may be found in the blood after administration of ethanol with disulfiram(64), pargyline (65), or pyrogallol (66). There are several similarities in the effects of chronic ethanol feeding and acetaldehyde on mitochondrial fatty acid oxidation. Acetate (1 to 3 mM) also depressed oxygen uptake and CO_2 production from palmitate, whereas it stimulated ketogenesis from palmitoyl-1-carnitine (39). Thus it is possible that metabolites of ethanol oxidation, as well as persisting structural damage to the mitochondria, may account for the impairment of fatty acid oxidation in mitochondria from chronically intoxicated rats.

Plasma Membranes

The effect of chronic ethanol administration on the plasmalemma of the hepatocyte is not well understood. Electron microscopically, occasional blebs are noted (4,5), and the serum levels of GOT almost invariably increase (5). Phospholipid transfer to other cytoplasmic organelles appears to be decreased (67). There is some controversy regarding the effect on ($Na^+ + K^+$)- activated ATPase. Whereas Israel's group has reported almost a tripling of this enzyme activity (68), Gang et al (69) and Gordon (70), have not found a significant increase. Whether this is an effect of the diet or analytical techniques remains to be elucidated.

SUMMARY

Chronic ethanol administration leads to changes in many organelles of the hepatocyte. Adaptive changes occur in the smooth endoplasmic reticulum and the Golgi complex. Injury is noted in the rough endoplasmic reticulum and especially the mitochondria. The effects on the plasma membrane are not well understood.

ACKNOWLEDGEMENT

This work was supported in part by USPHS Grant AA 287.

REFERENCES

1.   CONNEY AH: Pharmacological implications of microsomal enzyme induction. Pharmacol Rev 19: 317-366, 1967

2.   ISERI OH, LIEBER CS, GOTTLIEB LS: The ultrastructure of fatty liver induced by prolonged ethanol ingestion. Am J Path 48: 535-555, 1966

3.   RUBIN E, LIEBER CS: Fatty liver, alcoholic hepatitis and cirrhosis produced by alcohol in primates. New Eng J Med 29: 128-135, 1974

4.   RUBIN E, LIEBER CS: Experimental hepatic injury in man: Ultrastructural changes. Fed Proc 26: 1458-1467, 1967

5.   RUBIN E, LIEBER CS: Alcohol-induced hepatic injury in non-alcoholic volunteers. New Eng J Med 278: 869-876, 1968

6.   MISRA PS, LEFEVRE A, ISHII H, RUBIN E, LIEBER CS: Increase of ethanol, meprobamate and pentobarbital metabolism after chronic ethanol administration in man and rat. Am J Med 51: 346-351, 1971

7.   RUBIN E, LIEBER CS: Alcohol, alcoholism and drugs. Science 172: 1097-1102, 1971

8.   LIEBER CS, DECARLI LM: Hepatic microsomal ethanol oxidizing system: In vitro characteristics and adaptive properties in vitro. J Biol Chem 245: 2505-2512, 1970

9.   LIEBER CS, DECARLI LM: The role of the hepatic microsomal ethanol oxidizing system for ethanol metabolism in vivo. J Pharmacol Exp Ther 181: 279-287, 1972

10. MEZEY E: Duration of the enhanced activity of the microsomal ethanol-oxidizing enzyme system and rate of ethanol degradation in ethanol-fed rats after withdrawal. Biochem Pharmacol 21: 137-142, 1972

11. MAHLEY RW, HAMILTON RL, LEQUIRE VS: Characterization of lipoprotein particles isolated from the Golgi apparatus of rat liver. J Lipid Res 10: 433-439, 1969

12. MOLLENHAUER HH, MORRE DJ, KOGUT C: Dietary modification of the stability of rat liver Golgi apparatus. Exp Molec Path Vol. II: 113-122, 1969

13. RUBIN E, POPPER H: The evolution of human cirrhosis as deduced from observations in experimental animals. Med 46: 163-183, 1967

14. LO CHAI-HO, MARCH JB: Biosynthesis of plasma lipoproteins. Incorporation of ^{14}C-glucosamine by cells and subcellular fractions of rat liver. J Biol Chem 245: 5001-5006, 1970

15. ACHACHTER H, INDERJIT J, HUDGIN RL, PINTERIC L: Intracellular localization of liver sugar nucleotide glycoprotein glycosyltransferases in a Golgi-rich fraction. J Biol Chem 245: 1090-1100, 1970

16. GANG H, LIEBER CS, RUBIN E: Ethanol increases glycosyl transferase activity in the hepatic Golgi apparatus. Nature 243: 123-125, 1973

17. FLEISCHER B, FLEISCHER S, OZAWA H: Isolation and characterization of Golgi membranes from bovine liver. J Cell Biol 43: 59-79, 1969

18. LEELAVATHI DE, ESTES LW, FEINGOLD DS, LOMBARDI B: Isolation of a Golgi-rich fraction from rat liver. Biochem Biophys Acta 211: 124-128, 1970

19. DECARLI LM, LIEBER CS: Fatty liver in rat after prolonged intake of ethanol with a nutritionally adequate new liquid diet. J Nutr 91: 331-336, 1967

20. ORATZ M, ROTHSCHILD MA: The influence of alcohol and altered nutrition on albumin synthesis. In Alcohol and Abnormal Protein Synthesis. M.A. Rothschild, M. Oratz and S.S. Schreiber (eds.). Pergamon Press, N.Y., 1974. pp 343

21. LIEBER CS, JONES DP, MENDELSON J, DECARLI LM: Fatty liver, hyperlipemia and hyperuricemia produced by prolonged alcohol consumption, despite adequate dietary intake. Trans Assoc Am Physicians 76: 289-300, 1963

22. LIEBER CS, JONES DP, DECARLI LM: Effect of prolonged ethanol intake. Production of fatty liver despite adequate diets. J Clin Invest 44: 1009-1021, 1965

23. LIEBER CS, DECARLI LM, GANG H, WALKER G, RUBIN E: Hepatic effects of long term ethanol consumption in primates. In Medical Primatology Vol III.   K.K. Goldsmith and J. Moor-Jankowski (eds.). Basel, Karger, 1972. pp 270-278

24. LIEBER CS, DECARLI LM: Quantitative relationship between amount of dietary fat and severity of alcoholic fatty liver. Am J Clin Nutr 23: 474-478, 1970

25. LIEBER CS, SCHMID R: The effect of ethanol on fatty acid metabolism; stimulation of hepatic fatty acid synthesis in vitro. J Clin Invest 40: 394-399, 1961

26. LIEBER CS, SPRITZ N, DECARLI LM: Role of dietary, adipose and endogenously synthesized fatty acids in the pathogenesis of the alcoholic fatty liver. J Clin Invest 45: 51-62, 1966

27. KIESSLING KH, TOBE V: Degeneration of liver mitochondria in rats after prolonged alcohol consumption. Exp Cell Res 33: 350-354, 1974

28. RUBIN E, BEATTIE DS, LIEBER CS: Effect of ethanol on the biogenesis of mitochondrial membranes and associated mito-chondrial functions. Lab Invest 23: 620-627, 1970

29. FRENCH SW: Fragility of liver mitochondria in ethanol-fed rats. Gastroenterol 54: 1106-1114, 1968

30. CEDERBAUM AI, LIEBER CS, RUBIN E: Effect of chronic ethanol treatment on mitochondrial functions: Damage to coupling site I. Arch Biochem Biophys 165: 560-569, 1974

31. HEDLUND SG, KIESSLING KG: The physiological mechanism involved in hangover. The oxidation of some lower aliphatic fusel alcohols and aldehydes in rat liver and their effect in the mitochondrial oxidation of various substrates. Acta Pharmacol et Toxicol 27: 381-396, 1969

32. MARJANEN L: Intracellular localization of aldehyde dehydrogenase in rat liver. Biochem J 127: 633-639, 1972

33. GRUNNET N: Oxidation of acetaldehyde by rat liver mitochondria in relation to ethanol oxidation and the transport of reducing equivalents acros the mitochondrial membrane. Eur J Biochem 35: 236-243, 1973

34.   KIESSLING KH: The effect of acetaldehyde on mitochondrial respiration. Exp Cell Res 30: 569-576, 1963

35.   LINDROS KO: Role of the redox state in ethanol-induced suppression of citrate cycle flux in the perfused liver of normal, hyper- and hypo-thyroid rats. Eur J Biochem 26: 338-346, 1972

36.   YEH Z, BYINGTON KH: Interactions of acetaldehyde, ethyl alcohol and oxybarbiturates affecting mitochondrial functions. Biochem Pharmacol 22: 2045-2057, 1973

37.   CEDERBAUM AI, LIEBER CS, RUBIN E: The effect of acetaldehyde on mitochondrial function. Arch Biochem Biophys 161: 26-39, 1974

38.   CEDERBAUM AI, LIEBER CS, RUBIN E: Effect of chronic ethanol consumption and acetaldehyde on partial reactions of oxidative phosphorylation and CO_2 production from citric acid cycle intermediates. Arch Biochem Biophys: In press, 1976

39.   CEDERBAUM AI, RUBIN E: Differential effects of acetate on palmitate and octanoate oxidation: Segregation of acetyl CoA pools. Arch Biochem Biophys 166: 618-628, 1975

40.   CEDERBAUM AI, LIEBER CS, RUBIN E: Effect of acetaldehyde on fatty acid oxidation and ketogenesis by hepatic mitochondria. Arch Biochem Biophys 169: 29-41, 1975

41.   CEDERBAUM AI, LIEBER CS, BEATTIE DS, RUBIN E: Effect of chronic ethanol ingestion on fatty acid oxidation by hepatic mitochondria. J Biol Chem 250: 5122-5129, 1975

42.   CEDERBAUM AI, LIEBER CS, TOTH A, BEATTIE DS, RUBIN E: Effects of ethanol and fat on the transport of reducing equivalents into mitochondria. J Biol Chem 248: 4977-4986, 1973

43.   WHITE A, HANDLER P, SMITH EL: Principles of Biochemistry. McGraw Hill, N.Y., 1973. pp 349

44.   ONTKO JA: Effects of ethanol on the metabolism of free fatty acids in isolated liver cells. J Lipid Res 14: 78-86, 1973

45.   CHAPPELL JB: Systems used for the transport of substrates into mitochondria. Br Med Bull 24: 150-157, 1968

46.   ROBINSON BH, WILLIAMS GR, HALPERIN ML, LEZNOFF C: The sensitivity of the exchange reactions of tricarboxylate, 2-oxoglutarate and dicarboxylate transporting systems of rat liver mitochondria to inhibition by 2-pentylmalonate, p-iodobenzyl-malonate and benzene 1,2,3 tricarboxylate. Eur J Biochem 20: 65-71, 1971

47.   TUBBS PK, GARLAND PB: Membranes and fatty acid metabolism. Br
       Med Bull 24: 158-164, 1968

48.   VAN TOL A, HULSMANN WC: Dual localization and properties of
       ATP-dependent long chain fatty acid activation in rat liver
       mitochondria and the consequences for fatty acid oxidation.
       Biochim Biophys Acta 223: 416-428, 1970

49.   FRITZ IB, HUE KTN: Long chain carnitine acyltransferase and the
       role of acylcarnitine derivatives in the catalytic increase of fatty
       acid oxidation induced by carnitine. J Lipid Res 4: 279-288, 1963

50.   NORUM KR, FARSTAD M, BREMER J: The submitochondrial
       distribution of acid: CoA ligase (AMP) and palmityl CoA:
       Carnitine palmityltransferase in rat liver mitochondria. Biochem
       Biophys Res Commun 24: 797-804, 1966

51.   PADE SV: On rate-controlling factors of long chain fatty acid
       oxidation. J Biol Chem 246: 5384-4390, 1971

52.   LEFEVRE A, ADLER H, LIEBER CS: Effect of ethanol on ketone
       metabolism. J Clin Invest 49: 1775-1782, 1970

53.   GORDON ER: Mitochondrial functions in an ethanol-induced fatty
       liver. J Biol Chem 248: 8271-8280, 1973

54.   WILLIAMSON JR, SCHOLZ R, BROWNING ET, THURMAN RG,
       FUKAMI MH: Metabolic effects of ethanol in perfused rat liver.
       J Biol Chem 244: 5044-5054, 1973

55.   WILLIAMSON JR, OLSON MS: Control of citrate and acetoacetate
       synthesis in rat liver. Biochem Biophys Res Commun 32: 794-
       799, 1968

56.   GARLAND PB: Some kinetic properties of pig-heart oxoglutarate
       dehydrogenase that provide a basis for metabolic control of the
       enzyme activity and also a stoichiometric assay for coenzyme A
       in tissue extracts. Biochem J. 92: 10P, 1964

57.   PLAUT GW, AOGAICHI T: Purification and properties of diphospho-
       pyridine nucleotide-linked isocitrate dehydrogenase of mammalian
       liver. J Biol Chem 243: 5572-5583, 1968

58.   PARILLA R, OHKAWA K, LINDROS KO, ZIMMERMAN UJ,
       KOBAYASHI K, WILLIAMSON JR: Functional compartmentation
       of acetaldehyde oxidation in rat liver. J Biol Chem 249: 4926-
       4933, 1974

59. TOTTMAR SO, PETTERSSON H, KIESSLING KH: The subcellular distribution and properties of aldehyde dehydrogenases in rat liver. Biochem J 135: 577–586, 1973

60. HORTON AA, BARRETT MC: The subcellular localization of aldehyde dehydrogenase in rat liver. Arch Biochem Biophys 167: 426–436, 1975

61. CEDERBAUM AI, RUBIN E: The oxidation of acetaldehyde by isolated rat liver mitochondria. Submitted for publication.

62. LANOUE KF, NICKLAS WJ, WILLIAMSON JR: Control of citric acid cycle activity in rat heart mitochondria. J Biol Chem 245: 102–111, 1970

63. LANOUE KF, BRYLA J, WILLIAMSON JR: Feedback interactions in the control of citric acid cycle activity in rat heart mitochondria. J Biol Chem 247: 667–679, 1972

64. TRUITT EB, WALSH MJ: The role of acetaldehyde in the actions of ethanol. In Biology of Alcoholism, Vol I. Plenum Press, 1971. pp 161–195

65. MACNAMEE D, DEMBIEC D, COHEN G: Pargyline elevates blood acetaldehyde in ethanol intoxicated mice. Fed Proc 34: 663, 1975

66. COLLINS MA, GORDON R, BIGDELI MG, RUBENSTEIN JA: Pyrogallol potentiates acetaldehyde blood levels during ethanol oxidation in rats. Chem Biol Interactions 8: 127–130, 1974

67. KAMATH SA, RUBIN E: Effects of carbon tetrachloride and phenobarbital on plasma membranes; enzymes and phospholipid transfer. Lab Invest 30: 494–499, 1974

68. BERNSTEIN J, VIDELA L, ISRAEL Y: Metabolic alterations produced in the liver by chronic ethanol administration. Biochem J 134: 515–521, 1973

69. GANG H, LIEBER CS, RUBIN E: Effect of chronic ethanol administration on ATPase activity of the liver. In preparation.

70. GORDON ER: ATP metabolism in an ethanol-induced fatty liver. Alcoholism-Clinical and Research Studies, 1977. In press.

DISCUSSION

CHAIRMAN: M.J. PHILLIPS

POPPER: The mitochondria form a heterogeneous population and it is
       likely that some mitochondria are damaged more than others. Would
       it not be essential to prove that these changes do not just represent
       the spectrum of changes in this heterogeneous population?

RUBIN: We have measured in isolated fractions of heavy and light
       mitochondria obtained by differential centrifugation several para-
       meters including amino acid uptake and oxidation of various
       substrates. We were not able to find any differences. But I don't
       know how any differences could be correlated with changes measured
       by morphometric techniques anyway. It is very hard to tell on
       electron micrographs where the changes are. Our results probably do
       represent an average of all the mitochondria. But when you separate
       mitochondria on density gradients you separate them according to
       both size and density and it is very hard to tell which ones you have.
       The question is well taken.

GORDON: Have you correlated your changes with changes in the redox
       state of the mitochondria? What is the redox state at the time you
       see these changes?

RUBIN: We have not measured the redox changes in these mitochondria.

GORDON: Some of your results, for example those in the acetaldehyde
       studies, could be explained by competition from another source of
       hydrogen ions.

RUBIN: Well, the oxidation of acetaldehyde itself leads to the production
       of reducing equivalents and competition with other substrates. So
       this does play a role. But it still represents one method by which
       acetaldehyde can interfere with mitochondria.

195

GORDON: If we drive these isolated mitochondria at maximal speed they are not able to respond. They are damaged. In vivo they can act at rates that are faster than those of normal control animals. If you give thyroid hormone to an animal, you also get megamitochondria, morphologically the same as you get in the alcohol-treated animal. The mitochondria of the animal treated with thyroid hormone are using just about every normal substrate at a faster rate.

RUBIN: I agree that the correlation of function and morphology is very imperfect.

PHILLIPS: You have published some very interesting reports on the effects of alcohol on contractile proteins and muscle cells. Have you extended these studies to the liver?

RUBIN: We have isolated liver contractile proteins on polyacrylamide gels. We have been able to extract actin, troponin and tropomyosin from liver. We have also extracted them from isolated liver cells in the absence of vascular smooth muscle. For some reason we have not been able to extract any myosin from the hepatocytes. I suspect that there is some myosin there but that it is not polymerized. We have reconstituted a complete contractile system using myosin from another source. The Ca-Mg ATPase activities are apparently intact with a normal response to ATP, ADP and all the other manipulations that we do with muscle contractile proteins. So there is a contractile system in the liver.

PATHOGENESIS OF ALCOHOLIC LIVER DISEASE: AN OVERVIEW

C. S. Lieber

Section and Laboratory of Liver Disease, Nutrition and
Alcoholism, Bronx Veterans Administration Hospital, Bronx,
New York, and Mt. Sinai School of Medicine of the City
University of New York, New York, N.Y.

INTRODUCTION

To carry out my assignment of giving an overview of the pathogenesis
of alcoholic liver injury, I shall summarize some of the progress made over
the last 20 years, and I shall also attempt to indicate current approaches and
trends for the future. Until 20 years ago it was generally believed that liver
disease of the alcoholic was due exclusively to malnutrition and not to direct
toxic effects of alcohol itself; characteristically cirrhosis of the alcoholic
was not called "alcoholic cirrhosis" but "fatty nutritional cirrhosis". At first
this concept of an exclusively nutritional origin appeared attractive because
alcoholics do undoubtedly suffer from malnutrition for a variety of reasons.
First of all alcohol represents a large caloric load but these are so-called
"empty" calories since alcoholic beverages are usually devoid of minerals,
vitamins and proteins. Because it fulfills the caloric needs of the alcoholic,
alcohol decreases the intake of other nutrients and therefore alcoholics
commonly suffer from primary malnutrition. In addition, in view of the
intestinal pathology associated with alcoholism, maldigestion and malabsorption may contribute to secondary malnutrition. In turn, malnutrition
is known to adversely affect the liver. Therefore it was natural to postulate
that malnutrition is the mechanism whereby alcoholics develop liver disease.
This concept had direct impact on the management of the alcoholic. When
reluctant to give up his habit, the alcoholic was told by his physician that he
could preserve normal liver function despite continuation of the alcohol
intake provided that he maintained a normal diet. Some twenty years ago I
became dissatisfied with this concept when I had the charge of treating a
group of alcoholics who had developed cirrhosis apparently because of heavy
drinking and despite an apparently adequate or even a very rich diet. I
therefore wondered whether in addition to nutritional factors alcohol itself
might have direct toxic effects upon the liver. This led to a number of

studies which showed that indeed ethanol affects the liver independently of malnutrition.

These effects on hepatic cellular metabolism and structure were found to depend mainly on the dose and duration of intake. Following the ingestion of a substantial amount of ethanol, its presence alters a number of hepatic functions either because of the change in the hepatic redox state (NADH/NAD ratio) (resulting for instance in reduction of lipid oxidation) or because ethanol when present at high concentrations will inhibit a variety of microsomal functions involving particularly drug metabolism. These effects are not observed at low ethanol concentrations. Furthermore chronic ethanol consumption, at least in its early stages, produces adaptive metabolic changes in the endoplasmic reticulum which result primarily in increased metabolism of drugs and accelerated lipoprotein production. More extended periods of ethanol intake result in damage to cell organelles in what can be considered a third stage of the alcohol effect namely that of injury. The injury involves primarily mitochondria, possibly as a consequence of effects of acetaldehyde, the first product of ethanol metabolism. Prolongation of ethanol induced injury eventually culminates in hepatic lesions such as alcoholic hepatitis and cirrhosis. The purpose of this paper is to describe the abnormalities which characterize each of these three stages of alcohol induced changes in the liver, namely those associated with the metabolism of ethanol itself, followed by adaptive changes, upon chronic consumption, a phase which then leads to and partially overlaps with liver injury.

METABOLIC DERANGEMENT DIRECTLY ASSOCIATED WITH THE OXIDATION OF ETHANOL

1.   Effect of Excessive Hepatic NADH Generation by the Alcohol Dehydrogenase Pathway

As shown in Figure 1 (1), the oxidation of ethanol results in the transfer of hydrogen to NAD. The resulting enhanced NADH/NAD ratio, in turn, produces a change in the ratio of those metabolites that are dependent for reduction on the NADH-NAD couple. It was therefore proposed that the altered NADH/NAD ratio is responsible for a number of metabolic abnormalities associated with alcohol abuse (2). These include impaired gluconeogenesis and hypoglycemia (3).

The enhanced NADH/NAD ratio also reflects itself in an increased lactate/pyruvate ratio that results in hyperlactacidemia (4,5) because of both decreased utilization and enhanced production of lactate by the liver. The hyperlactacidemia contributes to acidosis and also reduces the capacity of the kidney to excrete uric acid, leading to secondary hyperuricemia (5), an observation which has been confirmed more recently (6). Alcohol induced ketosis may also promote the hyperuricemia. The latter may be related to the common clinical observation that excessive consumption of alcoholic beverages frequently aggravates or precipitates gouty attacks (7). Alcoholic hyperuricemia can be readily distinguished from the primary variety by its reversibility upon discontinuation of ethanol abuse (5). A fascinating but as yet hypothetical consequence of the increased availability of lactate may be the stimulation of collagen production and increased hepatic collagen proline hydroxylase activity which conceivably play a role in collagen accumulation (8). The increased NADH/NAD ratio also raises the concentration of α-glycerophosphate (9) that favors hepatic triglyceride accumulation by trapping fatty acids (10). In addition, excess NADH promotes fatty acid synthesis (11,12) possibly by the elongation pathway or transhydrogenation to nicotinamide adenine dinucleotide phosphate (NADP). Theoretically, enhanced lipogenesis can be considered a means for disposing of the excess hydrogen. In vivo, acute administration of a high dose of ethanol did not enhance fatty acid synthesis (13). Chronic ethanol administration however resulted in enhanced lipogenesis and increased activities of enzymes involved in lipogenesis (14). Some hydrogen equivalents can be transferred into the mitochondria by various "shuttle" mechanisms. However, the activity of the citric acid cycle is depressed (15,16) partly because of a slowing of the reactions of the cycle that require NAD. Indeed, a major site of interaction of ethanol in the citric acid cycle was found to be on α-ketoglutarate oxidation (17). Moreover, the redox change associated with ethanol oxidation decreases hepatic concentration of oxaloacetate (18), the availability of which controls the activity of citrate synthetase. The mitochondria will therefore use the hydrogen equivalents originating from ethanol, rather than from oxidation through the citric acid cycle of two carbon fragments derived from fatty acids. Thus, fatty acids that normally serve as the main energy source for the liver (19) are supplanted by ethanol. Decreased fatty acid oxidation by ethanol has been demonstrated in liver slices (11,20), perfused liver (16) (Figure 2), isolated hepatocytes (17), human liver biopsy tissue (21) and in vivo (22). This results in the deposition in the liver of dietary fat, when available, or fatty acids derived from endogenous synthesis in the absence of dietary fat (23-26) and can be considered a major cause for the development of alcoholic fatty liver.

2. Interaction of Ethanol with Microsomal Functions

Interactions of the effects of ethanol and various drugs have been widely recognized (27). Intoxicated individuals are more susceptible to several medications (28). These various effects are usually attributed to additive or synergistic effects of alcohol and various drugs on the central nervous system. However, there exists an at least partially common microsomal system for ethanol and drug metabolism (MEOS) (29,30) and the increased susceptibility of the inebriated individual can be explained, at least in part, by the effect of ethanol on microsomal drug-detoxifying enzymes. It has indeed been found that ethanol inhibits the metabolism of a variety of drugs in vitro (31-34) (Figure 3). With some systems, such as aniline hydroxylase, this inhibition is of a competitive nature (34,35). For some drug metabolising systems (such as aniline hydroxylase) the inhibitory effect is observed at low ethanol concentrations whereas for others (such as aminopyrine demethylase) high ethanol concentrations are required (34). In

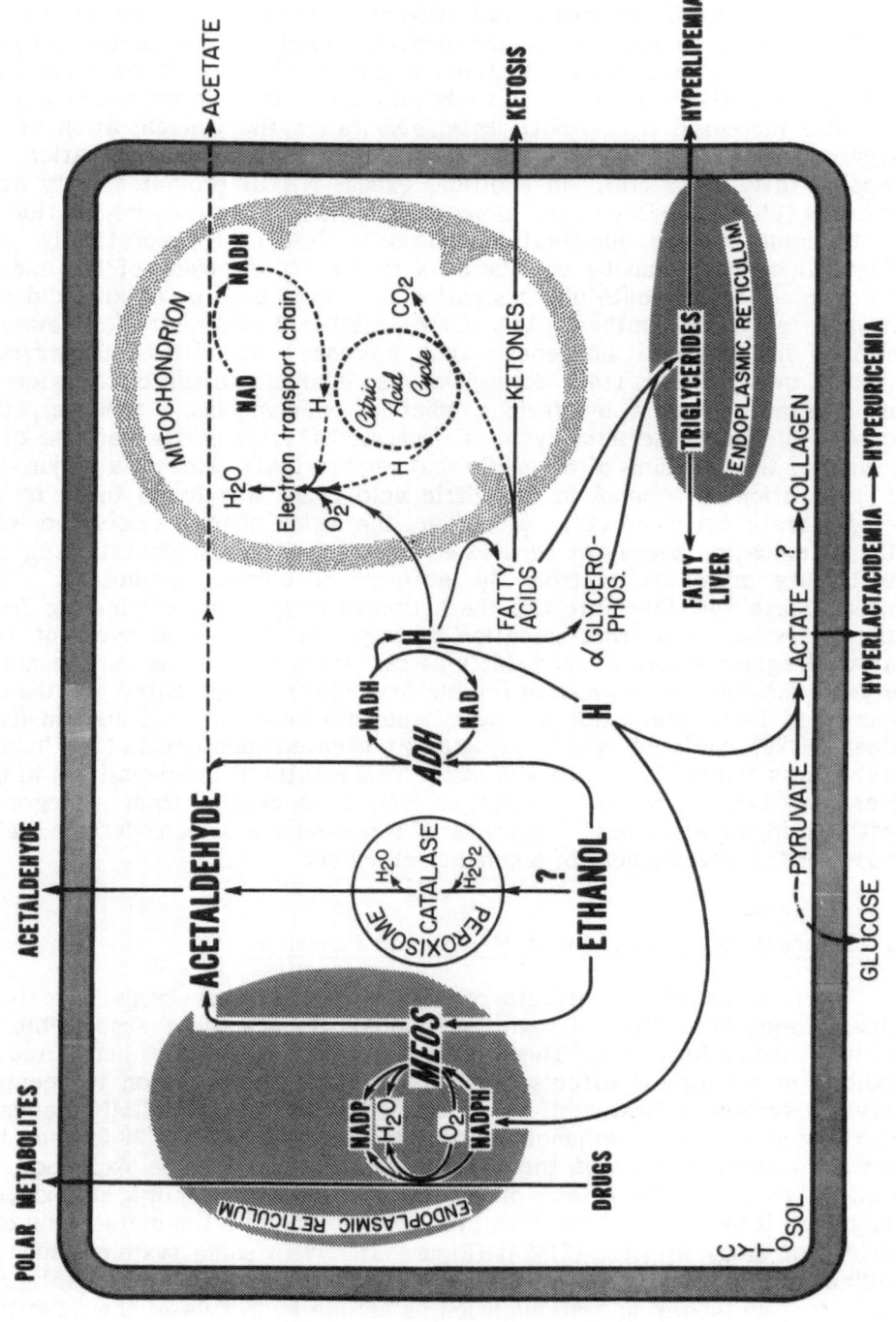

Fig. 1   *Metabolism of ethanol in the hepatocyte and schematic representation of its link to fatty liver, hyperlipemia, hyperuricemia, hyperlactacidemia, ketosis, and hypoglycemia. ADH, alcohol dehydrogenase; MEOS, microsomal ethanol-oxidizing system; NAD, nicotinamide adenine dinucleotide; NADH, nicotinamide adenine dinucleotide, reduced form; NADP, nicotinamide adenine dinucleotide phosphate; NADPH, nicotinamide adenine dinucleotide phosphate - reduced form. Pathways decreased by ethanol are represented by dashed lines (1).*

←——

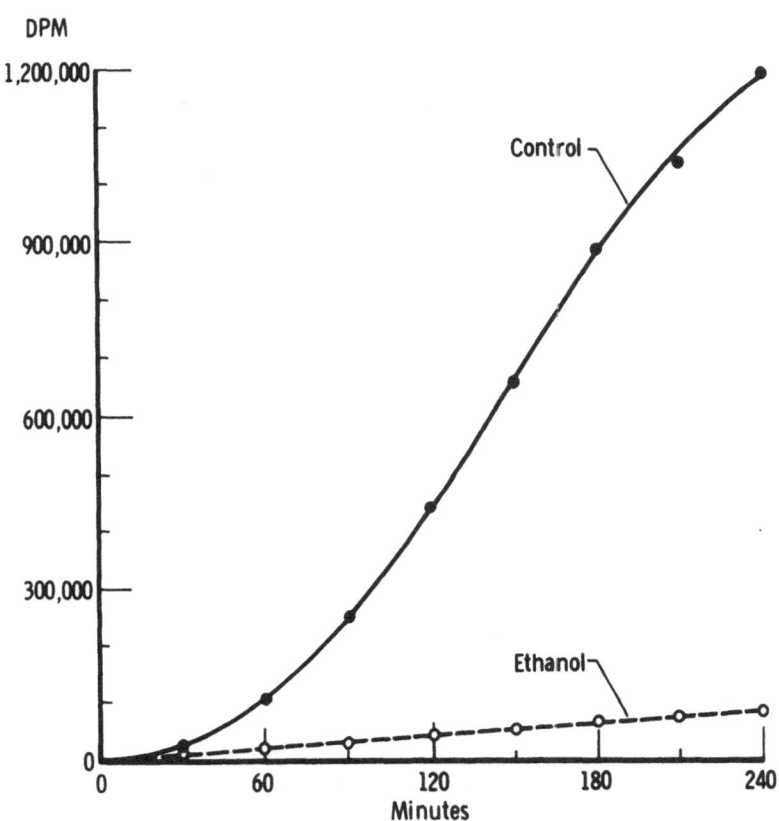

Fig. 2   *Effect of ethanol on total $^{14}CO_2$ production form ^{14}C-labelled chylomicrons in isolated perfused rat livers (16).*

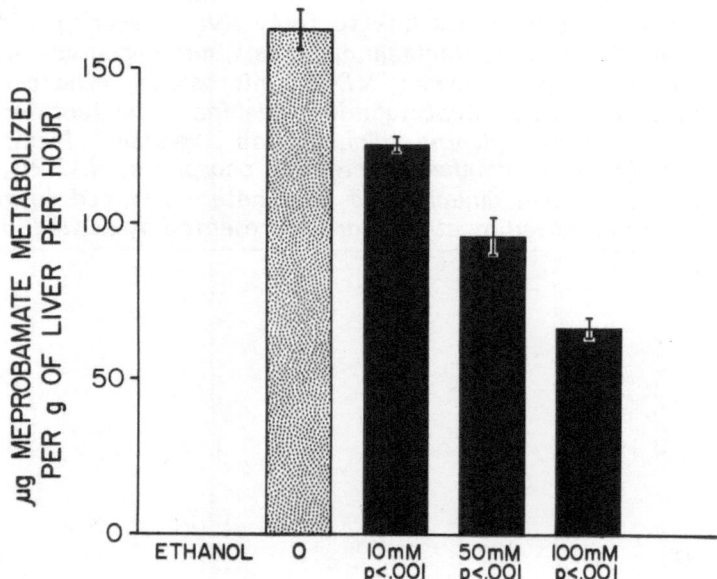

Fig. 3   Effect of ethanol on metabolism of meprobamate by rat liver
           slices. Each flask contained 500 mg liver and was incubated for
           120 minutes. Meprobamate concentration was 0.3 mM, includ-
           ing 1μc ^{14}C-meprobamate (34).

the latter case, low ethanol concentrations were even stimulatory (36),
possibly because of enhanced NADH and the likelihood that NADH may
serve as partial electron donor for microsomal drug detoxifying systems (37).
The inhibitory effects may explain the observation that, in vivo, simultaneous administration of ethanol and drugs slows the rate of drug
metabolism (34,38).   Conversely, drugs also inhibit ethanol oxidation by
microsomes in vitro in a way which has been considered as strong evidence
for a catalase independent fraction of ethanol metabolism in hepatic
microsomes (39).   At a low ethanol concentration, however, its metabolism
was stimulated by drugs (40) possibly because of increased reoxidation of
NADH again through microsomal utilization. In addition, some drugs inhibit
alcohol dehydrogenase (41).

3.   Effects of Acetaldehyde, the Metabolite of Ethanol

Acetaldehyde is the first major "specific" oxidation product of ethanol,
whether the latter is oxidized by the classic alcohol dehydrogenase of the
cytosol or by the more recently described microsomal system. Except after
Antabuse[R] administration, acetaldehyde concentrations after alcohol

ingestion are low, but it has long been speculated that they may contribute to the complications of alcoholism (42). Although the exact pathway of its metabolism is still the subject of debate, it is generally accepted that acetaldehyde oxidation proceeds via aldehyde dehydrogenase of which 80% of the activity is located in the mitochondria (43,44). Since metabolism of acetaldehyde via aldehyde dehydrogenase results in the generation of NADH, some of the acetaldehyde effects could be attributed to the NADH generation, as discussed before in the case of ethanol. Acetaldehyde however is a very reactive compound which may exert some toxic effects of its own.

Although the potential toxicity of acetaldehyde has been recognized for a number of years (42) little was known about blood acetaldehyde levels after alcohol consumption. Recently, Korsten et al. (45) showed a difference between alcoholic and non-alcoholic subjects in their blood acetaldehyde level after comparable ethanol challenges. Blood acetaldehyde and ethanol levels were measured in 11 subjects (six chronic alcoholic and five non-alcoholic controls) after alcohol had been given intravenously. Despite a progressive fall in blood ethanol concentration over a range of 54 to 33 mM, acetaldehyde did not decrease in any of the 11 subjects. The mean acetaldehyde plateau level was significantly ($p < 0.001$) higher in alcoholic (42.7 ± 1.2 μM) than in non-alcoholic (26.5 ± 1.5 μM) subjects (Figure 4). When the mean blood ethanol concentration reached 24 mM, the acetaldehyde plateau ended abruptly in each subject (Figure 5). The ethanol

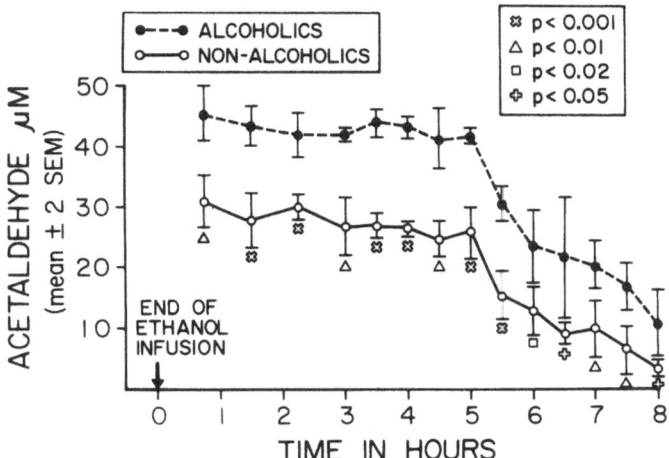

Fig. 4   *Comparison of blood acetaldehyde levels of alcoholic and nonalcoholic subjects after intravenous alcohol infusion. The significance level of the difference of the means is noted (45).*

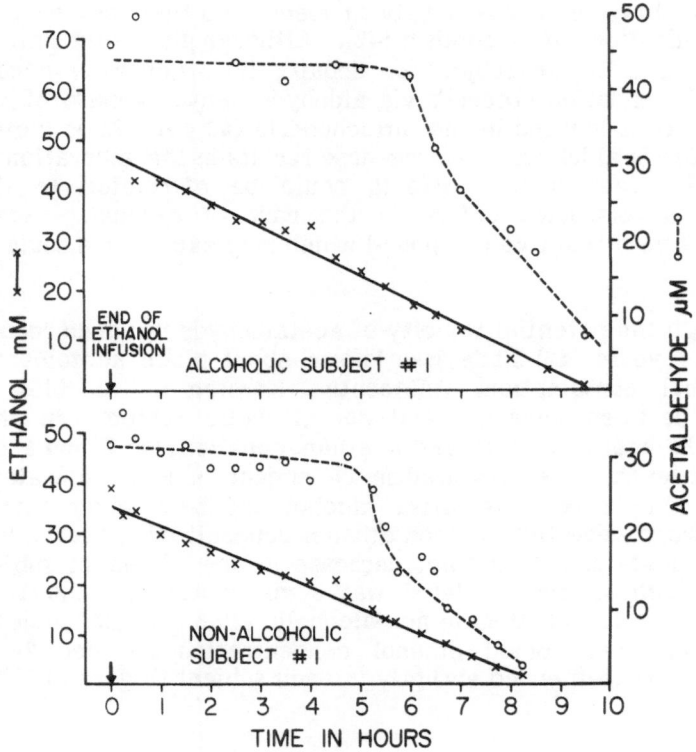

Fig. 5   *Blood acetaldehyde and ethanol levels after intravenous infusion*
in an alcoholic and nonalcoholic subject. The plateau acetalde-
hyde level of the former fluctuated around a higher mean than
that of the latter. In both, however, acetaldehyde sharply
declined at an ethanol concentration of 18 to 20 mM (45).

concentration at which this fall of blood acetaldehyde occurred suggests
desaturation of an ethanol oxidizing system other than alcohol deydrogenase
and indicates that at high ethanol blood levels, such a system contributes to
ethanol oxidation. If it is assumed that during the plateau period the
production and elimination of acetaldehyde are constant, it follows that
either decreased production or increased degradation could explain the
decline in acetaldehyde levels at a mean ethanol concentration of 24 mM.
Since a sudden increase in degradation is unlikely (43,46) and excretion of
acetaldehyde is minimal (47), it appears that production of acetaldehyde
must have decreased. Acetaldehyde production by alcohol dehydrogenase
should be unchanged since this system is fully saturated at ethanol levels
associated with the drop in acetaldehyde (48–50). On the other hand, the
MEOS, which has a K_m between 8 and 10 mM, would become desaturated,

and its activity would decrease at these ethanol levels (29,30). Higher levels of acetaldehyde may have been due to decreased catabolism, possibly in relation to alcohol-induced liver damage. Indeed, early structural and functional changes are induced by alcohol in liver organelles (51-54). Since these alterations primarily involve the mitochondrion, it is possible that defective acetaldehyde dehydrogenation, which is predominantly intramito-chondrial (43,44) delays acetaldehyde clearance and results in higher concentrations. Indeed, in rats fed ethanol chronically, Hasumura et al. (55) found that the liver mitochondria had a significantly reduced capacity to oxidize acetaldehyde. This was associated with decreased mitochondrial respiration with acetaldehyde as substrate.

The reduction of acetaldehyde metabolism observed in rats fed ethanol continuously over a long period might result in the accumulation of acetaldehyde in the liver as well as in the blood if the production rate of acetaldehyde is unchanged or increased, as discussed before. The enhanced blood acetaldehyde may in turn explain a number of ethanol related complications. Indeed, numerous neuro-toxic effects have been attributed to acetaldehyde (56). In addition to the release of catecholamines (57), acetaldehyde has been shown to participate in and favor the condensation reactions of biogenic amines (58,59). The products of these interactions could have addictive properties if sufficient amounts were generated in vivo. Acetaldehyde has also been shown to affect myocardial protein synthesis at concentrations (60,61) comparable to those found by Korsten et al. (43) in the blood. Acetaldehyde has also been shown to reduce the activity of various mitochondrial shuttles involved in the disposition of reducing equivalents and to inhibit oxidative phosphorylation (54). More recently, Cederbaum et al. (62) have shown that acetaldehyde depresses the capacity of liver mitochondria to oxidize fatty acids thereby mimicking defects associated with chronic alcohol consumption, (63). The concentrations of acetaldehyde required to achieve the hepatic effects in mitochondria of normal animals were greater than those seen in the blood. However, mitochondria of rats fed ethanol chronically were found to have an increased susceptibility to the effects of acetaldehyde; under these conditions, concentrations of acetaldehyde known to occur in the liver were found to depress mitochondrial functions (64). In view of the reactivity of acetaldehyde, a number of other metabolic effects of ethanol could be due to the action of this metabolite of ethanol. For instance, recent studies have indicated that individuals with chronic alcohol abuse frequently exhibited lowered plasma levels of pyridoxal 5' -phosphate, the coenzyme form of vitamin B_6. Veitch et al. (65) found that in rats fed ethanol (36% of total calories), there was a significant decrease in the hepatic pyridoxal phosphate content both in animals given a sufficient amount of vitamin B_6 in their diet and in those rendered B_6 deficient. In isolated perfused livers, the addition of 18 mM ethanol lowered the pyridoxal phosphate content of livers from vitamin B_6 deficient animals and decreased the net synthesis of pyridoxal phosphate from pyridoxine by the livers of vitamin B_6 deficient animals. Ethanol also diminished the rate of release of pyridoxal phosphate into the perfusate by the livers of vitamin B_6-deficient rats. These effects of ethanol, in vitro, were abolished by 4-methyl-pyrazole, an inhibitor of alcohol dehydrogenase. Thus the derangement of pyridoxal phosphate metabolism produced by ethanol is dependent upon its oxidation. One interpretation of these findings was that acetaldehyde may be the responsible agent, since in human erythrocytes, it has been shown that acetaldehyde acts to enhance the enzymatic hydrolysis of pyridoxal-5'-phosphate by cellular phosphatase (66). Similar observations were also made in isolated rat hepatocytes in preliminary studies thus far published only in abstract form (67). The latter study also reportedly showed that acetaldehyde can displace pyridoxal-5'-phosphate from its protein binding, thereby promoting its degradation. Thus, through a multitude of mechanisms, acetaldehyde may explain a variety of metabolic complications associated with alcohol abuse.

"ADAPTIVE" METABOLIC CHANGES FOLLOWING CHRONIC ETHANOL INTAKE

It is common knowledge that chronic alcohol consumption produces increased tolerance to ethanol. This is generally attributed to central nervous system adaptation. In addition, recent studies have shown the development of metabolic adaptation, that is an accelerated clearance of alcohol from the blood. Furthermore, there is an associated increased capacity to metabolize other drugs as well. Moreover, the liver acquires an enhanced capacity to rid itself of lipids through lipoprotein secretion into the blood stream. It is noteworthy that these functions which adaptively increase after chronic ethanol feeding involve to a large extent the activity of the hepatic smooth endoplasmic reticulum, which undergoes significant change after chronic alcohol consumption. It was indeed observed more than a decade ago that ethanol feeding results in a proliferation of the smooth membranes of the hepatic endoplasmic reticulum (68,69). This ultramicroscopic finding was subsequently confirmed (70-72) and established on a biochemical basis by the demonstration of an increase in both phospholipids and total protein content of the smooth membranes (73). Its functional counterparts include accelerated metabolism of drugs (including ethanol) and lipoprotein production.

1.   Accelerated Ethanol Metabolism After Chronic Ethanol Consumption

Regular drinkers tolerate large amounts of alcoholic beverages, mainly because of central nervous system adaptation. In addition, alcoholics develop increased rates of blood ethanol clearance, so-called metabolic tolerance (74,75). Experimental ethanol administration also results in an increased rate of ethanol metabolism (29,76,77). The mechanism of this acceleration has been discussed in detail in the paper by Matsuzaki et al. (64) which underlines the role of increased microsomal function.

2. Stimulation of the Microsomal Drug Metabolizing Enzymes

a) Enhanced drug metabolism (Drug tolerance): Repeated ethanol administration results in increased activities of a variety of microsomal drug–detoxifying enzymes (31,32,70,76,78). Some effects are already observed after a single ethanol dose (79). Ethanol consumption also increases the content of microsomal cytochrome P-450 and the activity of NADPH–cytochrome P-450 reductase (72,78,80). These increases occur in the smooth membranes (73,78). Moreover, it has been shown that microsomal cytochrome P-450, a reductase, and phospholipids play a key role in the microsomal hydroxylation of various drugs (81). Therefore, the increase in the activity of hepatic microsomal drug–detoxifying enzymes and in the content of cytochrome P-450 induced by ethanol ingestion offers a likely explanation for the recent observation that ethanol consumption enhances the rate of drug clearance in vivo. The tolerance of the alcoholic to various drugs has been generally attributed to central nervous system adaptation (82). However, there is sometimes a dissociation in the time course of the decreased drug sensitivity of the animals and the occurrence of central nervous system tolerance, the former preceding the latter (83). Thus, in addition to central nervous system adaptation, metabolic adaptation must be considered. Indeed, it has been shown that the rate of drug clearance from the blood is enhanced in alcoholics (84). Of course, this could be due to a variety of factors other than ethanol, such as the congeners and the use of other drugs so commonly associated with alcoholism. Controlled studies showed, however, that administration of pure ethanol with non–deficient diets either to rats or man (under metabolic ward conditions) resulted in a striking increase in the rate of blood clearance of meprobamate and pentobarbital (76), (Figure 6). Similarly, increases in the metabolism of aminopyrine (85), tolbutamide (70) and rifamycin (86) were found. Furthermore, the capacity of liver slices from animals fed ethanol to metabolize meprobamate was also increased (76) which clearly showed that ethanol consumption affects drug metabolism in the liver itself, independent of drug excretion or distribution. Failure to verify such an effect (87) was probably due to the very low dosage of ethanol administered.

b) Increased CCl_4 toxicity in alcoholics: The stimulation of microsomal enzyme activities also applies to those which convert exogenous substrates to toxic compounds. For instance, CCl_4 exerts its toxicity only after conversion in the microsomes. Alcohol pretreatment remarkably stimulates the toxicity of CCl_4 (88,89). The experiments of Hasumura et al. (88) were carried out at a time when the ethanol had disappeared from the blood to rule out the increase of the toxicity of CCl_4 due to the presence of ethanol (90). The potentiation of the CCl_4 toxicity by ethanol pretreatment may be accounted for by the increased production of toxic compounds of CCl_4 since the conversion of $^{14}CCl_4$ to $^{14}CO_2$ and covalent binding of CCl_4 metabolites to protein were significantly accelerated in microsomes of ethanol pretreated rats (88). Similarly, pretreatment of rats with phenobarbital, a well known inducer of the hepatic microsomal drug metabolizing system, increased CCl_4 hepatotoxicity (91) concomitant with an enhanced production of toxic metabolites of CCl_4 (92). Thus, the

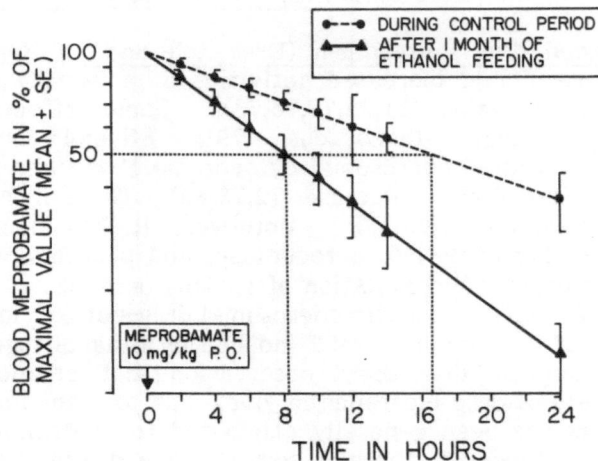

Fig. 6   Effect of ethanol consumption on clearance of meprobamate from blood. Four volunteer alcoholics were tested before and after one month of ethanol ingestion; half lives are shown by the dotted lines on x and y axes (76).

clinical observation of the enhanced susceptibility of alcoholics to the hepatotoxic effect of CCl_4 (93) may be, at least in part, due to an increased activation and biotransformation of CCl_4. It is likely that a larger number of other toxic agents will be found to display a selective injurious action in the alcoholic.   For instance, the observed increased hepatotoxicity of isoniazide in alcoholics (94) may well be due to increased production by the microsomes of an active metabolite of the acetyl derivative of the drug. Such side effect is possibly an undesirable consequence of the "adaptive" response to chronic ethanol consumption.

3.   Increase in Microsomal Functions Related to Lipid Metabolism

a)   Lipid peroxidation: A microsomal pathway requiring O_2 and NADPH is also capable of generating lipid peroxides.   Enhanced lipid peroxidation has been proposed as a mechanism for ethanol induced fatty liver (95), but its role is still controversial (96-99).   The accumulation of lipid peroxide may be secondary to the lipid accumulation (100), rather than represent its cause.   However, theoretically, increased activity of microsomal NADPH oxidase following ethanol consumption (101) could result in enhanced H_2O_2 production, thereby also favoring lipid peroxidation.   In any event, ethanol was found to exert a sparing action on vitamin E deficiency (102) which does not favor a lipoperoxidative mechanism for chronic ethanol hepatotoxicity.

b)   Cholesterol metabolism: The various functions of the endoplasmic reticulum include cholesterol synthesis.   Increased cholesterol synthesis after ethanol (103) may have a microsomal basis akin to that after barbiturate (104) and may explain, in part, the accumulation of cholesterol ester observed in the liver after feeding of alcohol (103, 105) especially with a cholesterol-free diet.   When ethanol is given with cholesterol-containing diets, decreased cholesterol catabolism, evidenced by a reduction in bile-acid production and turnover after alcohol feeding, plays a major part (103). Decreased hydrolysis of cholesterol ester may also be contributory (106). Upon cessation of alcohol feeding, increased bile secretion occurs (107), probably as a "rebound" phenomenon.

c)   Alcoholic hyperlipemia: In both man (108) and the rat (109) ethanol administration produces mild hyperlipemia, involving especially the very low density lipoproteins.   Incorporation into lipoprotein of intragastrically administered ^{3}H-palmitate and intravenously injected ^{14}C-lysine is increased (109) suggesting enhanced lipoprotein production. Fatty acids are esterified, and lipoproteins are formed in the endoplasmic reticulum.   Furthermore, chronic feeding of ethanol increases hepatic lipoprotein production, even when ethanol is not present at the time of testing, which suggests an increased capacity for lipoprotein synthesis (110) (Figure 7).   Moreover,

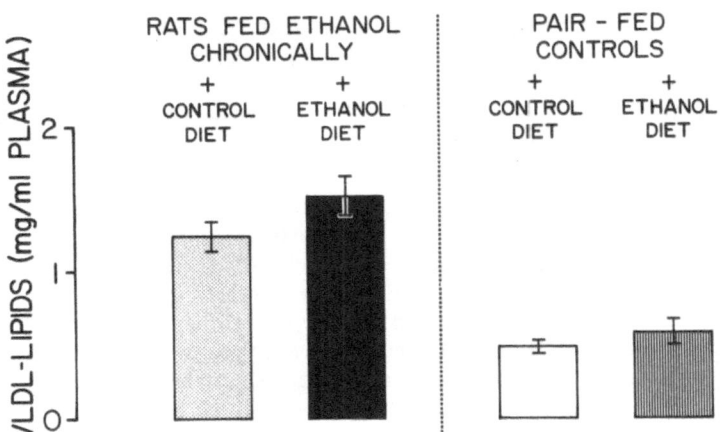

Fig. 7   Comparison between acute and chronic ethanol administration on postprandial lipemia in the rat. Animals were pair-fed liquid diets containing either ethanol (36% of total calories) or isocaloric carbohydrates (controls) for 3-4 weeks. Alcohol fed rats developed hyperlipemia in response to a load of diet with or without ethanol; by contrast, control fed rats did not develop hyperlipemia in response to an acute administration of ethanol containing diets (3 g ethanol per kg body weight). Data from Baraona et al. (110).

ethanol consumption enhances the activity of hepatic microsomal L-α-glycerophosphate acyltransferase (111). The mechanism of the alterations of these microsomal functions produced by ethanol has not been clarified. It could be linked directly to the fact that ethanol can be oxidized at this key metabolic site. Ethanol could also induce hepatic production of lipoproteins indirectly by enhancing the availability of fatty acids either by decreasing their oxidation or by enhancing synthesis, as alluded to before. Increased glycerolipid production has indeed been found after ethanol consumption (112). Ethanol feeding was observed to enhance the activity of glycosyl-transferase in the Golgi apparatus (113) and to increase the synthesis of the protein moiety of lipoproteins (109). In some individuals, the response is markedly exaggerated because of a fat rich diet (114-118) or because of some underlying abnormality of hyperlipemia (108,119,120), pancreatitis (121), diabetes or prediabetes (108,122) or an increased susceptibility to ethanol itself: indeed, whereas some subjects develop a comparable hyperlipemia after ethanol and carbohydrate (123), others have a selective response (116). The mechanism for the increased capacity of these patients to develop alcoholic hyperlipemia remains unknown. Since ethanol consumption results in an increased capacity to secrete lipoproteins in response to a lipid load (110) one may wonder whether the difference in response to ethanol between some alcoholics and some individuals with type IV hyperlipemia may be secondary, at least in part, to a difference in prior alcohol consumption.

Concerning the site of the ethanol effects, it is noteworthy that both in men and in rats, ethanol-induced hyperlipemia results in increased concentrations of the various serum lipoprotein fractions, but the main change occurs in the lipoproteins of d < 1.006. In the postprandial state, this fraction includes very low density lipoproteins and chylomicrons. In patients with alcoholic hyperlipemia, chylomicron-like particles have been observed in the fasting state (122). In the rat rendered hyperlipemic by ethanol feeding, the lipid/protein ratio of the d < 1.006 lipoproteins approaches that of chylomicrons (110). However, the site of origin of these particles cannot be deduced with certainty from physical or chemical characteristics. Indeed, in other states of accelerated lipoprotein production, such as carbohydrate-induced hyperlipemia, the lipid/protein ratio and particle size of the d < 1.006 lipoproteins increases even in the absence of dietary fat. The increase in serum lipoproteins of higher density both in man (119) and in rats (109) indicates that the hyperlipemia is not merely of intestinal origin and that the liver participates in this process.

The possibility still remains that, after alcohol feeding, the intestine releases more lipid into the lymph, either by decreasing oxidation of fatty acids or by increasing the synthesis of lipids from sources other than dietary fat (124,125). A decreased production of $^{14}CO_2$ from labelled fatty acids by intestinal slices after an acute load of alcohol (126) and an increased incorporation of these fatty acids into intestinal triglycerides by slices obtained from rats fed ethanol (127) have been reported. To what extent these alterations contribute to alcoholic hyperlipemia is unknown. Mistilis and Ockner (128) have shown that intraduodenal infusion of 10% ethanol to the fasted rat in a dose of 5 g/kg produces a mild increase in the very low density lipoprotein output in the lymph. They postulated that this increase in nondietary lymph lipid could contribute to the hyperlipemia, although the peak serum rise actually preceded the maximum increase in intestinal lymph lipids. Furthermore, lymph lipoproteins can derive in part from plasma lipoproteins (129).

Moreover, although a single intragastric administration of a diet containing ethanol (3 g/kg) increased both intestinal lymph flow and lipid output in rats not previously fed alcohol, postprandial hyperlipemia was not produced under these conditions (110). Actually, the acute load of an ethanol containing diet did not increase lymph lipid output in rats fed alcohol for several weeks, compared to their pair fed controls; however, marked hyperlipemia developed in these alcohol fed rats. Moreover, when a similar lymph lipid load was infused intravenously to alcohol pretreated and control rats with diversion of intestinal lymph, the alcohol fed rats developed hyperlipemia. If lymph depletion was not prevented by intravenous replacement, hepatic and plasma lipids decreased, and alcoholic hyperlipemia did not occur. This indicates that, although an adequate supply of dietary lipids represents a permissive factor needed to induce alcoholic hyperlipemia in the rat, changes in lymph lipid output do not seem to play a major role in the lipemic effect of ethanol and that the site of origin of the increased production of serum lipoprotein is a non-intestinal one, most likely hepatic. Similarly, the contribution of lymph lipids to the steatosis appears to be a minor one (130).

The mechanism for the increase in lipids other than triglycerides in the course of alcoholic hyperlipemia remains unknown. This is due partly to the fact that the role of cholesterol and phospholipids in serum lipoproteins has not been clarified. The changes in the plasma concentration of these lipids could be a reflection of variations in the mass of serum lipoprotein secondary to changes in triglyceride transport. As discussed before, ethanol also increases cholesterogenesis in the liver (103) and in the small intestine (131).

After the initial development of fatty liver associated with hyperlipemia, the blood lipids return towards normal (105) (Figure 8). Progressive deterioration of liver function, including lipoprotein production and secretion, could be responsible, and may secondarily aggravate fat accumulation in the liver. Indeed, high concentrations of ethanol exert depressive effects on lipoprotein secretion (contrasting to the adaptive response to the lower ones) which may be a reflection of a hepatotoxic effect and will be discussed in the following section.

4. Miscellaneous Changes in Microsomal Functions

Hepatic microsomes are responsible for a large number of metabolic functions some of which have been found to be affected by either acute or chronic ethanol consumption. For instance, some (132) report that ethanol

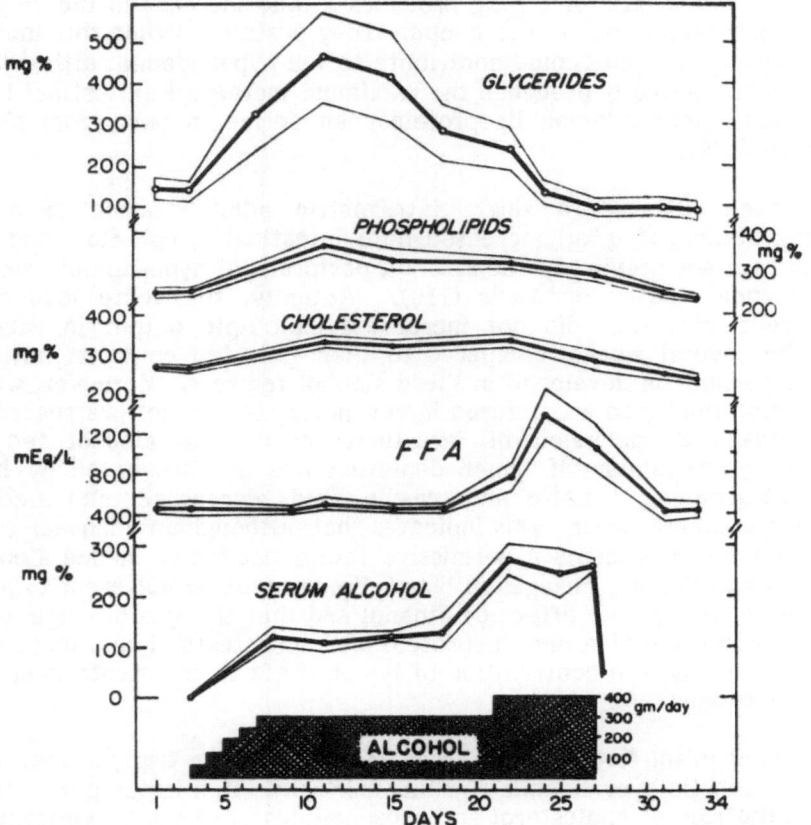

*Fig. 8   Effect of prolonged alcohol intake on serum lipids in 7 chronic
alcoholic individuals (average results ± S.E. of the mean) (105).*

prevents hyperbilirubinemia of the newborn, an effect attributed to
induction of microsomal uridine–diphosphate–glucuronyl transferase (133).
Others found no bilirubin change (134,135); in any event, practical
applications are limited by possible toxic effects of ethanol on the fetus
(fetal alcohol syndrome).

As discussed before, alcohol ingestion may also severely affect glucose
metabolism. Contrasting with the lack of effect of other microsomal
inducers on microsomal glucose-6-phosphatase, both short (136) and long

term (137) ethanol feeding significantly increased this activity. Another study (138), failed to reveal such an effect, but this may have been due to the diet used. Indeed, as discussed elsewhere (137) diets high in fructose or sucrose increase glucose-6-phosphatase activity. Fitch and Chaikoff (139) pointed out the importance of the type of carbohydrate: a 60% fructose diet increased glucose-6-phosphatase activity, but a 60% glucose diet did not. In the study of Ishii et al. (137) the carbohydrate preparation used (Dextri-Maltose), is broken down to glucose, and was expected not to interfere with the assessment of the effect of ethanol on glucose-6-phosphatase activity whereas in the study of Carter and Isselbacher (138) sucrose was used, and it provided 41% of total calories in the control diet, but only 5% in the ethanol diet. This difference may account for a high glucose-6-phosphatase activity in control animals and an apparent lack of ethanol effect. Thus, when the carbohydrate content is taken into account, it is clear that ethanol feeding increases glucose-6-phosphatase activity, but the significance of this effect with regard to carbohydrate metabolism has not been established.

INJURIOUS MANIFESTATIONS OF THE ALTERATIONS OF LIVER METABOLISM ASSOCIATED WITH ALCOHOLISM

In its milder form, alcoholic liver disease is characterized by accumulation of excess fat in the liver, so-called fatty liver. When a number of liver cells die and this necrosis causes inflammation, one is dealing with alcoholic hepatitis, a more severe form of alcoholic liver injury associated with a mortality ranging from 10-30% depending on the series. Eventually, scarring by fibrous tissue occurs and its excess distorts the normal architecture of the liver, fibrous bands dissect the organ and alter its function. The term cirrhosis characterizes this more severe, irreversible form of alcoholic liver injury.

Because the fatty liver is a very common complication of alcoholism and usually fully reversible, it has been considered as benign. However, already at the fatty liver stage, signs of hepatic injury are evident particularly in the mitochondria and in the capacity of the liver to export proteins. One must therefore wonder whether the fatty liver must be considered as a serious condition which in predisposed individuals may be a precursor to the hepatitis and cirrhosis. Furthermore it has now become clear that the entire spectrum of alcohol induced liver injury can be attributed to ethanol itself, in part, through the metabolic derangements produced by this compound, rather than to the malnutrition associated with alcoholism which was originally thought to be exclusively the cause of liver injury observed in the alcoholic.

1.   Alcoholic Fatty Liver

a)   Origin and mechanisms of fat deposition in the liver: Lipids which accumulate in the liver can originate from 3 main sources: dietary lipids, which reach the bloodstream as chylomicrons; adipose tissue lipids, which are transported to the liver as free fatty acids (FFA); and lipids synthesized in the liver itself. These fatty acids of various sources can accumulate in the liver because of a large number of metabolic disturbances, primarily a) increased peripheral fat mobilization, b) decreased hepatic lipoprotein release, c) decreased lipid oxidation in the liver, d) enhanced hepatic lipogenesis. Depending on the experimental conditions, any of the 3 sources and the 4 mechanisms can be implicated.

During consumption of ethanol with lipid containing diets, the fatty acids which accumulate in the liver are derived primarily from dietary fatty acids, whereas when ethanol is given with a low fat diet endogenously synthesized fatty acids are deposited in the liver (23-25). Some of these effects can be considered as consequences of the metabolism of ethanol in the liver. Depending on the metabolic state of the animal both decreased lipid oxidation and enhanced lipogenesis can be linked to ethanol oxidation and the associated increased generation of NADH as discussed before in this chapter.

In fasted rats, ethanol did not stimulate fatty acid synthesis (140). Moreover, in rats given one large, sublethal dose of ethanol, it was observed that fatty acids resembling those of adipose tissue accumulate in the liver (24,141). Experimental procedures or agents which reduce the normal rate of peripheral fat mobilization, i.e. adrenalectomy, spinal cord transection, or ganglioplegic drugs, prevent or decrease this type of hepatic fat accumulation (141,143). More direct approaches, however, such as studies in rats with prelabelled epididymal fat pads yielded conflicting information, with evidence for increased (144) or unchanged (145) fatty acid mobilization. Similarly, in rats, one large dose of ethanol has been reported to result in increased (141, 146) or unchanged (147) circulating levels of free fatty acids. In man, even with amounts of ethanol as large as 300 g/day, the concentration of circulating free fatty acids did not increase; it rose only after ingestion of very large doses of ethanol (400 g/day) (105) (Figure 8). In short term studies, ethanol administration produced a fall in the level of circulating free fatty acids in man (4,148) with reduced peripheral venous-arterial differences in free fatty acids (4), decreased free fatty acid turnover (149), and concomitant reduction in circulating glycerol (150). This effect of ethanol upon free fatty acid mobilization from adipose tissue was found to be mediated by acetate (151). Acetate is the end product of ethanol metabolism in the liver (Figure 1) and is released into the bloodstream. Since stressful doses of ethanol probably both stimulate fatty acid mobilization (via catecholamine release) and depress it (via the acetate produced), the net effect may depend upon the particular experimental conditions. This may account for some of the apparent contradictions of the literature.

Actually, whether or not enhanced peripheral fat mobilization is responsible for hepatic fat accumulation after one large sublethal dose of ethanol in the rat is of little clinical relevance after chronic ethanol consumption. Under the latter conditions, the fatty acids deposited in the liver do not derive primarily from adipose tissue (23,24).

Thus, the main events leading to the development of the alcoholic fatty liver can be summarized as follows: ethanol, which has an almost "obligatory" hepatic metabolism, replaces the fatty acids as a normal fuel for the hepatic mitochondria. This results in fatty acid accumulation, directly because of decreased lipid oxidation and indirectly because one way for the liver to dispose of excess hydrogen generated by ethanol oxidation is to synthesize more lipids. Fatty acids derived from adipose tissue accumulate in the liver only when very large amounts of ethanol are given. The lipids increase in the liver despite the fact that the transport mechanism via release of lipoproteins from the liver into the bloodstream is stimulated by ethanol, at least during the initial state of intoxication.

b) Alcohol as a direct cause of the fatty liver: Each gram of ethanol provides 7.1 calories, which means that 20 ounces (or 586 ml) of 86 proof (43% v/v) beverage represents about 1500 calories or 1/2 to 2/3rds of the normal daily caloric requirement. Therefore, the alcoholic has a much reduced demand for food to fulfill his caloric needs. Since alcoholic beverages do not contain significant amounts of protein, vitamins and minerals, the intake of these nutrients may become readily borderline or insufficient. Economic factors may also reduce the consumption of nutrient rich food by the alcoholic. In addition to acting as "empty" or "naked" calories, alcohol can result in malnutrition by interfering with the normal processes of food digestion and absorption (152). For all these reasons, deficiency diseases readily develop in the alcoholic. In rodents, severely deficient diets result in liver damage even in the absence of alcohol. Extrapolation from these animal results to man led to the belief that in alcoholics the liver disease is due not to ethanol but solely to the nutritional deficiencies and that given an adequate diet alcohol is merely acting by its caloric contribution and that it is not more toxic than a similar caloric load derived from fats or starches (153). This opinion prevailed, despite some statistical evidence gathered both in France (154) and in Germany (155) which indicated that the incidence of liver disease correlated with the amount of alcohol consumed rather than with deficiences in the diet. A major challenge to the concept of the exclusively nutritional origin of alcoholic liver disease arose from an improvement in the method of alcohol feeding to experimental animals. Indeed, when the conventional alcohol feeding procedure is used, namely when ethanol is given as part of the drinking water, rats usually refuse to take a sufficient amount of ethanol to develop liver injury, if the diet is adequate. This aversion of rats to ethanol was counteracted by the introduction of the new technique of feeding ethanol as part of a nutritionally adequate totally liquid diet (105,156,157). With this procedure, ethanol intake was sufficient to produce a fatty liver despite an adequate diet. This technique is now widely adopted for the study of the pathogenesis of the fatty liver in the rat. In addition to the fatty liver, ethanol dependence developed in these rats, as witnessed by typical withdrawal seizures after cessation of alcohol intake (158).

Having established an etiologic role for ethanol in the pathogenesis of the experimental fatty liver, the question of its importance for the development of human pathology remained. To determine whether ingestion

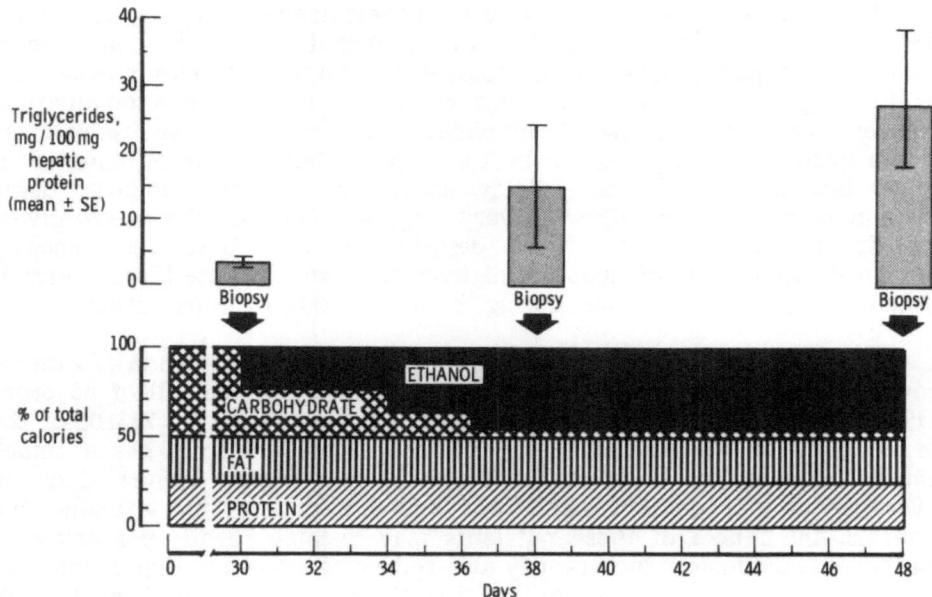

Fig. 9   Effect of ethanol on hepatic triglycerides in five volunteers given a high-protein, low-fat diet (159).

of alcohol, in amounts comparable to those consumed by chronic alcoholics, is capable of injuring the liver. even in the absence of dietary deficiencies, volunteers (with or without a history of alcoholism) were given a variety of nondeficient diets under metabolic ward conditions, with ethanol either as a supplement to the diet or as an isocaloric substitution for carbohydrates (71,105,156). In all these individuals, ethanol administration resulted in fatty liver development which was evident on both morphologic examination and by direct measurement of the lipid content of the liver biopsies which revealed a rise in triglyceride concentration up to 15 fold (Figure 9).

c)   The influence of dietary factors

    i) Role of dietary fat

    As discussed before, alcohol ingestion leads to deposition in the liver of dietary fat. This observation prompted an investigation into the role of the amount and kind of dietary fat in the pathogenesis of alcohol induced liver injury. Rats were given liquid diets containing a normal amount of protein for rodents (18% of total calories), with varying amounts of fat. Reduction in dietary fat to a level of 25% (or less) of total calories was accompanied by a significant decrease in the steatosis induced by ethanol (160). The importance of dietary fat was confirmed in volunteers: for a given alcohol intake, much more steatosis developed with diets of normal fat content than with a low fat diet (23). In addition to the amount, the chain length of the dietary fatty acid is also important for the degree of fat deposition in the liver after alcohol feeding. Replacement of dietary triglycerides containing long chain fatty acids (LCT) by fat containing medium chain fatty acids (MCT) markedly reduced the capacity of alcohol to produce a fatty liver in rats (16). The propensity of medium chain fatty acids to oxidation rather than to esterification most likely explains the reduction in alcoholic steatosis upon replacement of dietary long chain fatty acids by medium chain fatty acids.

ii) Role of protein and lipotropic factors (choline and methionine)

In perfused livers, ethanol was shown to increase choline uptake (161) but this was found to be unrelated to lipid accumulation (162). In growing rats. deficiencies in dietary protein and lipotropic factors (choline and methionine) can produce fatty liver (153) but primates are far less susceptible to protein and lipotrope deficiency than rodents (163). Clinically, treatment with choline of patients suffering from alcoholic liver injury has been found to be ineffective in the face of continued alcohol abuse (164) and, experimentally, massive supplementation with choline failed to prevent fatty liver produced by alcohol in volunteer subjects (165). This is not surprising, since there is no evidence that a diet which is deficient in choline is deleterious to adult man. Unlike rat liver, human liver contains very little choline oxidase activity which may explain the species difference with regard to choline deficiency. The phospholipid content of the liver represents another key difference between the ethanol and choline deficiency fatty liver. After the administration of ethanol, hepatic phospholipids increase (156) whereas in the fatty liver produced by choline deficiency, they decrease (166). Moreover, orotic acid which prevents the phospholipid decrease and the development of fatty liver due to choline deficiency, had no such effects after ethanol (167). Furthermore, hepatic ATP decreased after chronic ethanol feeding (168-170), but was unaffected in choline deficiency (171). Conversely, hepatic carnitine is decreased by choline deficiency (172) but increased after ethanol feeding (173). Moreover, ethanol induced fatty liver is associated with increased circulatory lipoproteins and enhanced incorporation of ^{14}C lysine into lipoproteins (109) whereas the opposite occurs with choline deficiency (174). Ultrastructurally, the lesions also differ (69,175). Thus, hepatic injury induced by choline deficiency appears to be primarily an experimental disease of rats with little, if any, relevance to alcoholic liver injury particularly in humans. Even in the rats, massive choline supplementation failed. to prevent fully the ethanol induced lesion, whether alcohol was administered acutely (176) or chronically (177). Alcohol has been reported to either aggravate (178) or attenuate (179) choline induced liver injury.

Protein deficiency may affect the liver but this has not yet been clearly delineated in human adults. In children, protein deficiency leads to steatosis, one of the manifestations of Kwashiorkor. In adolescent baboons, however, protein restriction to 7% of total calories (as part of a low fat diet, 14% of calories) did not result in liver injury on either biochemical analysis or light and electron microscopic examination even after 19 months (180). Conversely, an excess of protein was not capable of preventing ethanol from producing fat accumulation in human volunteers, as illustrated in Figure 9. In that study, dietary protein represented 25% of total calories, or 2½ times the recommended amount. Thus, even in the absence of protein deficiency, ethanol is capable, in man, of producing striking changes in the liver. Severe protein deficiency (4% of total calories) also produced steatosis in the baboon (180). Similar lesions were reported in the Rhesus monkey (181). When protein deficiency is present, it could potentiate the effect of ethanol. Indeed administration of ethanol with a diet deficient in protein and lipotropic factors had more pronounced effects than that of either factor alone (25,182), at least in rodents. Possible interactions of ethanol and protein nutrition were also suggested by the observation that ethanol feeding increases the activities of hepatic cystathionine synthetase and S-methyl-tetra-hydrofolate homocysteine methyltransferase, which may impair mechanisms for methionine conservation in protein deficiency (183). To what extent such abnormalities contribute to the ethanol induced liver lesions remains to be assessed. In any event, the ultrastructural abnormalities produced by protein deficiency (184,185) differ from those resulting from alcohol (53,69). Furthermore clinical protein malnutrition is associated with characteristic plasma amino acid abnormalities, including a depression of branched chain amino acids (186) whereas the alcohol induced liver injury in the well fed baboon was associated with opposite amino acid changes (186). Of course, in chronic alcoholic patients plasma amino acid abnormalities may reflect a complex interaction of many factors: nutrition, alcoholic liver disease, alcohol induced injury in other organs and associated disease states. The frequent concurrence of chronic alcoholism and nutrional deficiency makes the separation of these variables especially difficult. However, whereas branched chain amino acids (BCAA) and alpha amino-n-butyric acid (AANB) were found to be increased 2-3 fold and 7 fold respectively in the plasma of baboons fed alcohol as 50% of total calories (187), these amino acids are all depressed when measured in protein deficiency. Following intestinal bypass for obesity, decreased absorption of dietary protein is observed (188). In such patients, plasma BCAA, phenylalanine, threonine and lysine are decreased while plasma serine and glycine, both non-essential amino acids, are increased.

In patients studied at the Bronx Veterans Administration Hospital with a diagnosis of chronic alcoholism and alcoholic liver disease, plasma amino acid patterns similar to those described in patients by Zinnemen et al. (189), Ning et al. (190) and Siegel et al. (191) were found with depressions of BCAA, normal levels of AANB and slight depressions of plasma proline (192). The combination of low BCAA and relatively increased AANB was considered characteristic of changes of plasma amino acids in alcoholic liver disease (192), and the ratio of plasma AANB/leucine was found to reflect chronic alcohol consumption independent of liver injury or malnutrition (193).

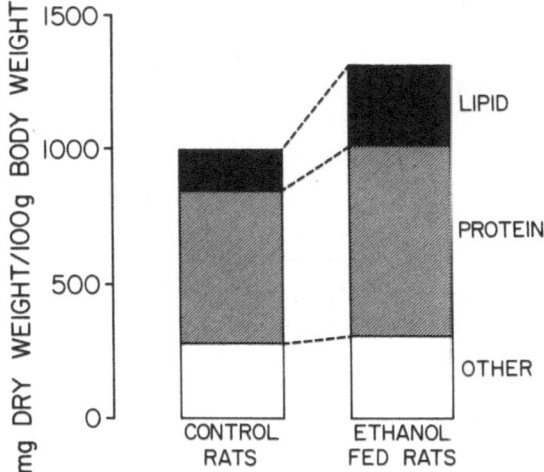

Fig. 10   *Effect of ethanol feeding on hepatic dry weight, lipid and protein contents (194).*

2.   Transitional Lesions From Alcohol Fatty Liver to Hepatitis

    a)   Accumulation of proteins in the alcoholic fatty liver and impair-
        ment of lipoprotein and protein export: Recent studies have
indicated that in addition to fat accumulation, the alcoholic fatty liver is
characterized by striking deposition of protein (194). In the early stages of
fatty liver development, this protein accumulation was found to be as
important quantitively as that of fat and contributed to a similar extent to
the hepatomegaly which developed after chronic alcoholism (Figure 10).
Although increasing organelle proteins (mitochondria and microsomes) do
contribute to the total increase, the major fraction of the proteins is
deposited in the cytosol. The nature of all the proteins which accumulate in
the cytosol has not been elucidated but up to now, increases have been found
in export proteins such as albumin and transferrin (195) but not in
constituent proteins of the cytosol. This observation led to the hypothesis
that one of the early lesions induced by chronic alcoholism may be the
interference with the capacity of the liver to export proteins. Consistent
with this concept was the finding of a decrease in hepatic microtubulin
believed to be implicated in the export of proteins from the liver (195) and
delayed serum albumin labelling after administration of labelled amino acids
(195). The retention of protein may be responsible for the "ballooning" of
the hepatocytes, a common morphologic alteration found in alcohol liver
injury, and the decrease in plasma transferrin in alcoholics with or without
cirrhosis (196).

In addition to protein release, lipoprotein secretion is also affected. Contrasting with the hyperlipemia, which is commonly associated with the administration of moderate to large amounts of ethanol, an extremely high dose has been reported to decrease serum triglycerides (197), very low density lipoproteins (198), high density lipoproteins (199), and the incorporation of glucosamine into the carbohydrate moiety of serum lipoproteins (200) in the rat.

In volunteers, chronic ethanol administration resulted in initial hyperlipemia (105). However, blood lipid content declined after 2-3 weeks (Figure 8), implying that lipoprotein output falls with progressing alcoholic liver disease. This concept is supported by the study of Marzo et al (201) who correlated serum lipids with histologic stage in 90 alcoholics. Peak serum lipid values were found during the stage of fatty metamorphosis. During the succeeding stages of steatosis and interstitial chronic hepatitis, a progressive decrease in serum lipids occurred. The decrease was predominantly in the triglyceride and cholesterol fractions. In well established cirrhosis, circulating lipoproteins are generally low (202). In addition, alpha lipoproteins are absent by electrophoresis in sera from cirrhotic patients (203), which illustrates another lipoprotein abnormality.

The progression of liver injury to alcoholic hepatitis in primates is associated with an enhancement of the steatosis (204). Our preliminary observations also indicate that serum lipoproteins decrease with advancing liver damage (205), suggesting the disappearance of the compensatory role that alcoholic hyperlipemia exerts on the development of fatty liver.

b) Alterations in protein synthesis: After chronic alcohol consumption, the membranes of the rough endoplasmic reticulum (RER) appear decreased on electron microscopy (53,69,71,206), and this reduction has now been substantiated by chemical fractionation (73). One of the main functions of the rough endoplasmic reticulum is protein synthesis. The subject of the interaction of ethanol with protein synthesis is complex and not fully elucidated, especially after chronic ethanol consumption. The effects may actually differ after acute and chronic ethanol administration. The administration of a single dose of ethanol to naive rats and the incubation of liver tissue in ethanol-containing media generally result in inhibitory effects on the production of liver and plasma proteins. Sometimes, these acute effects can be attributed to a direct action of high ethanol concentrations (207,208) or they depend on the route of administration (209). In other experimental situations, in which the ethanol concentrations achieved are compatible with moderate intoxication, the inhibitory effects appear to be associated with relative lack of amino acids (210-214): this inhibition of hepatic production of plasma proteins mimics that of fasting, is aggravated by fasting and is abolished by amino acid supplementation (210-213). A third experimental situation in which ethanol was shown to exert inhibitory effects on protein synthesis was obtained when liver slices (from fed or fasted rats) were incubated in a medium containing ethanol and only trace amounts of amino acids (214). The decreased incorporation of amino acid into the liver protein could result from reduced uptake (215,217) and/or decreased synthesis. Chronic ethanol consumption has been reported to be accompanied by enhanced liver protein synthesis (207,218). Only when ethanol feeding was associated with obvious signs of undernutrition was decreased protein production observed (219,220). Under those conditions ethanol feeding failed to sustain body growth and did not produce fatty liver and hepatic enlargement. Those results, therefore, are not directly relevant to the prevailing clinical situation of the alcoholic characterized by fatty liver and hepatomegaly. However, this clinical combination of fatty liver and hepatomegaly was reproduced with the administration of ethanol in liquid diets (156,157). As discussed before, the hepatomegaly is due to the retention of both fat and protein. Alteration of protein synthesis under these conditions is still being investigated.

c) Development of mitochondrial injury: In addition to the alterations of the rough endoplasmic reticulum, alcoholics are known to have profound hepatic mitochondrial changes (51) which are associated with increased serum activity of the intramitochondrial enzyme glutamate dehydrogenase (221). From these clinical observations, however, it was impossible to assess whether the mitochondrial changes were a direct result of chronic ethanol intake or were secondary to other factors such as dietary deficiencies. Recent studies have incriminated alcohol itself as the responsible agent and have clarified some functional counterparts of the ultrastructural lesions.

i) Ultrastructural changes of mitochondria

Chronic alcohol consumption results in striking mitochondrial alterations which include swelling and disfiguration of mitochondria, disorientation of the cristae, and intramitochondrial crystalline inclusions (51,52). Similarly, in the rat, isocaloric substitution of ethanol for carbohydrate in otherwise adequate diets leads to enlargement and alterations of the configurations of the mitochondria (69) indicating that ethanol itself or one of its metabolites causes the alterations rather than dietary deficiencies. Mitochondrial changes similar to those seen in chronic alcoholics were also produced by isocaloric substitution of ethanol for carbohydrate in baboons (180) and in man, both in alcoholics (53,71) and in non-alcoholics (165). Degenerated mitochondria were conspicuous and the debris of these degraded organelles was also found within autophagic vacuoles and residual vacuolated bodies (206). The striking structural changes of the mitochondria are associated with corresponding functional abnormalities.

ii) Alterations of mitochondrial functions; alcoholic ketoacidosis

These injured mitochondria have a reduction in cytochrome a and b content (222) and in succinic dehydrogenase activity (222,223) although in one study (224) succinic dehydrogenase activity measured in total liver homogenates was reported to be increased in ethanol-fed rats. The respiratory capacity of the mitochondria was found to be depressed (55,225 227) using pyruvate succinate and acetaldehyde as substrates. Oxidation of other substrates was also found to be reduced in mitochondria of ethanol-fed rats, except for α-glycerophosphate, the oxidation of which was reported by

some to be increased (228) or unchanged (229) whereas others found it to be
decreased (226).

Oxidative phosphorylation was found to be selectively altered at site I
(230). Since the structural changes of the mitochondria persist, the question
arose as to whether these in turn could be responsible for some alterations in
lipid metabolism beyond those which were attributed to the altered redox
change. The first indication that ethanol consumption may result in more
persistent metabolic changes came from the observation that alcohol
ingestion is associated with a progressive increase in ketonemia and
ketonuria, which was most pronounced in the fasting state (231) (Figures 11
and 12). The ketonemia may aggravate the acidosis of the hyperlactacidemia (105) and on occasion, may lead to severe alcoholic ketoacidosis
(232,233). The capacity for ethanol to produce ketonemia was found to be
greater than that of fat itself, provided however that fat was present in the
diet. Thus, fat seems to play a permissive role (231) (Table I). Mitochondria
obtained from ethanol-fed rats, when incubated in vitro, even in the absence
of ethanol, display decreased capacity to oxidize fatty acids, but enhanced
β-oxidation which is possibly responsible for the increased ketogenesis (63).

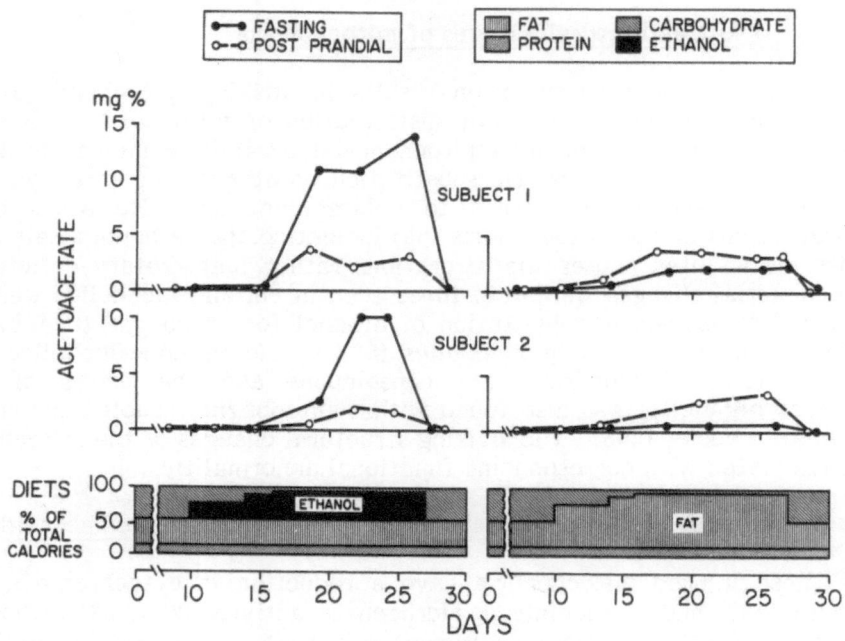

Fig. 11   The effect of isocaloric replacement of dietary carbohydrate
             (by either alcohol or fat) on blood acetoacetate concentration in
             two subjects, both in the fasting and postprandial states (231).

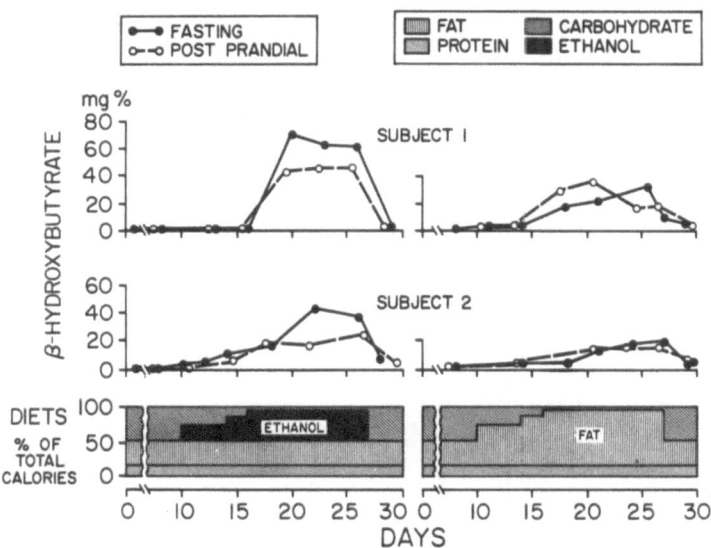

Fig. 12   The effect of isocaloric replacement of dietary carbohydrate
(by either alcohol or fat) on blood β-hydroxybutyrate concentration in two subjects, both in the fasting and postprandial states
(231).

Decreased fatty acid oxidation, whether as a function of the reduced citric
acid cycle activity (secondary to the altered redox potential), as discussed
before or whether as a consequence of permanent changes in mitochondrial
structure (as emphasized in this paragraph) offers the most likely explanation for the deposition of fat in the liver after chronic alcohol ingestion,
especially fat derived from the diet (23-26).   It is noteworthy that high
concentrations of acetaldehyde, the product of ethanol metabolism, mimic
the defects produced by chronic ethanol consumption on oxidative phosphorylation at site I (54).   One may wonder to what extent chronic exposure
to acetaldehyde is the cause for the defect observed after chronic ethanol
consumption, especially since it was found recently that after chronic
ethanol consumption, mitochondria become more susceptible to the toxic
effects of acetaldehyde; the latter were manifest already at 0.2 mM
acetaldehyde (234), a concentration reported in the liver in vivo after
ethanol administration.   As has been pointed out alcoholics may exhibit
higher acetaldehyde levels than non-alcoholics for a given ethanol load and
blood level. It is therefore not unreasonable to speculate that exposure to
high acetaldehyde levels may in turn affect mitochondrial function and
result in a vicious cycle depicted in Figure 13.

There are of course other possible mechanisms for increased acetaldehyde levels and aggravation of mitochondrial injury. Several studies of blood

TABLE I

EFFECT OF ETHANOL AND (OR) DIETARY FAT ON BLOOD KETONES (mg/100 ml) (231)

Diet composition (% of total calories)				No. of Subjects	β-Hydroxybutyrate		Acetoacetate	
Ethanol	Fat	Carbo-hydrate	Protein		Fasting	Postprandial	Fasting	Postprandial
–	36	49	15	4	1.8±0.4	2.1±0.2	0.27±0.06	0.26±0.05
46	36	3	15	4	49.9±6.3	27.4±4.9	7.6±0.9	1.7±0.2
–	82	3	15	4	15.8±3.0	16.2±2.1	2.2±0.5	2.3±0.3
–	5	80/70	15/25	6	1.2±0.4	1.7±0.6	0.26±0.07	0.29±0.08
46	5	34	15	3	2.9±0.5	3.6±0.5	0.27±0.07	0.17±0.02
60	5	10	25	3	5.2±0.9	4.2±0.8	0.44±0.10	0.29±0.12
66	5	4	25	1	9.5±0.5	7.1±1.9	1.0±0.4	0.53±0.18

Chronic ethanol consumption

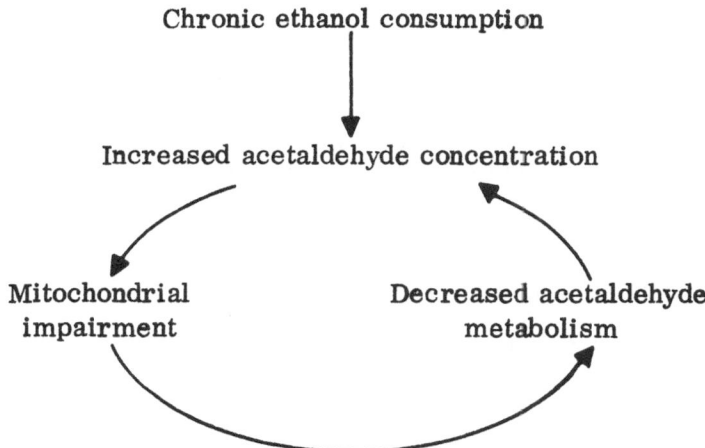

Fig. 13   *Possible relation between ethanol consumption, altered acetaldehyde levels, and mitochondrial impairment (55).*

acetaldehyde levels following oral ingestion of various alcoholic beverages have been performed.   Majchrowicz and Mendelson (235) showed that acetaldehyde levels in the blood of chronic alcoholic patients were higher after bourbon ingestion than after grain ethyl alcohol and attributed this difference to the acetaldehyde content of the bourbon. Truitt (236) followed levels of acetaldehyde after oral administration of vodka that resulted in modest elevations of blood ethanol; slightly higher levels of acetaldehyde were found in alcoholic subjects when compared with nonalcoholics. However, Freund (237) could find no measureable amounts of serum acetaldehyde after oral ingestion of an aqueous acetaldehyde solution ten times in excess of the concentration found in most bourbons.

Since the amount of acetaldehyde in even the "dirtiest" of alcoholic beverages is about one thousandth the amount produced by ethanol oxidation in the liver, it is probably not the acetaldehyde in the beverage that leads to higher blood acetaldehyde levels after ingestion, but more likely an effect of other congeners of the beverages. These congeners may somehow interfere with acetaldehyde metabolism initiating a vicious cycle of mitochondrial impairment which further decreases acetaldehyde catabolism. For example, Rubenstein et al. (238) found that pyrogallol (1 and 10 mM concentrations), a metabolic product of gallic acid found in tannins, inhibits rat liver aldehyde dehydrogenase activity in vitro. In vivo, Collins et al. (239) have shown that pyrogallol (250 mg/kg, i.p.) increases acetaldehyde blood levels in rats when it is given one hour before ethanol (3 gm/kg, i.p.).   Higher aliphatic aldehydes were found to inhibit mitochondrial acetaldehyde metabolism (240).   Thus elevated acetaldehyde levels following ingestion of alcoholic beverages (discussed above) when compared with acetaldehyde levels following ethanol-acetaldehyde mixture suggest an effect of congeners on acetaldehyde metabolism. When taken in relatively moderate amounts for a short period of time, the congener content of alcoholic beverages did not appear to affect the degree of steatosis (241) but the effects of higher amounts of congeners in conjunction with a greater alcohol intake over a longer period of time have not been extensively studied. Some evidence was recently presented that prolonged consumption of whiskey might exert more striking undesirable effects on the liver than pure ethanol (242) and that certain alcoholic beverages, particularly brandy, were more toxic to liver cell cultures than pure ethanol (243).

d)   Various effects of alcohol upon liver and serum enzymes: Alcohol abuse is often associated with reciprocal liver and serum enzyme changes, which again illustrates the hepatotoxicity of ethanol and suggests that parenchymal injury often complicates so-called "simple fatty liver". Indeed, serum isocitric dehydrogenase and ornithine carbamyltransferase activities are increased after ethanol ingestion (244) whereas hepatic isocitric dehydrogenase is reduced (245). Serum glutamyl transpeptidase activity is commonly found increased in alcoholics (246-249), probably as a nonspecific witness of liver injury, since this enzyme is increased in many types of liver diseases (250). In man, serum transaminases are also increased after ethanol administration (165, 251) reflecting either liver or muscle damage, or both. In rats given ethanol, hepatic glutamic-pyruvic transferase activity is also found to be decreased (252). Hepatic tryptophan oxygenase increased after acute ethanol administration in vivo (253,254), but decreases after chronic ethanol consumption (254), or when isolated livers are perfused with ethanol in vitro (255). The latter effect may be secondary to the acidosis produced by ethanol (256). Hepatic glucagon-responsive adenyl cyclase (but not the epinephrine-responsive component) is activated by ethanol (256). Hepatic coenzyme A is found to be reduced after ethanol by some (257) but not by others (258,259).

e)   Alterations of the immune system in alcoholic liver injury: Serum immunoglobulins are usually increased in patients with alcoholic liver disease (260) and they include some autoantibodies (261). In the last few years an increased body of evidence suggests that lymphocytes play an important role in tissue damaging immune reactions and autoimmunity. A cell-mediated mechanism has also been implicated in some chronic liver diseases. Changes in cellular immunity that have been documented in chronic alcoholic liver disease include loss of delayed hypersensitivity (262) decreased "active" T rosette formation (263), decreased lymphocyte response to phytohemagglutinin (264), and a pronounced decrease in peripheral blood T lymphocytes in patients with alcoholic hepatitis (265), suggesting that there is a basic impairment in cell-mediated immunity in alcoholic liver diseases. The pathogenetic role of the stimulation of lymphocytic transformation by ethanol in patients with alcoholic hepatitis (266) has not been clarified; it is relatively nonspecific since ethanol produces a similar change in patients with chronic active hepatitis (266). The observation of increased in vitro lymphocytic transformation in response to Australian antigen in patients with chronic alcoholic liver disease (267) is intriguing. In rats fed ethanol for 3 months, a delayed hypersensitivity to dinitrochlorobenzene was found (268). However, it is not known whether immunological reactions actually play any role in the induction and perpetuation of alcoholic liver disease. An altered cell-mediated immunity to liver antigens has been described in patients with alcoholic hepatitis using either autologous liver (266), normal human liver (269) or alcoholic hyaline (270). Finally it has recently been shown that lymphocytes from baboons with alcoholic hepatitis are cytotoxic against autologous liver cells in tissue culture (271). These observations suggest that immunological mechanisms may be involved in the perpetuation of hepatic damage produced by alcohol and while they do not provide direct support for this possibility they justify further investigation directed at determining the role of immunological factors in the development and progression of alcoholic liver disease, keeping in mind however that ethanol has more than one effect on the human immune system, as demonstrated by the inhibition, by alcohol, of bone marrow granulocyte colonies (272).

3.   Alcoholic Hepatitis and Cirrhosis

It has been known for a long time that alcoholics may display liver complications of a varying degree of severity ranging from the still reversible fatty liver to alcoholic hepatitis and finally irreversible cirrhosis. The relationship between alcoholic fatty liver and alcoholic hepatitis and cirrhosis (characterized by extensive scarring or fibrosis) may be, at least in part, a consequence of the necrosis and inflammation associated with the alcoholic hepatitis. Whether the fatty liver is a precursor for the hepatitis has been less well accepted (Figure 14). As has been pointed out, although hepatic fat accumulation by itself may be harmless, it reflects severe metabolic disturbance in the liver. It is possible that this disturbance, when exaggerated, may eventually engender irreversible damage of the hepatocyte possibly through one of the mechanisms described under "Transitional lesions from fatty liver to alcoholic hepatitis". Necrosis in turn could lead

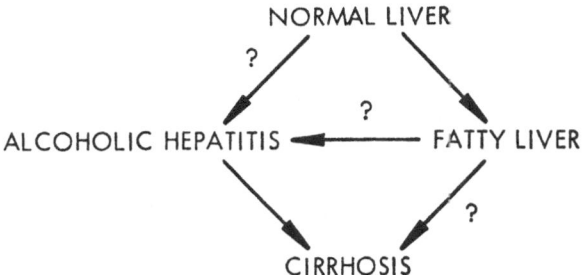

Fig. 14   Possible links between the three types of liver injury in the alcoholic (1).

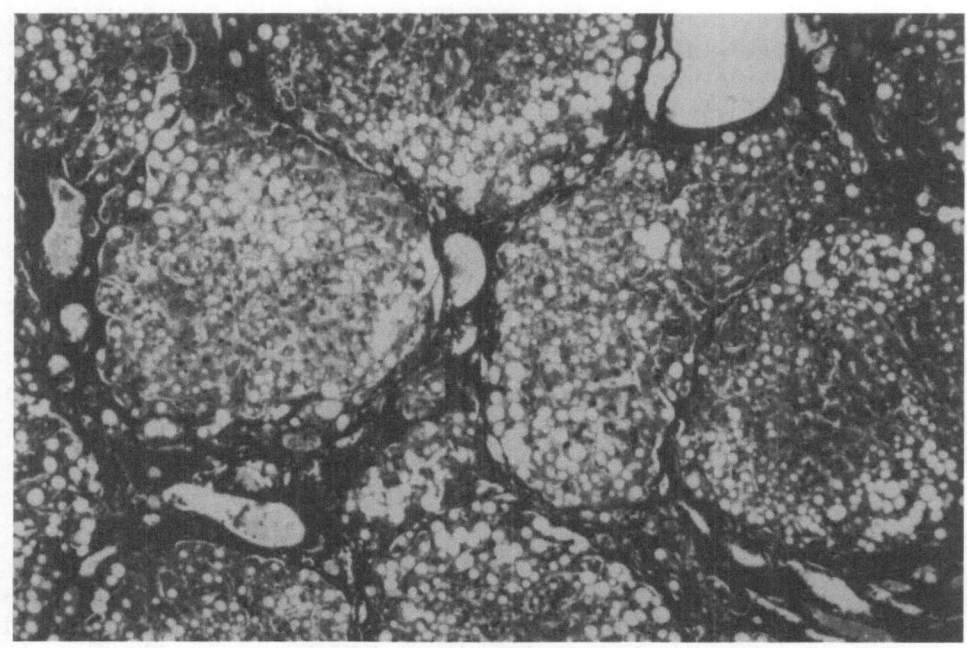

Fig. 15   Cirrhosis in a baboon fed alcohol for four years.   Fat is
               regularly distributed through hepatic nodules surrounded by
               connective tissue septa. (Chromotrope-aniline blue; x60) (204).

to inflammation, resulting in alcoholic hepatitis.   Indeed, comparable
electron microscopic changes of the mitochondria accompany alcoholic
hepatitis (51) and the fatty liver, as described in a preceding section.
Alteration of the rough endoplasmic reticulum was also found in patients
with alcoholic hepatitis (51).   Although the alcoholic fatty liver is not an
inflammatory condition, and is distinguishable from alcoholic hepatitis by
light microscopy, the remarkable similarity of the ultrastructural features in
the hepatocytes suggests that the former may represent the precursor of the
latter.   Other fatty livers, however, such as that of Kwashiorkor, do not
undergo transformation to cirrhosis (273).   Moreover, rats fed alcohol in
liquid diets, though they get a fatty liver, do not develop the more severe
forms of liver injury seen in alcoholics, namely hepatitis and cirrhosis. Thus
although the fatty liver could clearly be attributed to ethanol itself, in the
case of cirrhosis, the question remained whether factors other than ethanol
may play a key role, particularly malnutrition.

        The long standing debate whether the liver injury so commonly observed
in the alcoholic is due to malnutrition rather than alcohol per se was

rekindled by a report of Patek et al. (274). In this epidemiological study of 304 alcoholic patients, alcohol intake and dietary habits were evaluated. There were 195 patients with hepatic cirrhosis, 40 precirrhotics and 69 noncirrhotics. By history, alcohol contributed 50-58% of total calories. Two-thirds of the patients drank for more than twenty years. Duration and degree of alcohol abuse was comparable in all three groups. Dietary intake however differed. Over the two year period preceding the presenting illness, noncirrhotics had high food caloric intake and higher protein intake than the cirrhotics. This type of retrospective study, however, is complicated by the difficulty in differentiating cause and effect. It is well known that complications of severe liver disease, particularly cirrhosis, can by themselves be reasons for poor dietary intake. It is therefore not clear whether the differences in dietary intake between cirrhotics and noncirrhotics is the cause rather than a consequence of that disease.

The etiologic role of alcohol per se (in the absence of dietary deficiency) in the pathogenesis of alcoholic liver injury was assessed in experimental studies carried out in the baboon. Indeed failure to produce hepatitis and cirrhosis with alcohol in the rat might be due to the fact that in that species, even when alcohol is given as part of a liquid diet, its intake does not exceed 36% of total calories which corresponds to moderate consumption in man. Of potential importance was also the fact that whereas in the human, development of cirrhosis requires five to twenty years of steady drinking, the rat only lives about two years. To overcome this difficulty, we turned to the baboon, a species which is long-lived and phylogenetically closer to man than the rat. First, baboons were given a dose of ethanol similar to that of the rat (that is 36% of total calories) and again a fatty liver developed but no hepatitis or cirrhosis (180). The dose of alcohol was then increased to 50% of the total calories, taking advantage of the liquid diet technique first developed in the rat and now applied to the baboon (204). With this diet alcohol intake was sufficient to result in periods of obvious inebriation. Upon interruption of alcohol administration, some withdrawal symptoms (such as seizures) were observed. These experiments are still in progress but at the writing of this paper the following results have been observed: 16 baboons fed the isocaloric control diet retained normal livers, whereas the animals given ethanol all developed excessive fat accumulation. In addition, 5 showed mild alcoholic hepatitis and in 6 baboons studied for 2-4 years, cirrhosis evolved (Figure 15). However, severe inflammatory lesions sometimes seen in patients with a fulminant type of alcoholic hepatitis were not observed. The diagnosis of alcoholic hepatitis was based on necrosis and inflammation; although sometimes present, alcoholic hyaline of Mallory was not a required feature.

It has been widely postulated that the hepatitis, through the necrosis and inflammation, may in turn initiate scarring (or fibrosis) and, eventually cirrhosis. The earliest deposition of fibrous tissue appears to occur in the central zones of the hepatic lobule leading to what has been called "central hyaline sclerosis", a lesion commonly associated with alcoholic hepatitis (275). The appearance of this lesion appears to bridge the gap between alcoholic hepatitis and cirrhosis, and supports the theory that one is a precursor of the other. Similar lesions were present already at the fatty liver stage in the baboons fed alcohol. The magnitude of central hyaline sclerosis correlated with the degree of portal hypertension (276). Thus, for the first time an experimental model has now been developed (204) which reproduces all the liver lesions observed in the alcoholic namely the fatty liver, the hepatitis and the cirrhosis (277).

This study, by showing that animals which display fatty liver with a moderate alcohol intake developed hepatitis and cirrhosis when the alcohol content of the diet was increased supports the possibility that the fatty liver may be a precursor state for the hepatitis and cirrhosis. In addition, it was found that in the fatty liver phase there was an increase in chemically detectable collagen (8), the protein which is the hallmark for the fibrosis characteristic of cirrhosis and central sclerosis (276). This was associated with enhanced activity of peptidylproline hydroxylase, an enzyme active in the initial steps of fibrogenesis (8). Increased activity of this enzyme was confirmed in livers of alcoholics (278,279). This was associated with increased urinary hydroxy proline excretion in the case of alcoholic hepatitis (280).

Not all baboons fed ethanol progressed to cirrhosis; similarly, not all alcoholics develop this complication: the incidence varies depending on duration and dose of alcohol intake (281). Regardless of possible predisposing factors, the baboon study clarifies the respective role of malnutrition and alcohol itself in the pathogenesis of alcoholic hepatitis and cirrhosis. As discussed before, the fatty liver can be produced by ethanol per se in the absence of dietary deficiencies (71,105,156,165). Thus, one may conclude from our studies that despite the evidence produced before indicating that malnutrition can cause liver damage, alcohol itself is an indispensable etiologic agent for the development of the typical complications observed in the alcoholic. An important corollary of this finding is the fact that adequate diet did not prevent the development of the alcoholic lesions. The therapeutic implication of this observation is that alcoholics cannot fully prevent the development or the aggravation of liver injury by maintaining an adequate diet unless they also control the degree of alcohol intake. It has been shown in the past by others and our own group that alcohol ingestion results in impaired digestion, malabsorption and that it produces intestinal injury (282). It is unlikely however that the effects described are of sufficient magnitude to offset the large excess of nutrients present in our baboon diet. Moreover, preliminary studies have indicated the absence of protein and fat malabsorption under our experimental conditions (J. Lindenbaum and C.S. Lieber, unpublished observation). Furthermore, as discussed before, plasma amino acid changes observed in these baboons were the opposite of those produced by protein malnutrition (enhanced as opposed to depressed branch-chain amino acids) (187). The possibility that nutritional deficiencies may potentiate the effect of alcohol is presently being investigated in the baboon, since such a phenomenon was observed for the fatty liver in the rat (25). Whether this applies to clinical conditions and particularly the development of cirrhosis is less clear.

Epidemiologic studies of Lelbach (155,281) did not detect dietary insufficiency as a precondition for alcoholic cirrhosis: the incidence of cirrhosis correlated with the amount of alcohol consumed, not with history of dietary deficiencies; similar results were observed in France by Péquignot (154). Recently some have even suggested a lowered incidence of cirrhosis with dietary insufficiency (283), whereas others as discussed before reached the opposite conclusion (274). Regardless of the controversy surrounding the role of malnutrition in the pathogenesis of liver injury in the alcoholic, in our present state of knowledge, one is still justified in stressing the importance of correcting nutrient deficiencies when present.

SUMMARY

Alcohol induced liver changes proceed in three partially overlapping stages: metabolic effects directly associated with the oxidation of ethanol, followed, after chronic ethanol consumption, by an adaptive increase of some of the liver functions and persistent liver injury.

The changes linked to the metabolism of ethanol itself can be attributed mostly to the hydrogen generated by the oxidation of ethanol by the ADH pathway and the associated increase in NADH/NAD ratio. These effects include hyperlactacidemia and hyperuricemia, reduced gluconeogenesis (and hypoglycemia) and also enhanced lipogenesis and decreased lipid oxidation both of which promote steatosis. Ethanol is also oxidized via an accessory pathway, the microsomal ethanol oxidizing system (MEOS) which has now been reconstituted with cytochrome P-450, NADPH, cytochrome-c reductase and phospholipids, components of the microsomal drug metabolizing enzyme system. The oxidation of ethanol is associated with inhibition of the metabolism of some drugs, probably through competition for a partially common microsomal detoxification process.

Chronic ethanol consumption is followed by adaptive increases in the activity of various microsomal systems: MEOS (with enhanced rates of ethanol metabolism), drug detoxification (with accelerated drug metabolism) and lipoprotein formation (with the development of hyperlipemia). Side effects include increased activation of and susceptibility to some hepatotoxic agents (such as CCl_4) and a hypermetabolic state associated with energy wastage. Finally, hepatic injury develops. "Ballooning" of the hepatocyte results, at least in part, from an interference by ethanol with the export of proteins from the liver, leading to their accumulation in the cytosol, with swelling of the hepatocyte; hepatomegaly is caused as much by protein as by fat accumulation. In addition, structure and function of mitochondria deteriorate which secondarily promotes steatosis through decreased lipid oxidation. Blood acetaldehyde also increases because of decreased acetaldehyde oxidation by the affected mitochondria. In turn, the elevation of blood acetaldehyde may contribute to liver injury through direct toxic effects of acetaldehyde on various functions including those of the mitochondria, resulting in further elevation of blood acetaldehyde. Fibrosis can be caused by several mechanisms: enhanced collagen formation during the early stages of liver injury and as a response to necrosis and inflammation. Ethanol can be incriminated as a direct etiologic agent of the liver injury, since the entire spectrum of liver lesions has been reproduced experimentally in baboons fed alcohol, despite an adequate diet. Central sclerosis appeared at a precirrhotic stage and was associated with the development of early portal hypertension. Lymphocytes acquired cyto-toxicity against cultured liver cells. However, the inflammatory component in the liver was moderate and less pronounced than the "florid" alcoholic hepatitis sometimes observed in man. Thus, the baboon model closely mimics the clinical course of a majority of alcoholics who develop steatosis, moderate inflammation and necrosis and eventually cirrhosis.

REFERENCES

1.   LIEBER CS, DECARLI LM: Metabolic aspects of alcohol on the liver. In Metabolic Aspects of Alcoholism, Chapter 2. C.S. Lieber, (ed.). Lancaster,England, Medical and Technical Publishing Co., Ltd., 1976. In press.

2.   LIEBER CS, DAVIDSON CS: Some metabolic effects of ethyl alcohol. Am J Med 33: 319-327, 1962

3.   FREINKEL N, ARKEY RA: Effects of alcohol on carbohydrate metabolism in man. Psychosom Med 28: 551-563, 1966

4.   LIEBER CS, LEEVY CM, STEIN SW, GEORGE WS, CHERRICK GR, ABELMANN WH, DAVIDSON CS: Effect of ethanol on plasma free fatty acids in man. J Lab Clin Med 59: 826-832, 1862

5.   LIEBER CS, JONES DP, LOSOWSKY MS, DAVIDSON CS: Inter-relation of uric acid and ethanol metabolism in man. J Clin Invest 41: 1863-1870, 1962

6.   OLIN JS, DEVENYI P, WELDON KL: Uric acid in alcoholics. Quart J Stud Alcohol 34: 1202-1207, 1973

7.   NEWCOMBE DS: Ethanol metabolism and uric acid. Metabolism 21: 1193-1203, 1972

8.   FEINMAN L, LIEBER CS: Hepatic collagen metabolism: Effect of alcohol consumption in rats and baboons. Science 176: 795, 1972

9.   NIKKILA EA, OJALA K: Role of hepatic L-α-glycerophosphate and triglyceride synthesis in production of fatty liver by ethanol. Proc Soc Exp Biol Med 113: 814-817, 1963

10.   JOHNSON O: Influence of the blood ethanol concentration on the acute ethanol-induced liver triglyceride accumulation in rats. Scand J Gastroenterology 2: 207-213, 1974

11.   LIEBER CS, SCHMID R: The effect of ethanol on fatty acid metabolism; Stimulation of hepatic fatty acid synthesis in vitro. J Clin Invest 40: 394-399, 1961.

12.   GORDON ER: Effect of an intoxicating dose of ethanol on lipid metabolism in an isolated, perfused rat liver.   Biochem Pharmacol 21: 2991-3004, 1972

13.   GUYNN RW, VELOSO D, HARRIS RI, LAWSON JWR, VEECH RI: Ethanol administration and the relationship of malonyl-coenzyme A concentrations to the rate of fatty acid synthesis in rat liver. Biochem J 136: 639-647, 1973

14.   ARAKAWA M, TAKETOMI S, FURUNO K, MATSUO T, IWATSUKA H, SUZUOKI Z: Metabolic studies on the development of ethanol-induced fatty liver in KK-Ay mice. J Nutr 105: 1500-1508, 1975

15.   FORSANDER OA, MAENPAA PH, SALASPURO MP: Influence of ethanol on the lactate/pyruvate and β-hydroxybutyrate /acetoacetate ratios in rat liver experiments. Acta Chem Scand 19: 1770-1771, 1965

16.   LIEBER CS, LEFEVRE A, SPRITZ N, FEINMAN L, DECARLI LM: Difference in hepatic metabolism of long- and medium-chain fatty acids: The role of fatty acid chain length in the production of the alcoholic fatty liver. J Clin Invest 46: 1451-1460, 1967

17.   ONTKO JA: Effects of ethanol on the metabolism of free fatty acids in isolated liver cells. J Lipid Res 14: 78-86, 1973

18.   WILLIAMSON JR, SCHOLZ R, BROWNING ET, THURMAN RG FUKAMI MH: Metabolic effects of ethanol in perfused rat liver. J Biol Chem 244: 5044-5054, 1969

19.   FRITZ IB: Factors influencing the rates of long-chain fatty acid oxidation and synthesis in mammalian systems. Physiol Rev 41: 52-129, 1961

20.   BOMSTRAND R, KAGER L, LANTTO O: Studies on the ethanol-induced decrease of fatty acid oxidation in rat and human liver slices. Life Sci 13: 1131-1141, 1973

21.   FISCHEL P, OETTE K: Experimental Untersuchungen an menschlichen Leberpunktaten und Rattenleberschnitten zur Oxidation von Fettsäuren mit unterschiedlicher Kettenlänge und unterschiedlicher Zahl von Doppelbindungen. Res exp Med 163: 1-16, 1974

22.   BLOMSTRAND R, KAGER L: The combustion of triolein-1-^{14}C and
       its inhibition by alcohol in man. Life Sci 13: 113-123, 1973

23.   LIEBER CS, SPRITZ N: Effects of prolonged ethanol intake in man:
       Role of dietary, adipose, endogenously synthesized fatty acids in
       the pathogenesis of the alcoholic fatty liver. J Clin Invest 45:
       1400-1411, 1966

24.   LIEBER CS, SPRITZ N, DECARLI LM: Role of dietary, adipose and
       endogenously synthesized fatty acids in the pathogenesis of the
       alcoholic fatty liver. J Clin Invest 45: 51-62, 1966

25.   LIEBER CS, SPRITZ N, DECARLI LM: Fatty liver produced by
       dietary deficiencies: Its pathogenesis and potentiation by
       ethanol. J Lipid Res 10: 283-287, 1969

26.   MENDENHALL CL: Origin of hepatic triglyceride fatty acids:
       Quantitative estimation of the relative contribution of linoleic
       acid by diet and adipose tissue in normal and ethanol-fed rats. J
       Lipid Res 13: 177-183, 1972

27.   FORNEY RB, HUGHES FW: Combined effects of alcohol and other
       drugs. Springfield, Illinois. Charles C. Thomas, publisher, 1968.
       pp. 124

28.   SOEHRING K, SCHUPPEL R: Wechselwirkungen zwischen Alkohol
       und Arzneimittein. Deutsch Med Wschr 91: 1892-1898, 1966

29.   LIEBER CS, DECARLI LM: Hepatic microsomal ethanol oxidizing
       system: In vitro characteristics and adaptive properties in vivo.
       J Biol Chem 245: 2505-2512, 1970

30.   TESCHKE R, HASUMURA Y, LIEBER CS: Hepatic microsomal
       ethanol oxidizing system: Solubilization, isolation and character-
       ization. Arch Biochem Biophys 163: 404-415, 1974

31.   RUBIN E, LIEBER CS: Hepatic microsomal enzymes in man and rat:
       Induction and inhibition by ethanol. Science 162: 690-691, 1968

32.   ARIYOSHI T, TAKABATAKE E, REMMER H: Drug metabolism in
       ethanol induced fatty liver. Life Sci (Part II) 9: 361-369, 1970

33.   SCHUPPEI R: Wirkungen von Alkohol auf den Arzneistoffwechsel. In
       Alcohol and the Liver.   W. Gerok, K. Sickinger, H.H.
       Hennekeuser (eds.). New York, Schattauer Verlag, 1971. pp.
       227-242

34.   RUBIN E, GANG H, MISRA PS, LIEBER CS: Inhibition of drug
       metabolism by acute ethanol intoxication. A hepatic microsomal
       mechanism. Am J Med 49: 801-806, 1970

35.   COHEN GM, MANNERING GJ: Involvement of a hydrophobic site in
       the inhibition of the microsomal p-hydroxylation of aniline by
       alcohols. Molec Pharmacol 9: 383-397, 1973

36.   CINTI DI, GRUNDIN R, ORRENIUS S: The effect on drug oxidations
       in vitro and the significance of ethanol-cytochrome P-450
       interaction. Biochem J 134: 367-375, 1973

37.   COHEN BS, ESTABROOK RW: Microsomal electron transport
       reactions.   III. Cooperative interactions between reduced
       diphosphopyridine nucleotide and reduced triphosphopyridine
       nucleotide linked reactions. Arch Biochem Biophys 143: 54-65,
       1971

38.   WHITEHOUSE IW, PAUL CJ, COLDWELL BB, THOMAS BH: Effect
       of ethanol on diazepam distribution in rat. Res Commun Chem
       Path Pharmacol 12: 221-241, 1975

39.   HILDEBRANDT AG, SPECK M ROOTS I: The effects of substrates
       of mixed function oxidase on ethanol oxidation in rat liver
       microsomes. Naunyn-Schmiedeberg's Arch Pharmacol 281: 371-
       382, 1974

40.   GRUNDIN R: Metabolic interaction of ethanol and alprenolol in
       isolated liver cells. Acta Pharmacol Toxicol 37: 185-200, 1975

41.   SUTHERLAND VC, BURBRIDGE TN, ADAMS JE, SIMON A:
       Cerebral metabolism in problem drinkers under the influence of
       alcohol and chlorpromazine hydrochloride. J Appl Physiol 15:
       189-196, 1960

42.   TRUITT EB, DURTIZ G: The role of acetaldehyde in the actions of
       ethanol. In Biochemical Factors in Alcohol. R.P. Maickel (ed.).
       Pergamon Press, 1966. pp. 61-69

43.   MARJANEN L: Intracellular localization of aldehyde dehydrogenase
       in rat liver. Biochem J 127: 633-639, 1972

44.   GRUNNET N: Oxidation of acetaldehyde by rat-liver mitochondria in
       relation to ethanol oxidation and the transport of reducing
       equivalents across the mitochondrial membrane. Eur J Biochem
       35: 236-243, 1973

45.   KORSTEN MA, MATSUZAKI S, FEINMAN L, LIEBER CS: High blood
       acetaldehyde levels after ethanol administration in alcoholics.
       New Eng J Med 292: 386-389, 1975

46.   TOTTMAR SO, PETTERSSON H, KIESSLING K-H: The subcellular
       distribution and properties of aldehyde dehydrogenases in rat
       liver. Biochem J 135: 577-586, 1973

47.   FORSANDER OA: Variations in the acetaldehyde level of some tissues in hyper- and hypothyroid rats.   In Second International Symposium on Alcohol Intoxication and Withdrawal, Section of 20th International Institute on Alcoholism,   ICAA, vol 59. Manchester, England, 1974. pp. 139

48.   LUNDQUIST F, WOLTHERS H: The influence of fructose on the kinetics of alcohol elimination in man.   Acta Pharmacol 14: 290-294, 1958

49.   REYNIER M: Pyrazole inhibition and kinetic studies of ethanol and retinol oxidation catalyzed by rat liver alcohol dehydrogenase. Acta Chem Scand 23: 1119-1129, 1969

50.   MAKAR AB, MANNERING GJ: Kinetics of ethanol metabolism in the intact rat and monkey.   Biochem Pharmacol 19:   2017-2022, 1970

51.   SVOBODA DJ, MANNING RT: Chronic alcoholism with fatty metamorphosis of the liver: Mitochondrial alterations in hepatic cells. Amer J Pathol 44: 645-662, 1964

52.   KIESSLING K-H, PILSTROM L: Ethanol and the human liver. Structural and metabolic changes in liver mitochondria. Cytobiol 4: 339348, 1971

53.   LANE BP, LIEBER CS: Ultrastructural alterations in human hepatocytes following ingestion of ethanol with adequate diets. Amer J Pathol 49: 593-603, 1966

54.   CEDERBAUM AI, LIEBER CS, RUBIN E: The effect of acetaldehyde on mitochondrial function. Arch Biochem Biophys 161: 26-39, 1974

55.   HASUMURA Y, TESCHKE R, LIEBER CS: Acetaldehyde oxidation by hepatic mitochondria: Decrease after chronic ethanol consumption. Science 189: 727-729, 1975

56.   WALSH MJ: Role of acetaldehyde in the interactions of ethanol with neuroamines. In Biological Aspects of Alcohol. M.K. Roach, W.M. McIsaac, P.J. Creaven (eds.).   Austin and London, University of Texas Press, 1971. pp. 233

57.   EADE NR: Mechanism of sympathomimetic action of aldehydes. J Pharmacol Exp Ther 127: 29-34, 1959

58.   DAVIS VE, WALSH MJ: Alcohol, amines and alkaloids: A possible biochemical basis for alcohol addiction. Science 167: 1005-1007, 1970

59. COHEN G, COLLINS M: Alkaloids from catecholamines in adrenal tissue: Possible role in alcoholism. Science 167: 1749-1751, 1970

60. SCHREIBER SS, BRIDEN K, ORATZ M, ROTHCHILD MA: Ethanol, acetaldehyde and myocardial protein synthesis. J Clin Invest 51: 2808-2819, 1972

61. SCHREIBER SS, ORATZ M, ROTHSCHILD MA, REFF F, EVANS C: Alcoholic cardiomyopathy. II. The inhibition of cardiac microsomal protein synthesis by acetaldehyde. J Molec Cell Cardiol 6: 207-213, 1974

62. CEDERBAUM AI, LIEBER CS, RUBIN E: Effect of acetaldehyde on fatty acid oxidation and ketogenesis by hepatic mitochondria. Arch Biochem Biophys 169: 29-41, 1975

63. CEDERBAUM AI, LIEBER CS, BEATTIE DS, RUBIN E: Effect of chronic ethanol ingestion on fatty acid oxidation by hepatic mitochondria. J Biol Chem 250: 5122-5129, 1975

64. MATSUZAKI S, TESCHKE R, OHNISHI K, LIEBER CS: Accelerated ethanol metabolism at high ethanol concentrations and after chronic ethanol consumption. In Alcohol and the Liver. M.M. Fisher and J.G. Rankin (eds.). Plenum Press, New York, 1977

65. VEITCH RL, LUMENG L, LI TK: Vitamin B_6 metabolism in chronic alcohol abuse: The effect of ethanol oxidation on hepatic pyridoxal 5'-phosphate metabolism. J Clin Invest 55: 1026-1032, 1975

66. LUMENG L, LI T-K: Vitamin B_6 metabolism in chronic alcohol abuse. J Clin Invest 53: 693-704, 1974

67. VEITCH RL, LUMENG L, LI T-K: The effect of ethanol and acetaldehyde on vitamin B_6 metabolism in liver. Gastroenterology 66: 868, 1974

68. ISERI OA, GOTTLIEB LS, LIEBER CS: The ultrastructure of ethanol-induced fatty liver. Fed Proc 23: 579, 1974

69. ISERI OA, LIEBER CS, GOTTLIEB LS: The ultrastructure of fatty liver induced by prolonged ethanol ingestion. Am J Pathol 48: 535-555, 1966

70. CARULLI N, MANENTI F, GALLO M, SALVIOLI GF: Alcohol-drugs interaction in man; Alcohol and tolbutamide. Eur J Clin Invest 1: 421-424, 1971

71.   LIEBER CS, RUBIN E: Alcoholic fatty liver in man on a high protein
       and low fat diet. Am J Med 44: 200-206, 1968

72.   RUBIN E, HUTTERER F, LIEBER CS: Ethanol increases hepatic
       smooth endoplasmic reticulum and drug-metabolizing enzymes.
       Science 159: 1469-1470, 1968

73.   ISHII H, JOLY J-G, LIEBER CS: Effect of ethanol on the amount and
       enzyme activities of hepatic rough and smooth microsomal
       membranes. Biochim Biophys Acta 291: 411-420, 1973

74.   KATER RM, CARULLI N, IBER FL: Differences in the rate of
       ethanol metabolism in recently drinking alcoholic and nondrink-
       ing subjects. Am J Clin Nutr 22: 1608-1617, 1969

75.   UGARTE G, PEREDA T, PINO ME, ITURRIAGA H: Influence of
       alcohol intake, length of abstinence and meprobamate on the
       rate of ethanol metabolism in man. Quart J Stud Alcohol 33:
       698-705, 1972

76.   MISRA PS, LEFEVRE A, ISHII H, RUBIN E, LIEBER CS: Increase of
       ethanol, meprobamate and pentobarbital metabolism after
       chronic ethanol administration in man and in rats. Am J Med 51:
       346-351, 1971

77.   TOBON F, MEZEY E: Effect of ethanol administration on hepatic
       ethanol and drug-metabolizing enzymes and on rates of ethanol
       degradation. J Lab Clin Med 77: 110-121, 1971

78.   JOLY J-G, ISHII H, TESCHKE R, HASUMURA Y, LIEBER CS: Effect
       of chronic ethanol feeding on the activities and submicrosomal
       distribution of reduced nicotinamide adenine dinucleotide phos-
       phate (NADPH)-cytochrome P-450 reductase and the deme-
       thylases for aminopyrine and ethyl-morphine. Biochem
       Pharmacol 22: 1532-1535, 1973

79.   POWIS G: Effect of a single oral dose of methanol, ethanol and
       propan-2-ol on the hepatic microsomal metabolism of foreign
       compounds in the rat. Biochem J 148: 269-277, 1975

80.   LUOMA P, VORNE M: The combined effect of ethanol and
       phenobarbital on the activities of hepatic drug metabolizing
       enzymes in rats. Acta Pharmacol Toxicol 33: 442-448, 1973

81.   LU AY, JUNK KW, COON MJ: Resolution of the cytochrome P-450
       containing ω-hydroxylation system of liver microsomes into
       three components. J Biol Chem 244: 3714-3721, 1969

82.   KALANT H KHANNA JM, MARSHMAN J: Effect of chronic intake of ethanol on pentobarbital metabolism. J Pharmacol Exper Ther 175: 318-324, 1970

83.   RATCLIFFE F: The effect of chronic ethanol administration on the responses to amylobarbitone sodium in the rat. Life Sci 8: 1051-1061, 1969

84.   KATER RM, ROGGIN G, TOBON F, ZIEVE P, IBER FE: Increased rate of clearance of drugs from the circulation of alcoholics. Am J Med Sci 258: 35-39, 1969

85.   VESELL ES, PAGE JG, PASSANANTI GT: Genetic and environmental factors affecting ethanol metabolism in man. Clin Pharmacol Ther 12: 192-201, 1971

86.   GRASSI GG, GRASSI C: Ethanol-antibiotic interactions at hepatic level. J Clin Pharmacol Biopharm 11: 216-225, 1975

87.   IOANNIDES C, LAKE BG, PARKE DV: Enhancement of hepatic microsomal drug metabolism in vitro following ethanol administration. Xenobiotica 5: 665-767, 1975

88.   HASUMURA Y, TESCHKE R, LIEBER CS: Increased carbon tetrachloride hepatotoxicity, and its mechanism, after chronic ethanol consumption. Gastroenterology 66: 415-422, 1974

89.   MALING HM, STRIPP B, SIPES IG, HIGHMAN B, SAUL W, WILLIAMS MA: Enhanced hepatotoxicity of carbon tetrachloride, thioacetamide, and dimethyl-nitrosamine by pretreatment of rats with ethanol and some comparisons with potentiation by isopropanol. Toxicol Appl Pharmacol 33: 291-308, 1975

90.   TRAIGER GJ, PLAA GL: Relationship of alcohol metabolism to the potentiation of CCl_4 hepatotoxicity induced by aliphatic alcohols. J Pharmacol Exper Ther 183: 481-488, 1972

91.   GARNER RC, McLEAN AE: Increased susceptibility to carbon tetrachloride poisoning in the rat after pretreatment with oral phenobarbitone. Biochem Pharmacol 18: 645-650, 1969

92.   DIAZ GOMES MI, CASTRO JA, DE FERREYRA EC, D'ACOSTA N, DE CASTRO CR: Irreversible binding of ^{14}C from $^{14}CCl_4$ to liver microsomal lipids and proteins from rats pretreated with compounds altering microsomal mixed function oxygenase activity. Toxicol Appl Pharmacol 25: 534-541, 1973

93.   MOON HD: The pathology of fatal carbon tetrachloride poisoning with special reference to the histogenesis of the hepatic and renal lesions. Am J Pathol 26: 1041-1057, 1950

94.   MITCHELL JR, JOLLOWS DJ: Metabolic activation of drugs to toxic
      substances. Gastroenterology 68: 392-410, 1975

95.   DI LUZIO NR, HARTMAN AD: Role of lipid peroxidation in the
      pathogenesis of the ethanol-induced fatty liver. Fed Proc 26:
      1436-1442, 1967

96.   HASHIMOTO S, RECKNAGEL RO: No chemical evidence of hepatic
      lipid peroxidation in acute ethanol toxicity. Exper Molec Pathol
      8: 225-242, 1968

97.   SCHEIG R, KLATSKIN G: Some effects of ethanol and carbon
      tetrachloride in lipoperoxidation in rat liver. Life Sci 8: 855-
      865, 1969

98.   BUNYAN J, CAWTHORNE MA, DIPLOCK AT, GREEN J: Vitamin E
      and hepatotoxic agents. 2. Lipid peroxidation and poisoning with
      orotic acid, ethanol and thioacetamide in rats. Brit J Nutr 23:
      309-317, 1969

99.   COMPORTI M, BURDINO E, RAJA F: Fatty acid composition of
      mitochondrial and microsomal lipids of rat liver after acute
      ethanol intoxication. Life Sci 10: (Part II) 855-866, 1971

100. BLOOM RJ, WESTERFIELD WW: The thiobarbituric acid reaction in
      relation to fatty liver. Arch Biochem Biopys 145: 669-675, 1971

101. LIEBER CS, DECARLI LM: Reduced nicotinamide-adenine dinucleo-
      tide phosphate oxidase: Activity enhanced by ethanol con-
      sumption. Science 170: 78-80, 1970

102. LEVANDER OA, MORRIS VC, HIGGS DJ, VARMA RN: Nutritional
      interrelationships among vitamin E selenium, antioxidants and
      ethyl alcohol in the rat. J Nutr 103: 536-542, 1973

103. LEFEVRE AF, DECARLI LM, LIEBER CS: Effect of ethanol on
      cholesterol and bile acid metabolism. J Lipid Res 13: 48-55,
      1972

104. SCHOENFIELD LJ, BONORRIS GG, GANZ P: Induced alterations in
      the rate-limiting enzymes of hepatic cholesterol and bile acid
      synthesis in the hamster. J Lab Clin Med 82: 858-868, 1973

105. LIEBER CS, JONES DP, MENDELSON J, DECARLI LM: Fatty liver,
      hyperlipemia and hyperuricemia produced by prolonged alcohol
      consumption, despite adequate dietary intake. Trans Ass Amer
      Physicians 76: 289-300, 1963

106. TAKEUCHI N, ITO M, YAMAMURA Y: Esterification of cholesterol and hydrolysis of cholesteryl ester in alcohol induced fatty liver of rats. Lipids 9: 353-357, 1974

107. MADDREY WC, BOYER JL: The acute and chronic effects of ethanol administration on bile secretion in the rat. J Lab Clin Med 82: 215-225, 1973

108. LOSOWSKY MS, JONES DP, DAVIDSON CS, LIEBER CS: Studies of alcoholic hyperlipemia and its mechanism. Am J Med 35: 794-803, 1963

109. BARAONA E, PIROLA RC, LIEBER CS: Effects of chronic ethanol feeding on serum lipoprotein metabolism in the rat. J Clin Invest 49: 769-778, 1970

110. BARAONA E, PIROLA RC, LIEBER CS: The pathogenesis of postprandial hyperlipemia in rats fed ethanol-containing diets. J Clin Invest 52: 296-303, 1973

111. JOLY J-G, FEINMAN L, ISHII H, LIEBER CS: Effect of chronic ethanol feeding on hepatic microsomal glycerophosphate acyltransferase activity. J Lipid Res 14: 337-343, 1973

112. MENDENHALL CL, BRADFORD RH, FURMAN RH: Effect of ethanol on glycerolipid metabolism in rat liver. Biochim Biophys Acta 187: 501-509, 1969

113. GANG H, LIEBER CS, RUBIN E: Ethanol increased glycosyl transferase activity in the hepatic Golgi apparatus. Nature (New Biology) 243: 123-125, 1973

114. BARBORIAK JJ, MEADE RC: Enhancement of alimentary lipemia by preprandial alcohol. Am J Med Sci 255: 245-251, 1968

115. BREWSTER AC, LANKFORD HG, SCHWARTZ MG, SULLIVAN JF: Ethanol and alimentary lipemia. Am J Clin Nutr 19: 255-259, 1966

116. KUDZMA DJ, SCHONFELD G: Alcoholic hyperlipidemia; Induction by alcohol but not by carbohydrate. J Lab Clin Med 77: 384-395, 1971

117. VERDY M, GATTEREAU A: Ethanol, lipase activity and serum-lipid level. Am J Clin Nutr 20: 997-1003, 1967

118. WILSON DE, SCHREIBMAN PH, BREWSTER AC, ARKY RA: The enhancement of alimentary lipemia by ethanol in man. J Lab Clin Med 75: 264-274, 1970

119. MENDELSON JH, MELLO NK: Alcohol-induced hyperlipidemia and beta lipoproteins. Science 180: 1372-1374, 1973

120. GENSBERG H, OLEFSKY J, FARQUHAR JW, REAVEN GM: Moderate ethanol ingestion and plasma triglyceride levels. Ann Intern Med 80: 143-149, 1974

121. KESSLER JL, MILLER M, BARZA D, MISHKIN S: Hyperlipemia in acute pancreatitis. Metabolic studies in a patient and demonstration of abnormal lipoprotein-triglyceride complexes resistant to the action of lipoprotein lipase. Am J Med 42: 968-977, 1967

122. CHAIT A, FEBRUARY AW, MANCINI M, LEWIS BL: Clinical and metabolic study of alcoholic hyperlipidaemia. Lancet 2: 62-64, 1972

123. FRYMM, SPECTOR AA, CONNOR SL, CONNOR WE: Intensification of hypertriglyceridemia by either alcohol or carbohydrate. Am J Clin Nutr 26: 798-802, 1973

124. WINDMUELLER HG, LEVY RI: Production of β-lipoprotein by intestine in the rat. J Biol Chem 243: 4878-4884, 1968

125. OCKNER RK, HUGHES FB, ISSELBACHER KJ: Very low density lipoproteins in intestinal lymph. Origin, composition, and role in lipid transport in the fasting state. J Clin Invest 48: 2079-2088, 1969

126. BARAONA E, PIROLA RC, LIEBER CS: Acute and chronic effects of ethanol on intestinal lipid metabolism. Biochim Biophys Acta 388: 19-28, 1975

127. CARTER EA, DRUMMEY GD, ISSELBACHER KJ: Ethanol stimulates triglyceride synthesis by the intestine. Science 174: 1245-1237, 1971

128. MISTILIS SP, OCKNER RK: Effects of ethanol on endogenous lipid and lipoprotein metabolism in small intestine. J Lab Clin Med 80: 34-46, 1972

129. WINDMUELLER HG, HERBERT PN, LEVY RI: Biosynthesis of lymph and plasma lipoprotein apoproteins by isolated perfused rat liver and intestine. J Lipid Res 14: 215-223, 1973

130. OCKNER RK, MISTILIS SP, PEPPENHAUSEN RB, STIEHL AF: Ethanol-induced fatty liver: Effect of intestinal lymph fistula. Gastroenterology 64: 603-609, 1973

131. MIDDLETON WR, CARTER EA, DRUMMEY GD, ISSELBACHER KJ: Effect of oral ethanol administration on intestinal cholesterogenesis in the rat. Gastroenterology 60: 880-887, 1971

132. WALTMAN R BONURA F, NIGRIN G. PIPAT C: Ethanol in prevention of hyperbilirubinaemia in the newborn. Lancet 2: 1265-1267, 1969

133. IDEO G, DEFRANCHIS R, DEL NINNO E, DIOGUARDI N: Ethanol increases liver uridine-diphosphate-glucuronyltransferase. Experientia 27: 24-25, 1971

134. OKOLICSANYI L, CARTEI G, NACCARATO R: Effects of ethanol on Gilbert's hyperbilirubinaemia. Lancet 1: 450, 1972

135. JOUPPILA P, KOIVISTO M, SUONIO S: Ethanol in the prevention of neonatal hyperbilirubinaemia. Acta Paediat Scand 63: 501-504, 1973

136. NELSON P, TAN WC, WAGLE SR, ASHMORE J: Hepatic metabolism and enzyme activity in acute ethanol administration. Biochem Pharmacol 16: 1813-1819, 1967

137. ISHII H, JOLY J-G, LIEBER CS: Increase of microsomal glucose-6-phosphatase activity after chronic ethanol administration. Metabolism 22: 799-806, 1973

138. CARTER EA, ISSELBACHER KJ: The role of microsomes in the hepatic metabolism of ethanol. Ann NY Acad Sci 179: 282-294, 1971

139. FITCH WW, CHAIKOFF IL: Extent and patterns of adaptation of enzyme activities in liver of normal rats fed diets high in glucose and fructose. J Biol Chem 235: 554-557, 1960

140. OLIVECRANA T, HERNELL O, JOHNSON O, FEX G, WALLINDER L, SANDREN O: Effect of ethanol on some enzymes inducible by fat free refeeding. Quart J Stud Alcohol 33: 1-13, 1972

141. BRODIE BB, BUTLER WM, HORNING MG, MAICKEL RP, MALING HM: Alcohol induced triglyceride deposition in liver through derangement of fat transport. Am J Clin Nutr 9: 432-435, 1961

142. MALLOV S: Effect of adrenalectomy on ethanol and fat metabolism in the rat. Am J Physiol 189: 428-432, 1957

143. REBOUCAS G, ISSELBACHER KJ: Studies on the pathogenesis of the ethanol-induced fatty liver. I. Synthesis and oxidation of fatty acids by the liver. J Clin Invest 40: 1355-1362, 1961

144. KESSLER JI, YALOVSKY-MISHKIN S: Effect of ingestion of saline, glucose, and ethanol on mobilization and hepatic incorporation of epididymal pad palmitate-1-^{14}C in rats. J Lipid Res 7: 772-778, 1966

145. POGGI M, DI LUZIO NR: The role of liver and adipose tissue in the pathogenesis of the ethanol-induced fatty liver. J Lipid Res 5: 437-441, 1964

146. MALLOV S: Effect of ethanol intoxication on plasma free fatty acids in the rat. Quart J Stud Alcohol 22: 250-253, 1961

147. ELKO EE, WOOLES WR, DI LUZIO NR: Alterations and mobilization of lipids in acute ethanol-treated rats. Am J Physiol 201: 923-926, 1961

148. JONES DP, LOSOWSKY MS, DAVIDSON CS, LIEBER CS: Effects of ethanol on plasma lipids in man. J Lab Clin Med 62: 675-682, 1963

149. JONES DP, PERMAN ES, LIEBER CS: Free fatty acid turnover and triglyceride metabolism after ethanol ingestion in man. J Lab Clin Med 66: 804-813, 1965

150. FEINMAN L, LIEBER CS: Effect of ethanol on plasma glycerol in man. Am J Clin Nutr 20: 400-403, 1967

151. CROUSE JR, GERSON CD, DECARLI LM, LIEBER CS: Role of acetate in the reduction of plasma free fatty acids produced by ethanol in man. J Lipid Res 9: 509-512, 1968

152. LINDENBAUM J, LIEBER CS: Effects of chronic ethanol administration on intestinal absorption in man in the absence of nutritional deficiency. Ann NY Acad Sci 252: 228-234, 1975

153. BEST CH, HARTROFT WS, LUCAS CC, RIDOUT JH: Liver damage produced by feeding alcohol or sugar and its prevention by choline. Brit Med J II: 1001-1006, 1949

154. PEQUIGNOT G: Die Rolle des Alkohols bei der Atiologie von Leberzirrhosen in Frankreich. Munchen Med Wschr 103: 1464-1468, 1962

155. LELBACH WK: Leberschaden bei chronischem Alkoholismus. Acta Hepatosplen 14: 9-39, 1967

156. LIEBER CS, JONES DP, DECARLI LM: Effects of prolonged ethanol intake: Production of fatty liver despite adequate diets. J Clin Invest 44: 1009-1021, 1965

157. DECARLI LM, LIEBER CS: Fatty liver in the rat after prolonged intake of ethanol with a nutritionally adequate new liquid diet. J Nutr 91: 331-336, 1967

158. LIEBER CS, DECARLI LM: Ethanol dependence and tolerance: A nutritionally controlled experimental model in the rat. Res Commun Chem Path Pharmacol 6: 983-991, 1973

159. LIEBER CS: Chronic alcoholic hepatic injury in experimental animals and man: Biochemical pathways and nutritional factors. Fed Proc 26: 1443-1448, 1967

160. LIEBER CS, DECARLI LM: Quantitative relationship between the amount of dietary fat and the severity of the alcoholic fatty liver. Am J Clin Nutr 23: 474-478, 1970

161. BARAK AJ, TUMA DJ, SORRELL MF: Relationship of ethanol to choline metabolism in the liver: A review. Am J Clin Nutr 26: 1234-1241, 1973

162. MENDENHALL CL, WILSON NL: Observations on the relationship of hepatic choline uptake to ethanolic fatty liver in the rat. Can J Biochem 51: 1010-1013, 1973

163. HOFFBAUER FW, ZAKI FG: Choline deficiency in baboon and rat compared. Arch Pathol 79: 364-369, 1965

164. OLSON RE: Nutrition and alcoholism. In Modern Nutrition in Health and Disease. M.G. Wohl, R.S. Goodhart (eds.). Philadelphia, Lea & Febiger, 1964

165. RUBIN E, LIEBER CS: Alcohol-induced hepatic injury in non-alcoholic volunteers. New Eng J Med 278: 869-876, 1968

166. ASHWORTH CT, WRIGHTSMAN F, BUTTRAM V: Hepatic lipids. Arch Pathol 72: 620-624, 1961

167. EDREIRA JG, HIRSCH RL, KENNEDY JA: Production of fatty liver with dietary ethanol despite orotic acid supplementation. Quart J Stud Alcohol 35: 20-25, 1974

168. FRENCH SW: Effect of acute and chronic ethanol ingestion on rat liver ATP. Proc Soc Exper Biol Med 121: 681-685, 1966

169. WALKER JE, GORDON ER: Biochemical aspects associated with an ethanol-induced fatty liver. Biochem J 119: 511-516, 1970

170. BERNSTEIN J, VIDELA L, ISRAEL Y: Metabolic alterations produced in the liver by chronic ethanol administration. II. Changes related to energetic parameters of the cell. Biochem J 134: 515-522, 1973

171. SHULL KH, OLER A, LOMBARDI B: Hepatic adenosine triphosphate levels during acute choline deficiency in the rat. Proc Soc Exper Biol Med 140: 575-577, 1972

172. CORREDOR C, MANSBACHC, BRESSLER R: Carnitine depletion in the choline-deficient state. Biochim Biophys Acta 144: 366-374, 1967

173. KONDRUP J, GRUNNET N: The effect of acute and prolonged ethanol treatment on the contents of coenzyme A, carnitine and their derivatives in rat liver. Biochem J 132: 373-379, 1973

174. OLER A, LOMBARDI B: Further studies on a defect in the intracellular transport and secretion of proteins by the liver of choline-deficient rats. J Biol Chem 245: 1282-1288, 1970

175. RUEBNER BH, MOORE J, RUTHERFORD RB, SELIGMAN AM, ZUIDEMA GD: Nutritional cirrhosis in rhesus monkeys: Electron microscopy and histochemistry. Exper Molec Pathol 11: 53-70, 1969

176. DI LUZIO NR: Effect of acute ethanol intoxication on liver and plasma lipid fractions of the rat. Am J Physiol 194: 453-456, 1958

177. LIEBER CS, DECARLI LM: Study of agents for the prevention of the fatty liver produced by prolonged alcohol intake. Gastroenterology 50: 316-322, 1966

178. TAKEUCHI J, TAKADA A, HASUMURA Y, MATSUDA Y, IKEGAMI F: Acute alcoholic liver injury and choline deficiency. Meth Achievm Exper Pathol 6: 81-110, 1972

179. PATEK AJ, BOWRY SC, ANURAS S: Alcohol and sucrose in choline deficiency cirrhosis in the rat. Arch Pathol 96: 377-382, 1973

180. LIEBER CS, DECARLI LM, GANG H, WALKER G, RUBIN E: Hepatic effect of long-term ethanol consumption in primates. In Medical Primatology. E.I. Goldsmith, J. Moor-Jankowski (eds.). Basel, Karger, 1972. Part III, pp. 270-278

181. KUMAR V, DEO MG, RAMALINGASWAMI V: Mechanism of fatty liver in protein deficiency. Gastroenterology 62: 445-451, 1972

182. KLATSKIN G, KREHL WA, CONN HO: The effect of alcohol on the choline requirement. I. Changes in the rat's liver following prolonged ingestion of alcohol. J Exp Med 100: 605-614, 1954

183. FINKELSTEIN JD, CELLO JP, KYLE WE: Ethanol-induced changes in methionine metabolism in rat liver. Biochem Biophys Res Commun 61: 475-481, 1974

184. ERICSSON JL, ORRENIUS S, HOLM I: Alterations in canine liver cells induced by protein deficiency. Ultrastructural and biochemical observations. Exper Molec Pathol 5: 329-349, 1966

185. PATRICK RS, MACKAY AM, COWARD DG, WHITEHEAD RG: Experimental protein-energy malnutrition in baby baboons. Brit J Nutr 30: 171-179, 1973

186. HOLT JR LE, SNYDERMAN SE, NORTON PM, ROITMAN E: The plasma aminogram as affected by protein intake. In Protein Nutrition and Free Amino Acid Patterns. J.H. Leathem, N. Brunswick, N.J. Rutgers (eds.). University Press, 1968. pp. 32

187. SHAW S, LIEBER CS: Plasma amino acids in alcoholic liver injury; Contrast with protein malnutrition. Clin Res 23: 459A, 1975

188. MOXLEY RT, POZEFSKY T, LOCKWOOD DH: Protein nutrition and liver disease after jejunoileal bypass for morbid obesity. New Eng J Med 290: 921-926, 1974

189. ZINNEMAN HH, SEAL US, DOE RP: Plasma and urinary amino acids in Laennec's cirrhosis. Am J Dig Dis 14: 118-126, 1969

190. NING M, LOWENSTEIN LM, DAVIDSON CS: Serum amino acid concentrations in alcoholic hepatitis. J Lab Clin Med 70: 554-562, 1967

191. SIEGEL FL, ROACH MK, POMEROY LR: Plasma amino acid patterns in alcoholism: The effects of ethanol loading. Proc Nat Acad Sci USA 51: 605-611, 1964

192. SHAW S, LIEBER CS: Characteristic plasma amino acid abnormalities in the alcoholic: Respective roles of alcoholism, nutrition and liver injury. Clin Res 24: 291A, 1976

193. SHAW S, STIMMEL B, LIEBER CS: Plasma α-amino-n butyric acid/leucine: An empirical biochemical marker of alcoholism. Proc AMSA/NCA Conf (in press)

194. BARAONA E, LEO M, BOROWSKY SA, LIEBER CS: Alcoholic hepatomegaly: Accumulation of protein in the liver. Science 190: 794-795, 1975

195. BARAONA E, LEO MA, BOROWSKY SA, LIEBER CS: Hepatic accumulation of export proteins after chronic ethanol consumption. Gastroenterology 69: 806, 1975

196. LAMY J, LAMY J, ARON E, WEILL J: Profil biologique des premieres etapes se la cirrhose alcoolique: IgA, transferrine, haptoglobine, orosomucoide et α_1-antitrypsine. Pathologie Giologie Mai 22: 401-408, 1974

197. DAJANI RM, KOUYOUMJIAN C: A probable direct role of ethanol in the pathogenesis of fat infiltration in the rat. J Nutr 91: 535-539, 1967

198. MADSEN NP: Reduced serum very low-density lipoprotein levels after acute ethanol administration. Biochem Pharmacol 18: 261-262, 1969

199. KOGA S, HIRAYAMA C: Disturbed release of lipoprotein from ethanol induced fatty liver. Experientia 24: 438-439, 1968

200. MOOKERJEA S, CHOW A: Impairment of glycoprotein synthesis in acute ethanol intoxication in rats. Biochim Biophys Acta 184: 83-92, 1969

201. MARZO A, CHIRARDI P, SARDINI D: Serum lipids and total fatty acids in chronic alcoholic liver disease at different stages of cell damage. Heft Unfallheilk 48: 949-950, 1970

202. CACHERA R, LAMOTTE M, LAMOTTE-BARRILLON S: Etude Clinique, Biologique et Histologique des Steatoses du Foie Chez Les Alcooliques. Semaine Hop Paris 26: 3497-3514, 1950

203. PAPADOPOULOS NM, CHARLES MA: Serum lipoprotein patterns in liver disease. Proc Soc Exper Biol Med 134: 797-799, 1970

204. LIEBER CS, DECARLI LM: An experimental model of alcohol feeding and liver injury in the baboon. J Med Primatol 3: 153-163, 1974

205. BOROWSKY SA, PERLOW W, BARAONA E, LIEBER CS: Disappearance of alcoholic hyperlipemia as a sign of advancing liver damage. Gastroenterology 70: A-120, 1976

206. RUBIN E, LIEBER CS: Early fine structural changes in the human liver induced by alcohol. Gastroenterology 52: 1-13, 1967

207. KURIYAMA K, SZE PT, RAUSCHER GE: Effects of acute and chronic ethanol administration on ribosomal protein synthesis in mouse brain and liver. Life Sci 10: 181-189, 1971

208. JEEJEEBHOY KN, HO J, GREENBERG GR. PHILLIPS MJ, BRUCE-ROBERTSON A, SODTKE U: Albumin, fibrinogen and transferrin synthesis in isolated rat hepatocyte suspensions. Biochem J 146: 141-155, 1975

209. NADKARNI G-SD: Effect of acute ethanol administration on rat plasma protein synthesis. Biochem Pharmacol 23: 389-393, 1974

210. ROTHSCHILD M, ORATZ M, MONGELLI J, SCHREIBER S: Alcohol-induced depression of albumin synthesis: Reversal by tryptophan. J Clin Invest 50: 1812-1818, 1971

211. JEEJEEBHOY KN, PHILLIPS MJ, BRUCE-ROBERTSON A, HO J, SODTKE U: The acute effect of ethanol on albumin, fibrinogen and transferrin synthesis in the rat. Biochem J 126: 111-1126, 1972

212. KIRSCH RE, FRITH LO, STEAD RH, SAUNDERS SJ: Effect of alcohol on albumin synthesis by the isolated perfused rat liver. Am J Clin Nutr 26: 1191-1194, 1973

213. ORATZ M, ROTHSCHILD MA: The influence of alcohol and altered nutrition on albumin synthesis. In Alcohol and Abnormal Protein Biosynthesis. M.A. Rothschild, M. Oratz, S.S. Schreiber (eds.). New York, Pergamon Press, Inc. 1975. pp. 343

214. PERIN A, SCALABRINO G, SESSA A ARNABOLDI A: In vitro inhibition of protein synthesis in rat liver as a consequence of ethanol metabolism. Biochim Biophys Acta 366: 101-108, 1974

215. FREINKEL N, COHEN AK, ARKY RA: Alcohol hypoglycemia: II. A postulated mechanism of action based on experiments with rat liver slices. J Clin Endocrinol Metabol 25: 76-93, 1965

216. CHAMBERS JW, GEORG RH, BASS AD: The effect of ethanol on the uptake of α-aminoisobutyric acid by the isolated perfused rat liver. Life Sci 5: 2293-2300, 1966

217. CHAMBERS JW, PICCIRILLO VJ: Effects of ethanol on amino-acid uptake and utilization by the liver and other organs of rats. Quart J Stud Alcohol 34: 707-717, 1973

218. RENIS M, GIOVINC A, BERTOLINO A: Protein synthesis in mitochondrial and microsomal fractions from rat brain and liver after acute or chronic ethanol administration. Life Sci 16: 1447-1458, 1975

219. BANKS WL, KLINE ES, HIGGINS ES: Hepatic composition and metabolism after ethanol consumption in rats fed liquid purified diets. J Nutr 100: 581-594, 1970

220. MORLAND J: Incorporation of labelled amino acids into liver protein after acute ethanol administration. Biochem Pharmacol 24: 439-442, 1975

221. KONTTINEN A, HARTEL G, LOUHIJA A: Multiple serum enzyme analyses in chronic alcoholics. Acta med Scand 188: 257-264, 1970

222. RUBIN E, BEATTIE DS, LIEBER CS: Effects of ethanol on the biogenesis of mitochondrial membranes and associated mitochondrial functions. Lab Invest 23: 620-627, 1970

223. OUDEA MC LAUNAY AN, QUENEHERVE S, OUDEA P: The hepatic lesions produced in the rat by chronic alcoholic intoxication. Histological, ultrastructural and biochemical observations. Rev Europ Etudes Clin Biol 15: 748-764, 1970

224. VIDELA L, ISRAEL Y: Factors that modify the metabolism of ethanol in rat liver and adaptive changes produced by its chronic administration. Biochem J 118: 275-281, 1970

225. KIESSLING K-H, PILSTROM L: Effect of ethanol on rat liver. V. Morphological and functional changes after prolonged consumption of various alcoholic beverages. Quart J Stud Alcohol 29: 819-827, 1968

226. HASUMURA Y, TESCHKE R, LIEBER CS: Characteristics of acetaldehyde oxidation in rat liver mitochondria. J Biol Chem: 1976 (in press)

227. GORDON ER: Mitochondrial functions in an ethanol induced fatty liver. J Biol Chem 248: 8271-8280, 1973

228. KIESSLING KH: Effect of ethanol on rat liver. VI. A possible correlation between α-glycerophosphate oxidase activity and mitochondrial size in male and femal rats fed ethanol. Acta Pharmacol 26: 245-252, 1968

229. PILSTROM L, KIESSLING K-H: A possible localization of α-glycerophosphate dehydrogenase to the inner boundary membrane of mitochondria in livers from rats fed with ethanol. Histochemie 32: 329-334, 1972

230. CEDERBAUM AI, LIEBER CS, RUBIN E: Effects of chronic ethanol treatment on mitochondrial functions. Arch Biochem Biophys 165: 560-569, 1974

231. LEFEVRE A, ADLER H, LIEBER CS: Effect of ethanol on ketone metabolism. J Clin Invest 49: 1775-1782, 1970

232. JENKINS DW, ECKEL RW. CRAIG JW: Alcoholic ketoacidosis. JAMA 217: 177-183, 1971

233. LEVY LJ, DUGA J, GIRGIS M, GORDON EE: Ketoacidosis associated with alcoholism in nondiabetic subjects. Ann Intern Med 78: 213-219, 1973

234. MATSUZAKI S, LIEBER CS: Increased susceptibility of hepatic mitochondria to the toxicity of acetaldehyde after chronic ethanol consumption. Submitted for publication.

235. MAJCHROWICZ E, MENDELSON JH: Blood concentrations of acetaldehyde and ethanol in chronic alcoholics. Science 168: 1100-1102, 1970

236. TRUITT EB: Blood acetaldehyde levels after alcohol consumption by alcoholics and non-alcoholic subjects. In Biological Aspects of Alcohol. M.K. Roach, W.M. McIsaac, P.J. Creaven (eds.). Texas, University of Texas Press, 1971. pp 212

237. FREUND G: Alcohol, barbiturate, and bromide withdrawal syndrome in mice. In Recent Advances in Studies of Alcoholism. U.S. Dept. of Health, Education and Welfare, Health Services and Mental Health Administration, National Institute of Mental Health, National Institute on Alcohol Abuse and Alcoholism. U.S. Government Printing Office, Washington, D.C., 1971. pp. 453

238. RUBENSTEIN JA, COLLINS MA, TABAKOFF B: Inhibition of liver aldehyde dehydrogenase by pyrogallol and related compounds. Experientia 31: 414-415, 1975

239. COLLINS MA, GORDON R, BIDGELI MG, RUBENSTEIN JA: Pyrogallol potentiates acetaldehyde blood levels during ethanol oxidation in rats. Chem Biol Interactions 8: 127-130, 1974

240. HEDLUND SG, KIESSLING K-H: The physiological mechanism involved in hangover. I. The oxidation of some lower aliphatic fusel alcohols and aldehydes in rat liver and their effect on the mitochondrial oxidation of various substrates. Acta Pharmacol Toxicol 27: 381-396, 1969

241. DI LUZIO NR: Comparative study of the effect of alcoholic beverages on the development of the acute ethanol-induced fatty liver. Quart J Stud Alcohol 23: 557-561, 1962

242. JORDO L, OLSSON R: Effect of long-term administration of different hard liquors and red wine on the rat liver. Acta Pathol Microbiol Scand 83: 345-354, 1975

243. WALKER F, ELMSLIE W, FRASER RA, SNAPE PE, WATT GC: Cytotoxic effect of alcohol on liver cells and fibroblast in vitro. Scot Med J 19: 125-127, 1974

244. GOLDBERG DM, WATTS C: Serum enzyme changes as evidence of liver reaction to oral alcohol. Gastroenterology 49: 256-261, 1965

245. FIGUEROA RB, KLOTZ AP: Alterations of alcohol dehydrogenase and other hepatic enzymes following oral alcohol intoxication. Am J Clin Nutr 11: 235-239, 1962

246. ROLLASON JG, PINCHERLE G, ROBINSON D: Serum gamma glutamyl transpeptidase in relation to alcohol consumption. Clin Chim Acta 39: 75-80, 1972

247. ROSALKI SB, TAU D: Serum γ-glutamyl transpeptidase activity in alcoholism. Clin Chim Acta 39: 41-47, 197?

248. LAMY J, BAGLIN MC, ARON E, WEILL J: Diminution de la γ-glutamyltranspeptidase serique des cirrhotiques a la suite du sevrage. Clin Chim Acta 60: 97-101, 1975

249. LAMY J, BAGLIN M-C, FERRANT J-P, WEILL J: Emploi de la mesure de la glutamyltranspeptidase serique pour controler le succes des cures de desintoxication anti-alcoolique. Clin Chim Acta 60: 103-107, 1975

250. LUM G, GAMBINO SR: Serum gamma-glutamyl transpeptidase activity as an indicator of disease of liver, pancreas or bone. Clin Chem 18: 358-362, 1972

251. MENDELSON JH, STEIN S, McGUIRE MT: Comparative psycho-physiological studies of alcoholic and non-alcoholic subjects undergoing experimentally induced ethanol intoxication. Psychosom Med 28: 1-12, 1966

252. HENLEY KS, WIGGINS H, HIRSCHOWITZ B, POLLARD HM: The effect of oral ethanol on glutamic pyruvic and glutamic oxalacetic transaminase activity in the rat liver. Quart J Stud Alcohol 19: 54-68, 1958

253. SARDESAI VM, PROVIDO HS: The effect of ethyl alcohol on rat liver tryptophan oxygenase. Life Sci 11: 1023-1028, 1972

254. BADAWY AA, EVANS M: Alcohol addiction, porphyria and mental disorders. Lancet 2: 374-375, 1972

255. MORLAND J, CHRISTOFFERSEN T, OSNES JB, SEGLEN PO, JERVELL KF: An effect of ethanol administration on tryptophan oxygenase in the perfused rat liver. Biochem Pharmacol 21: 1849-1859, 1972

256. GORMAN RE, BITENSKY MW: Selective activation by short chain alcohols of glucagon responsive adenyl cyclase in liver. Endocrinol 87: 1075-1081, 1970

257. AMMON HP, ESTLER CJ, HEIM F: Inactivation of coenzyme A by ethanol. I. Acetaldehyde as mediator of the inactivation of coenzyme A following the administration of ethanol in vivo. Biochem Pharmacol 18: 29-33, 1969

258. BODE C, STAHLER E, KONO H, GOEBELL H: Effects of ethanol on free coenzyme A. Free carnitine and their fatty acid esters in rat liver. Biochim Biophys Acta 210: 448-455, 1970

259. BREEN KJ, SHAW J, LEVINSON JD, SCHENKER S: The acute effect of alcohol on hepatic coenzyme A and acetyl CoA concentrations. Proc Soc Exper Biol Med 138: 1096-1100, 1971

260. PARAF A, RENAULT G, RAUTUREAU J, FABIA F, DAMOUR LEBARD J: Modification immunitaires et infections dans les cirrhoses alcooliques. Sem Hosp Paris 51: 811-815, 1975

261. ZINNEMAN MD: Autoimmune phenomena in alcoholic cirrhosis. Dig Dis 20: 337-345, 1975

262. BERENYI MR, STRAUS B, CRUZ D: In vitro and in vivo studies of cellular immunity in alcoholic cirrhosis. Am J Dig Dis 19: 199-205, 1974

263. BERENYI MR, STRAUS B, AVILA L: T rosettes in alcoholic cirrhosis of the liver. JAMA 232: 44-46, 1975

264. LUNDY J, RAAF JH, DEAKINS S WANEBO HJ, JACOBS DA, LEE T, JACOBOWITZ D, SPEAR C, OETTGEN HF: The acute and chronic effects of alcohol on the human immune system. Surg Gynec Obstet 141: 212-218, 1975

265. BERNSTEIN IM, WEBSTER KH, WILLIAMS RC, STRICKLAND RG: Reduction in circulating T lymphocytes in alcoholic liver disease. Lancet 2: 488, 1974

266. SORRELL MF, LEEVY CM: Lymphocyte transformation and alcoholic liver injury. Gastroenterology 63: 1020-1025, 1972

267. PETTIGREW NM, GOUDIE RB, RUSSELL RI, CHAUDHURI AK: Evidence for a role of hepatitis virus B in chronic alcoholic liver disease. Lancet 2: 724-725, 1972

268. TENNENBAUM JI, RUPPERT RD, ST PIERRE RL, GREENBERGER NJ: The effect of chronic alcohol administration on the immune responsiveness of rats. J Allergy 44: 272-281, 1969

269.   MIHAS AA, BULL DM DAVIDSON CS: Cell-mediated immunity to liver in patients with alcoholic hepatitis. Lancet 1: 951-953, 1975

270.   ZETTERMAN RK, CHEN T, LEEVY CM: Role of altered lymphocyte function in alcoholic liver disease. Gastroenterology 67: 837, 1974

271.   PARONETTO F, LIEBER CS: Alcoholic liver injury in baboons: Cytotoxicity of lymphocytes. Clin Res 24: 434A, 1976

272.   TISMAN G, HERBERT V: In vitro myelosuppression and immuno-suppression by ethanol. J Clin Invest 52: 1410-1414, 1973

273.   McLAREN DS, FARIS R, ZEKAIN B: The liver during recovery from protein-calorie malnutrition. J Trop Med Hyg 71: 271-281, 1968

274.   PATEK AJ, TOTH IG, SAUNDERS MG, CASTRO GA, ENGEL JJ: Alcohol and dietary factors in cirrhosis. Arch Intern Med 135: 1053-1057, 1975

275.   EDMONDSON HA: Tumors of the liver and intrahepatic bile ducts. In Atlas of Tumor Pathology. Armed Forces Institute of Pathology, Section VII, Fascicle 25, 1958. pp. 49

276.   LIEBER CS, ZIMMON D, KESSLER R, DECARLI LM: Portal hypertension in experimental alcoholic liver injury. Clin Res 24: 478A, 1976

277.   LIEBER CS, DECARLI LM, RUBIN E: Sequential production of fatty liver, hepatitis and cirrhosis in sub-human primates fed ethanol with adequate diets. Proc Nat Acad Sci USA 72: 437-441, 1975

278.   PATRICK RS: Alcohol as a stimulus to hepatic fibrogenesis. J Alcoholism 8: 13-27, 1973

279.   McGEE JO'D, PATRICK RS, RODGER MC, LUTY CM: Collagen proline hydroxylase activity and ^{35}S sulphate uptake in human liver biopsies. Gut 15: 260-267, 1974

280.   RESNICK RH, CERDA JC, BOITNOTT J, ARON J, IBER FL: Urinary hydroxyproline excretion in hepatic disorders. Am J Gastro-enterology 60: 576-584, 1973

281.   LELBACH WK: Cirrhosis in the alcoholic and its relation to the volume of alcohol abuse. NY Acad Sci 252: 85-105, 1975

282.   BARAONA E, LINDENBAUM J: Metabolic aspects of alcoholism in the intestine. In Metabolic Aspects of Alcoholism, Chapter 3. C.S. Lieber (ed). Lancaster, England, Medical and Technical Publishing Co., Ltd., 1976. In press

283.   KYOSOLA K, SALORINNE Y: Liver biopsy and liver function tests in
       28 consecutive long-term alcoholics. <u>Ann Clin Res</u> 7: 80-84,
       1975

DISCUSSION

CHAIRMAN: K.J. ISSELBACHER

ISSELBACHER: What numbers do you now have in terms of baboons with cirrhosis versus those just with alcoholic hepatitis?   What are the data at the moment?

LIEBER: A total of 17 baboons have been fed alcohol, as 50% of total calories.   17 controls did not develop any lesions.   Of the 17 alcohol fed animals five have developed mild hepatitis and six have developed cirrhosis, one incomplete.   One out of three developed cirrhosis.

ISSELBACHER: And that's over what period of time?

LIEBER: 2-5 years.   The shortest time for the development of the early cirrhosis was 2 years.   The shortest time for the appearance of hepatitis was 9 months.

ISSELBACHER: You and others have emphasized malabsorption as a potential cause of malnutrition in alcoholism.   Your baboons did not have evidence of impaired absorption.   How does this fit into your overall concept?

LIEBER: The effects of alcohol on the gut are striking if we study segments of the intestine.   But if we study the overall balance of the body it apparently takes more severe alcohol ingestion and perhaps a different diet to produce an imbalance.   If we had put down a tube in these baboons and studied segmental amino acid absorption or segmental thiamine absorption, we may well have found an impairment of that segment.   But in terms of the overall body metabolism we found that these animals were still capable of absorbing their protein and fat.

ROTHSCHILD: The use of specific activity to measure protein synthesis demands that the precursor specific activity be known. Otherwise one can only measure relative rates of protein synthesis. A second point I want to make is that we have never found a retention of precursor radioactivity within or without albumin in our acute studies with the alcohol perfused liver. There is no evidence of retention of labelled protein within a liver acutely perfused with alcohol.

LIEBER: The point was not to emphasize protein synthesis here because what you have shown is decreased protein synthesis and what we have found after chronic ethanol feeding is protein accumulation. Acute alcohol feeding does not produce this latter condition. Protein accumulation in the liver is seen only after chronic alcohol feeding. There is essentially no disagreement between your data obtained after an acute perfusion of alcohol in vitro and our long term ethanol feeding studies.

TAMBURRO: If one looks at the liver biopsies of individuals who consume more than a fifth of whisky or its equivalent each day, one finds that one third of these individuals have very limited damage, another third has fatty liver with or without necrosis and another third has cirrhosis. Another observation is that if individuals with a severely fatty liver without necrosis are de-fatted and then return to drinking, they commonly return with a fatty liver rather than with a more advanced disease even if they have been drinking for a longer period of time. Similarly those with alcoholic hyaline tend to have repeated admissions with alcoholic hyaline. The third observation is that if you look at individuals who develop fatty liver with necrosis, you find evidence of collagen deposition and early cirrhosis. The question is whether there might not be two pathogenetic mechanisms, the first involving the direct toxicity of alcohol and the second involving immunological toxicity. Lymphocytes from individuals with alcoholic hepatitis can be induced and in culture they produce a factor which stimulates fibroblasts to produce more collagen. Leevy's group has purified alcoholic hyaline. The lymphocytes of alcoholics with fatty liver do not respond to this material but the lymphocytes of individuals with alcoholic hepatitis do. There appears to be a double mechanism for necrosis, one immunological and the other chemical. We have been doing some HLA tissue typing on individuals with alcoholic liver disease. There appear to be two separate HLA tissue types differing in blacks and whites which are associated with the development of severe injury.

LIEBER: I agree that there is more than one pathogenetic mechanism. All I was trying to point out was that you don't have to have hyaline to develop a full blown cirrhosis.

ISRAEL: We started a primate colony and found that we were plagued with infections, respiratory and intestinal. We wanted to see if the lesions would develop faster in the presence of hypoxia but we dropped the project because too many of the animals were hypo-xaemic to start with. Have you had upper respiratory diseases in your animals?

LIEBER: Which type of animal did you use?

ISRAEL: The Rhesus monkey.

LIEBER: It took me exactly five years to develop this model and we considered several species of sub-human primates and several feeding procedures. One does run into a number of problems. We finally selected a baboon from the highlands rather than the lowlands of Ethiopia. We have developed some pulmonary infections but primarily after the animals already have cirrhosis. In other words, once we get cirrhosis, we have trouble with these animals. We now use very careful techniques with complete surgical isolation, and strictly synthetic diets. So I am not surprised that you had difficulties initially; I had five years with them before I could get the system to work. But I would be happy to give you the secret.

RAISFELD: Dr. Lelbach has developed a good dose response curve in man for alcoholic liver injury including cirrhosis. But there has been difficulty in developing other animal models, even in animals with apparently similar ethanol metabolism. Would you comment on this difficulty in finding an appropriate animal model?

LIEBER: What distinguishes the human from other primates is not our metabolism of alcohol but our appetite for alcohol. Our challenge is to induce the animal to take an amount of alcohol comparable to the human species without impairment of nutrition. To do this we have to go to the liquid diet and even in the rat all we could get was 36% of total calories as alcohol, which is moderate drinking. Heavy drinking is 50% or more and this we achieved in the baboon. In this sense the baboon is closer to man. So it is the appetite, not the metabolism which accounts for the difficulty.

ALCOHOLIC HEPATITIS

S. W. French, J. S. Sim, K. E. Franks, E. J. Burbige, T. Denton
and M. G. Caldwell

Departments of Pathology and Medicine,
Martinez V. A. Hospital and
University of California School of Medicine, Davis, California

INTRODUCTION

The pathogenesis of alcoholic hepatitis (AH) is, as yet, unknown. Our approach to the problem has been to start with a study of the AH lesion in order to search for clues which would suggest the pathogenesis. Subsequent experiments have been designed to pursue the leads derived from the morphologic observations.

In a prior study French and Davies (1) noted that hepatocytes in AH underwent a number of changes in the region of the liver lobule around the terminal hepatic veins. These changes included the formation of Mallory bodies (MBs), a maldistribution of subcellular organelles, and the accumulation of fat. These findings led us to postulate that the hepatocellular injury was due to a colchicine-like effect of chronic alcohol ingestion, i.e. alcohol caused a loss of microtubular function which interfered with the transport and secretory functions of the liver cells.

The important observations of Baraona et al (2) support this hypothesis. These workers reported that chronic ethanol-fed rats retained export proteins (i.e. albumin and transferrin) in the soluble fraction of the liver and at the same time colchicine binding protein was decreased. The latter change reflects a decrease in the functional state of the microtubules. The loss of microtubular function could explain the retention of export protein and fat by the liver cells. Thus, there is both morphologic and biochemical evidence to support the microtubular failure hypothesis of liver injury caused by chronic alcohol ingestion.

This report deals with studies which further delineate the nature of liver cell injury in AH including the nature of MBs and the possible role played by lymphocytes in the progression of AH.

MATERIAL AND METHODS

Survey of Liver Morphology in AH

All liver biopsies at the MVAH for the years 1974 and 1975 (202 cases) were reviewed in a retrospective study. The slides were reviewed without knowledge of clinical information or diagnosis. The cases were categorized according to the morphologic diagnosis. The diagnosis of AH was made according to the criteria of Brunt et al (3). The presence of MBs, piecemeal necrosis, focal parenchymal lymphocytic infiltrate, fatty change and cirrhosis was also recorded. After the morphologic diagnoses were made the charts were reviewed to determine which patients had a history of alcoholism. In a prospective study electronmicroscopy examination was performed on selected cases.

Experimental Induction of MBs

MBs were produced experimentally in mice by administration of griseofulvin in the food according to the method of Denk et al (4). Twenty adult male C3H strain mice weighing between 25-29 g were fed a semisynthetic complete standard diet (Teklad Test Diet, Madison, Wis.) which contained 30% casein (5) and 2.5% griseofulvin (provided by Schering Corp., Ltd., Quebec, Canada). Five control mice were fed the diet without griseofulvin added. The mice were sacrificed after five months and a portion of liver was fixed in 10% formalin for light microscopy, a portion was fixed in 3% glutaraldehyde in 0.1 M phosphate buffer and post-fixed in 1% osmium tetroxide for electronmicroscopy, a portion was frozen for immunofluorescent studies and the remainder was used for salt and urea extractions to isolate intermediate filament protein.

Experimental Induction of Microfilament Hyperplasia

Microfilament hyperplasia was induced in the liver of male C3H mice according to the method of Gabbiani et al (6). Ten adult mice were fed Purina laboratory chow ad lib. Five mice were given Phalloidin (generously supplied by Th. Wieland, Heidelberg, Germany,) intraperitoneally once daily at a dose of 1 mg/kg of body weight in one ml of 0.9% saline. Five control animals were injected with saline alone. Two experimental mice and two controls were sacrificed at 19 days and at 40 days. Liver was examined by light and electronmicroscopy. Samples were also frozen in liquid nitrogen for immunofluorescent studies.

Immunologic Characterization of MBs

Tissue slices containing MBs obtained from three cases of AH were examined by indirect immunofluorescent techniques utilizing human smooth muscle antibody (SMA) (generously supplied by Dr. H. J. Smith, BioScience Laboratories) and anti-MB antibody. Horseradish peroxidase-antiperoxidase (PAP) binding was also studied using light microscopy (7). Frozen sections of liver obtained from griseofulvin fed mice and Phalloidin-injected mice were similarly studied.

Antiserum to MB protein was prepared in rats. MB protein was isolated (8) and further purified in 5% deoxycholate as previously described. Lyophilized MB (8.8 mg) as antigen was dispersed in 0.5 ml saline and mixed with an equal volume of Freunds complete adjuvant. The antigen emulsion was injected intramuscularly three times at two week intervals. Antiserum was obtained two weeks after the last injection. The antiserum was inactivated at 53°C and stored at -18°C prior to use.

Specificity of the antiserum for MB protein was established using both the double immunodiffusion technique (9) and indirect immunofluorescent techniques (11). The lyophilized MB protein extract (solubilized in 1% SDS, 8 M urea) and control protein were solubilized in 1 M urea in 0.01 M phosphate buffer, pH 7.4. Antisera and control sera were absorbed with lyophilized tissue powder from control human liver. The absorption mixtures were left overnight in the cold (10) and the supernatants were utilized in immunodiffusion against MB and control antigens. Precipitating antibodies to MB protein persisted in the absorbed MB antisera.

Immunofluorescent staining of MBs in human AH livers and griseofulvin-fed mice livers was done using MB antisera and SMA. Control livers, Phalloidin-treated mice livers and isolated MBs were similarly studied. Staining was performed with fluorescein isothiocyanate (FITC)-conjugated anti-rat and anti-human IgG sera using the indirect technique (11). The MB antiserum and SMA were absorbed with purified actin (Worthington) in order to distinguish MB antibody from actin antibody (21).

Identification of MB Protein by Slab Gel Co-electrophoresis

Protein extracts of isolated MB fractions, livers containing MBs from griseofulvin-fed mice, control mouse liver and chicken gizzard were co-electrophoresed on polyacrylamide slab gels using the discontinuous sodium dodecyl sulfate (SDS) buffer system of Laemmli (12). The protein was extracted from the tissues to selectively concentrate intermediate filament (IF) protein according to the method of Cooke (13). Actomyosin was first extracted from the tissue by three daily changes of 0.6 M KC1 in 0.5 M Tris pH 8.8. The residual pellets were then dispersed in 8 M urea for 24 hours and the supernatant was dialyzed against 50 mM phosphate buffer, pH 7.5 containing 1 mM mercaptoethanol. The MB fractions were isolated by the two-phase polymer system (14) modified so as to remove collagen by incubating the liver homogenate for five hours in five volumes of 0.05 Tris buffer, pH 7.5, containing 0.1% DNA-ase (Sigma Chemical Co.), clostridial collagenase (Worthington Enzymes), 0.36 mM $CaCl_2$, 0.1 mM magnesium sulfate, 50 units mycostatin and 0.25 mg/ml tetracycline at 37°C. Purity of the isolated MB fractions was monitored by light and electronmicroscopy. The MB protein samples were solubilized by boiling (2 min.) in a solution containing 1 M Tris, pH 6.8, 1% SDS, 1% mercaptoethanol and 8 M urea and 20% glycerol. Bromophenol blue was used as a dye reference. Protein concentrations were 8-10 μg for each protein standard and 70-100μg of the MB extract as determined by the Lowry method. The samples were applied to the gel wells and electrophoresis was performed at 50 ma/gel for 1.5 to 2 hours. The gels were stained by the method of Fairbanks et al (15). The separating gels consisted of a 10% running and a 4% stacking gel. Both gels were prepared from a stock solution of 30g of acrylamide and 0.8g of Bis in 100 ml of water. SDS (0.1%) was in both gels and buffers. Gels (1.5 mm) were poured with a 10 well comb utilizing the system of Ames (16).

Distribution of T and B Lymphocytes in AH

T and B lymphocytes were isolated from peripheral and hepatic venous blood and liver biopsy specimens in patients with AH and control subjects (approved by Human Use Committee; informed consent obtained). Lympho-cytes from blood were isolated on a Ficoll-Isopaque density gradient and washed two times with phosphate buffered saline (PBS). Lymphocytes were retrieved from liver biopsy specimens after enzyme digestion using a modification of the Van Boxel and Paget technique (19). The liver tissue digest was layered onto 5 ml of Ficoll-Isopaque and centrifuged. The interface was washed once. The isolated lymphocytes from blood and liver were assayed for viability with trypan blue (0.1%) and counted in a hemocytometer. For T-cell rosettes (E) the method of Wybran and Fudenberg (17) was used. For B-cell quantitation the method of Giuliano et al (18) was used.

RESULTS

Survey of Liver Morphology in AH

Of 202 consecutive liver biopsies 27, or 13.3%, filled the morphologic criteria for the diagnosis of AH. Other diagnoses were: chronic aggressive hepatitis 14.4%, idiopathic cirrhosis 8%, fatty liver 5.4%, normal liver 17.8% and miscellaneous 41.1%. MBs were found in all cases of AH with cirrhosis and in 62% without cirrhosis (Table I) for an overall frequency of 77%. Other features of AH included fibrosis around the terminal hepatic veins (Fig. 1), cholestasis, fatty change and inflammatory infiltrates including PMNε, lymphocytes and macrophages. The most prominent and consistent hepatocellular change was the swelling of single (Fig. 1) or clusters of liver cells (Fig. 2). The swollen cells showed maldistribution of organelles and loss of the normal polyhedral cell shape. The cytosol was often filled with amorphous material which was relatively devoid of organelles or completely occupied by countless, small lipid droplets (Fig. 3). Degenerative changes in

TABLE I

FREQUENCY OF ALCOHOLISM, MALLORY BODIES AND PIECEMEAL NECROSIS*

DIAGNOSIS	No. of Cases	Average Age	% of Alcoholics	% With Mallory Bodies	% With Piecemeal Necrosis
Alcoholic Hepatitis	27	53	96	77	44
- With Cirrhosis				100	64
- Without Cirrhosis				62	31
Chronic Aggressive Hepatitis	29	45	46	3	100
- With Cirrhosis				6	100
- Without Cirrhosis				0	100
Cirrhosis, Idiopathic	16	55	69	0	12
Fatty Liver	11	-	–	0	18

*Piecemeal necrosis includes both periportal and parenchymal invasion by lymphocytes with liver cell drop-out.

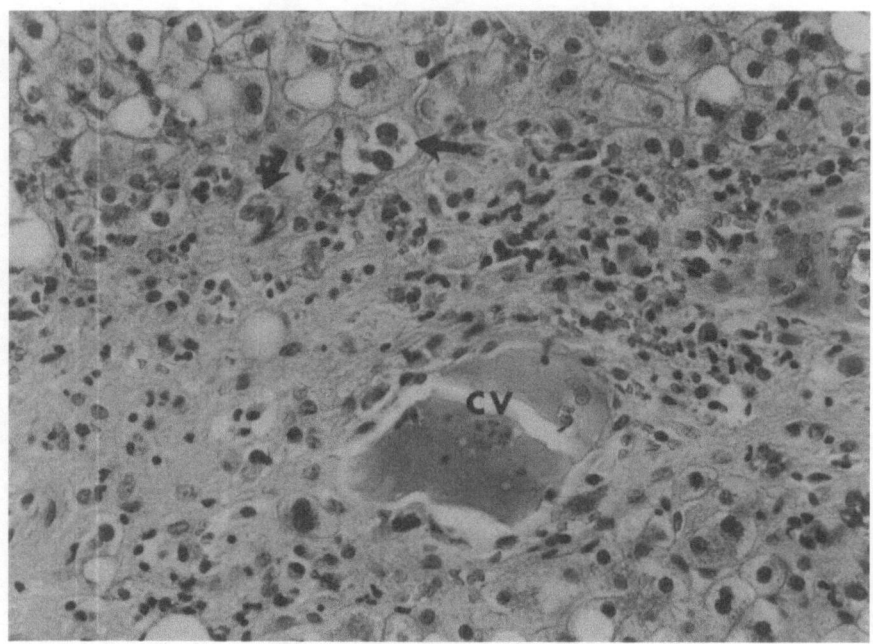

Fig. 1   *Alcoholic hepatitis.   Note the scarring around the terminal hepatic vein (CV).   Numerous plasma cells and lymphocytes are noted among the fibroblasts.   At the interface between the scar and liver cells are rounded liver cells with clear cytoplasm containing MBs (arrows).   Note the lymphocytes and plasma cells. Hematoxylin and eosin X250.*

mitochondria were often noted and both lymphocytes and PMNs appeared to invade the affected liver cells. Like PMNs, lymphocytes were occasionally seen in close opposition to hepatocytes (Fig. 4).

Focal lymphocytic infiltration and piecemeal necrosis (Fig. 5) were frequently encountered (Table I) making it sometimes difficult to distinguish AH from chronic aggressive hepatitis. This change was more conspicuous in more advanced disease since it was seen in 18% of fatty liver, 31% of AH and 64% of AH with cirrhosis.

Experimental Induction of MBs

The livers of griseofulvin-fed mice were markedly enlarged (20.8g/100g body weight) compared to controls (6.5g/100g). All mice fed griseofulvin had MBs in the liver cells (Fig. 6). Affected cells were enlarged, swollen and rounded so as to closely resemble the swollen hepatocytes seen in AH (Fig.

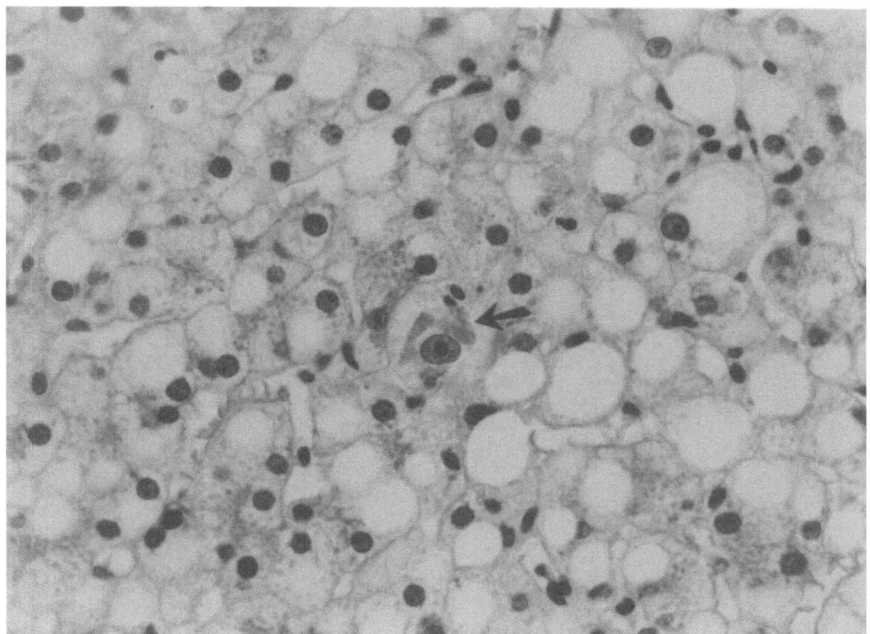

*Fig. 2   Alcoholic hepatitis. A single round swollen liver cell containing a
           MB (arrow) is seen among unaffected liver cells containing fat.
           No fibrosis is present.   Characteristically, such swollen cells
           contain an enlarged nucleus with an enlarged nucleolus. Note the
           lymphocyte abutting against the swollen liver cell. Hematoxylin
           and eosin X400.*

2). Electronmicroscopic (EM) examination (Fig. 7) revealed that MBs were
indeed present in the affected cells confirming the results of Denk et al (4).
The MB filaments branched in a manner indistinguishable from that seen in
AH. The smooth endoplasmic reticulum appeared very prominent in these
cells.   No change in the microfilaments (MFs) in the ectoplasm was
observed.

Experimental Induction of MF Hyperplasia

      Phalloidin injections induced marked hyperplasia of the pericanalicular
MFs as visualized by light (Fig. 8) and by EM (Fig. 9) thus confirming
findings of Gabbiani et al (6).   These filaments were increased in the
ectoplasm bordering on the space of Disse as well (Fig. 9).   French and
Davies (20) found that MFs normally occur at this location. Rounded masses
of filaments filled Kupffer cells. No MBs were encountered. Control livers
showed no increase in the pericanalicular MFs (Fig. 10).

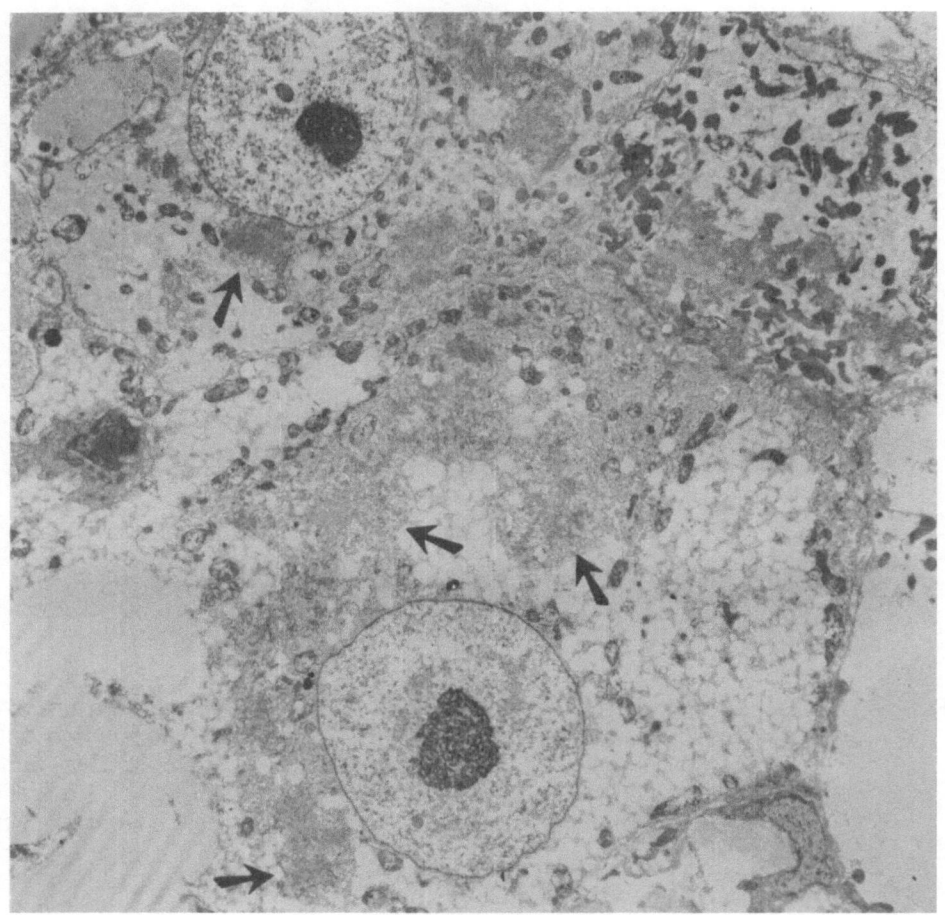

Fig. 3   *Alcoholic hepatitis. Note the rounded contour of the hepatocyte
containing numerous small fat globules and MBs (arrows).
Organelles are maldistributed and decreased in number. Note the
lymphocyte within the cytoplasm of a liver cell containing fat.
Uranyl acetate and lead citrate X4100.*

Immunologic Characterization of MBs

The rat MB antiserum bound MBs from human liver (Fig. 11) and mouse
liver. Absorption of MB antiserum with purified actin did not diminish the
fluorescent antibody staining of MBs with the MB antiserum. Absorption
with MB extract eliminated the staining of MBs with MB antiserum. Both
the MB antiserum and SMA bound to the hyperplastic MFs of Phalloidin-
treated mice. This immunofluorescent reaction was almost completely
eliminated by absorption of the MB antiserum or SMA with actin. SMA did

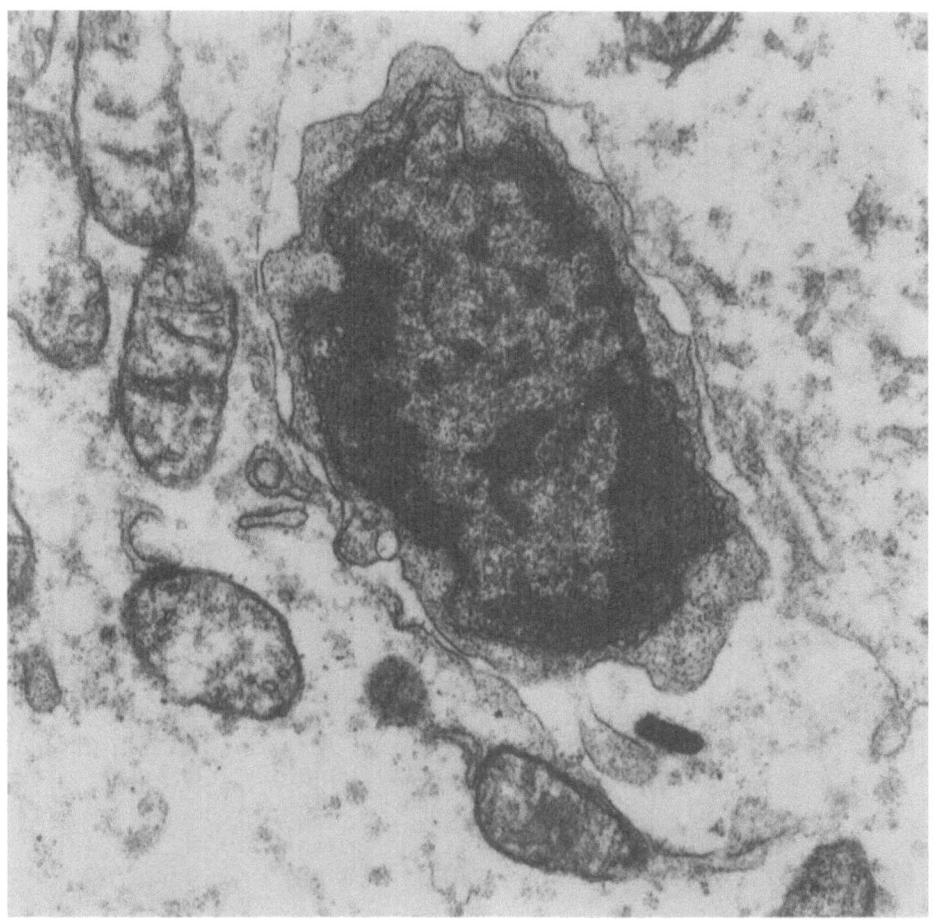

*Fig. 4   Alcoholic hepatitis.   A lymphocyte is seen to be wedged between
two hepatocytes.   Uranyl acetate and lead citrate X39,000.*

not bind human MBs; thus, we could not confirm Nenci's findings (21). It is
concluded that the rat MB antiserum contained two antibodies, one which
bound MFs and one which bound MB protein.   The SMA contained one
antibody which bound MFs (actin). MBs from AH and griseofulvin-fed mice
both bound PAP whereas the Phalloidin-induced microfilaments did not.
Thus, the MBs from the two species were antigenically the same and shared
a nonspecific binding characteristic.

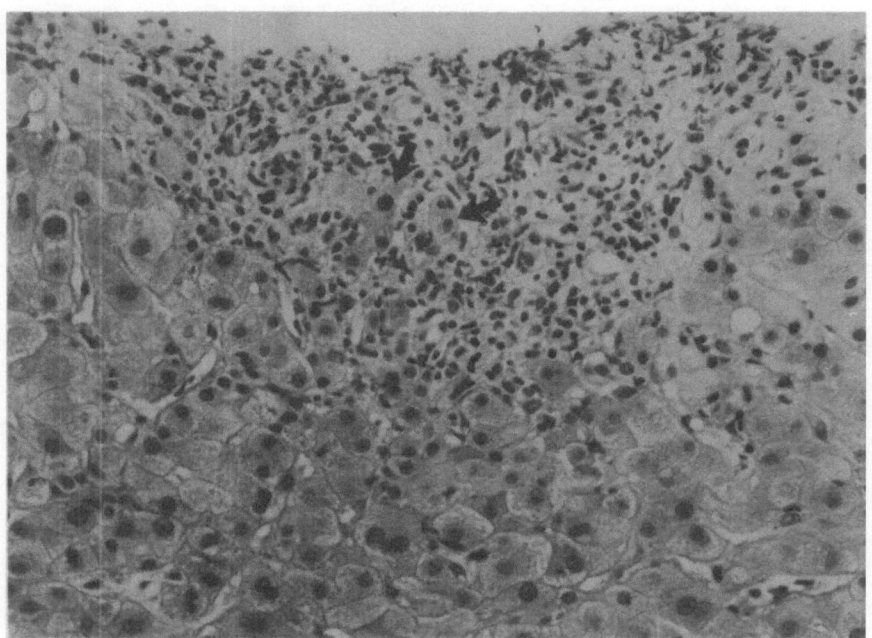

*Fig. 5   Alcoholic hepatitis.   Piecemeal necrosis is evident in that
lymphocytes and fibroblasts are seen disrupting the limiting plate
and entrapping liver cells (arrows). Hematoxylin and eosin X275.*

Identification of the MB Protein by Slab Gel Co-electrophoresis

The extracts of chicken gizzard smooth muscle, the human MB
griseofulvin-fed mice livers and control liver all had one protein band which
had the same electrophoretic mobility (Fig. 12). This protein was dominant
in the extracts and corresponded to the protein derived from IFs from
smooth muscle identified by Cooke (13).   This protein had a molecular
weight of 53,800 as determined by comparing the relative mobilities of the
proteins with standard proteins of known molecular weight. These findings
contrast with the results of Okamura et al (14) who reported 5 major MB
protein bands on gel electrophoresis.

Distribution of T and B Lymphocytes in AH

Human T and B lymphocytes were identified by rosette formation with
sheep red blood cells and enumerated.   For B cells antibody-coated
erythrocytes were used (purified goat anti-human F (ab') Subtype 2). Only a
few patients have been studied so far so no conclusions are possible (Table

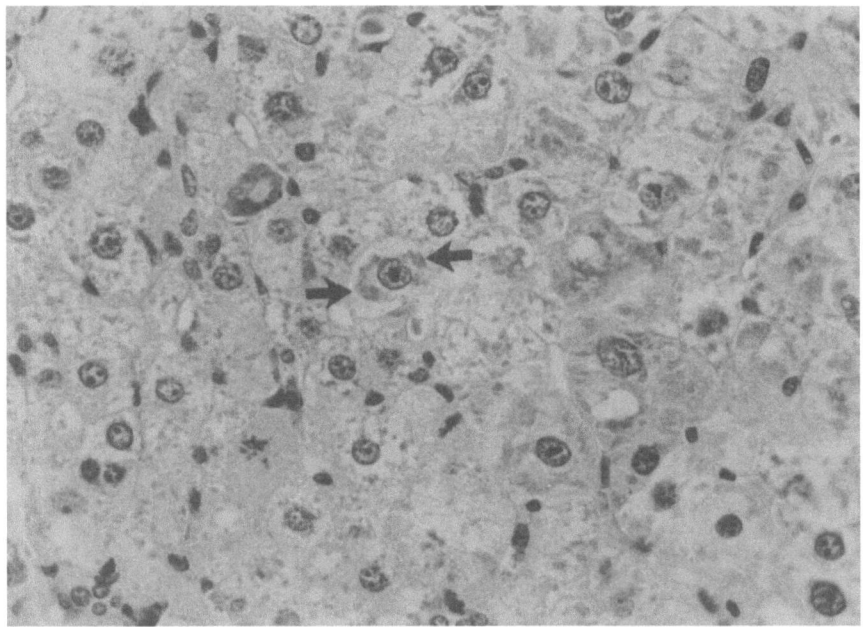

*Fig. 6   Griseofulvin-fed mouse liver. After 5 months of feeding griseo-
fulvin (2.5%) mice developed MBs within their swollen hepatocytes
(arrows). Hematoxylin and eosin X400.*

II). The lymphocytes in the liver were mostly T cells in AH. The number of
lymphocytes obtained from the liver was high enough to do a differential
count.

DISCUSSION

The morphologic changes in the liver cells noted in AH included swelling
and rounding up of cells, loss and disorganization of cytoplasmic organelles,
formation of MBs and cell death.   These changes have been described in
previous reports. Edmondson et al (22) described swollen hydropic liver cells
which were characterized by organelle disorganization in one-third of
hospitalized chronic alcoholic patients that had been drinking heavily. Biava
(23) and Yokoo et al (24) illustrated the accumulation of small fat droplets
associated with MB formation. Horvath et al (25) noted no abnormalities in
hepatocellular organelles in cells containing a small amount of MB but when
the MB material increased signs of advanced injury in the form of dilatation
of endoplasmic reticulum, increase in cytosegresomes and accumulation of

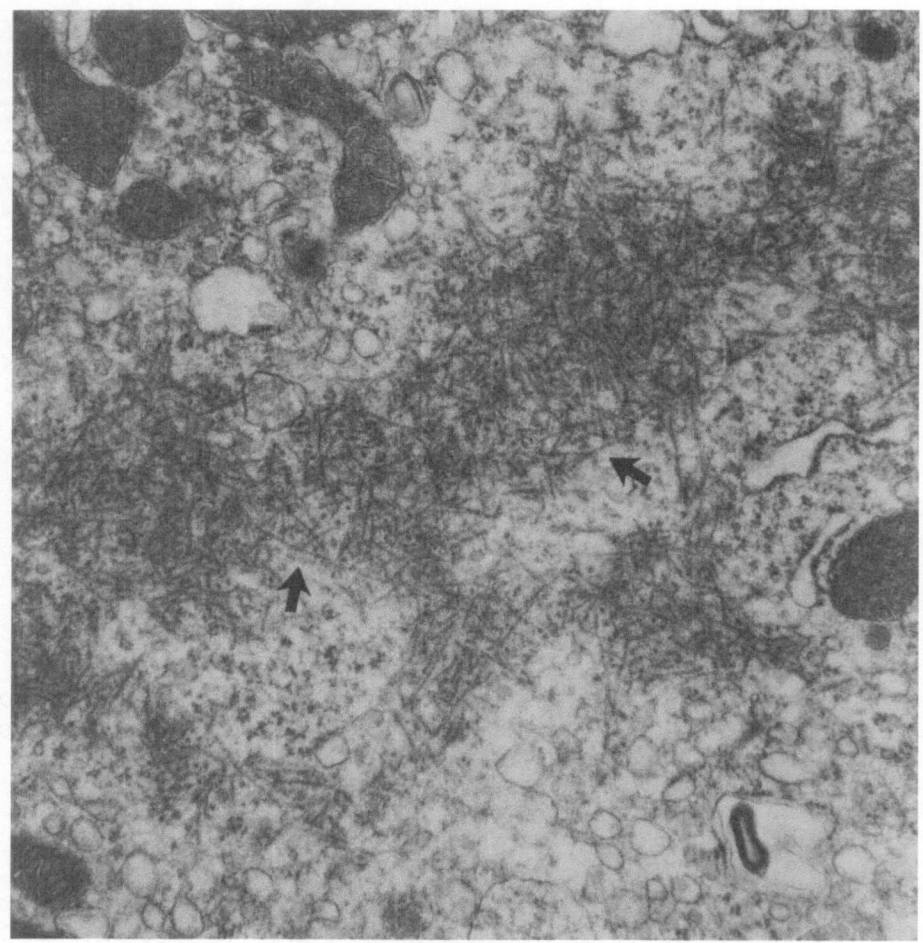

Fig. 7   Griseofulvin-fed mouse liver. The MB filaments are arranged at angles with frequent branching (arrows) identical to MB filaments seen in AH. Uranyl acetate and lead citrate X38,900.

lipid droplets developed.   Thus, there is a progression from minimal MB formation to hepatocellular enlargement and degeneration to cell death. This swelling and necrosis of hepatocytes around the terminal hepatic veins is the hallmark of AH (3).

Many of the morphologic changes that occur in the hepatocytes could result from the failure of the microtubular system of the cell to function normally; i.e. secretion of export proteins and low density lipoproteins into

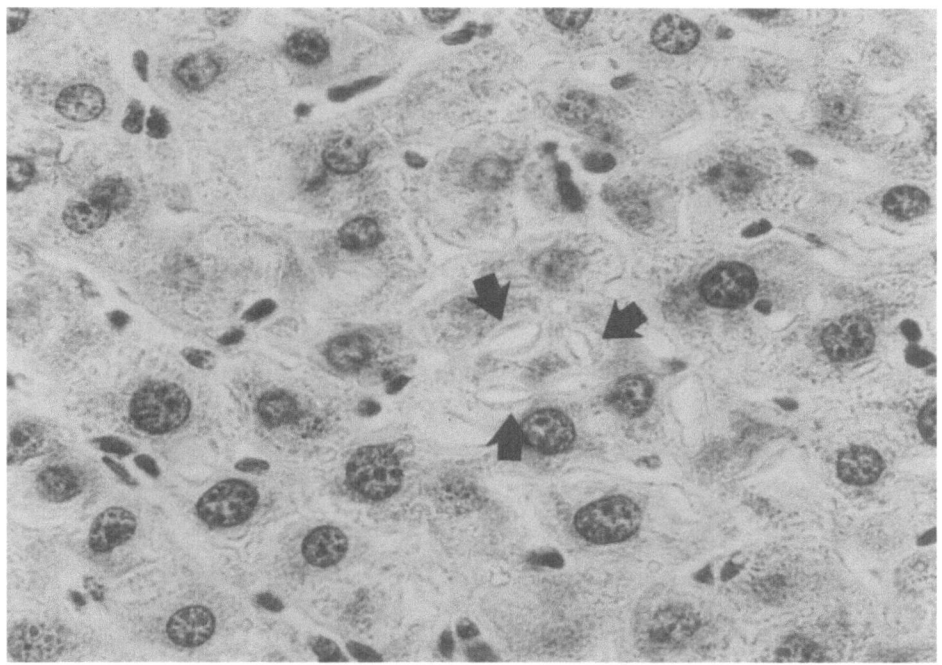

Fig. 8   Phalloidin-injected mouse liver. The bile canaliculi are dilated, rigid and slit-shaped and are surrounded by a thickened wall (arrows). Hematoxylin and eosin X400.

the blood and dispersion of IFs. Failure to secrete could account for the retention of albumin and transferrin (2), the accumulation of multiple small fat globules in the cytosol and the enlargement of individual hepatocytes. Failure to disperse IFs could account for MB formation and the loss of cell shape.

Much of the evidence supporting the microtubular failure hypothesis of liver injury in AH is based on the known effects of antitubulins such as colchicine and griseofulvin. Denk et al (4) have shown, and we have confirmed, that griseofulvin induces MB formation. Griseofulvin, like colchicine, stops mitoses in metaphase (26). Like colchicine, griseofulvin inhibits the directional movement of leukocytes (27) presumably through its antitubulin action.

The possibility that microtubules play a role in MB formation hinges on the identity of MB protein as IF protein by demonstration that MB protein has the same electrophoretic mobility as IF protein derived from chicken

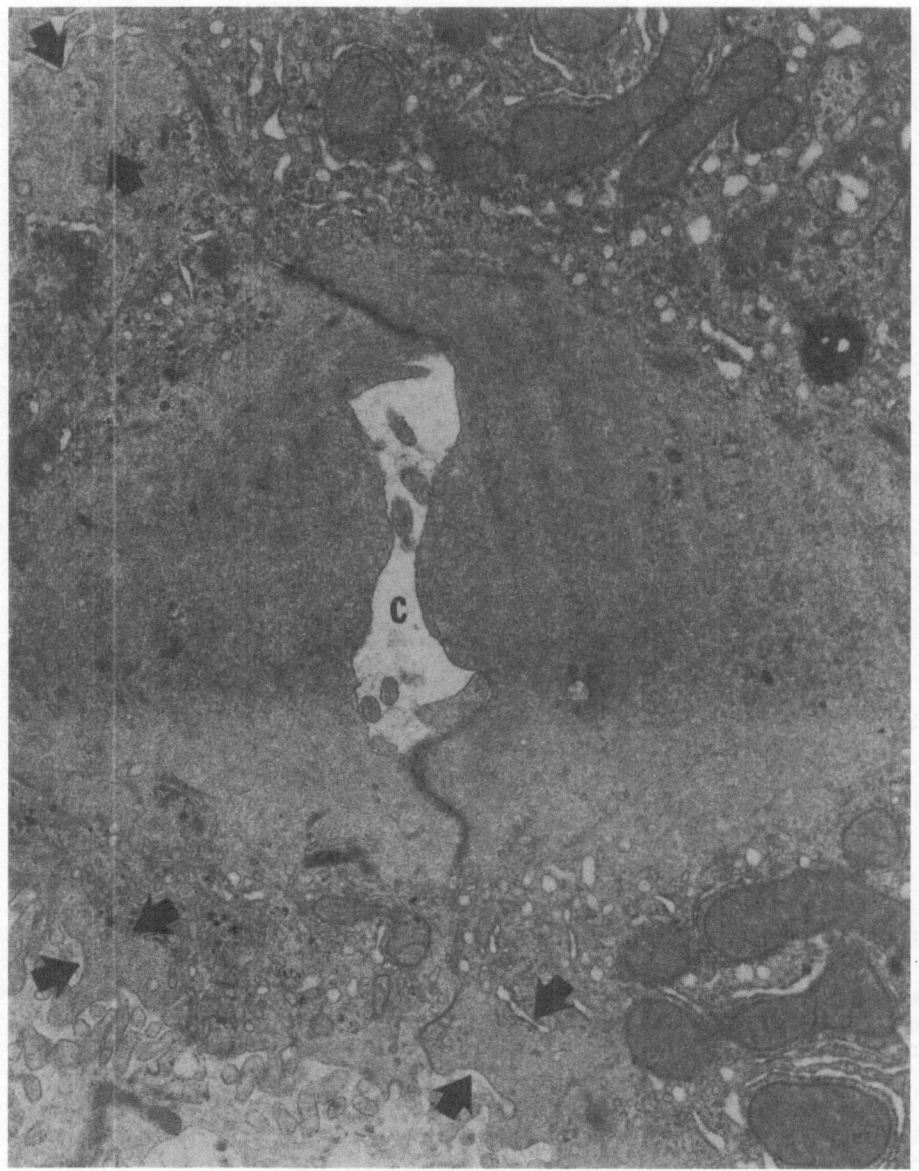

Fig. 9   Phalloidin-injected mouse liver. Note the partial loss of microvilli
          and the extreme thickening of the microfilament pericanalicular
          ectoplasm.   The ectoplasm facing the sinusoids is also thickened
          (between the arrows). Uranyl acetate and lead citrate X20,600.

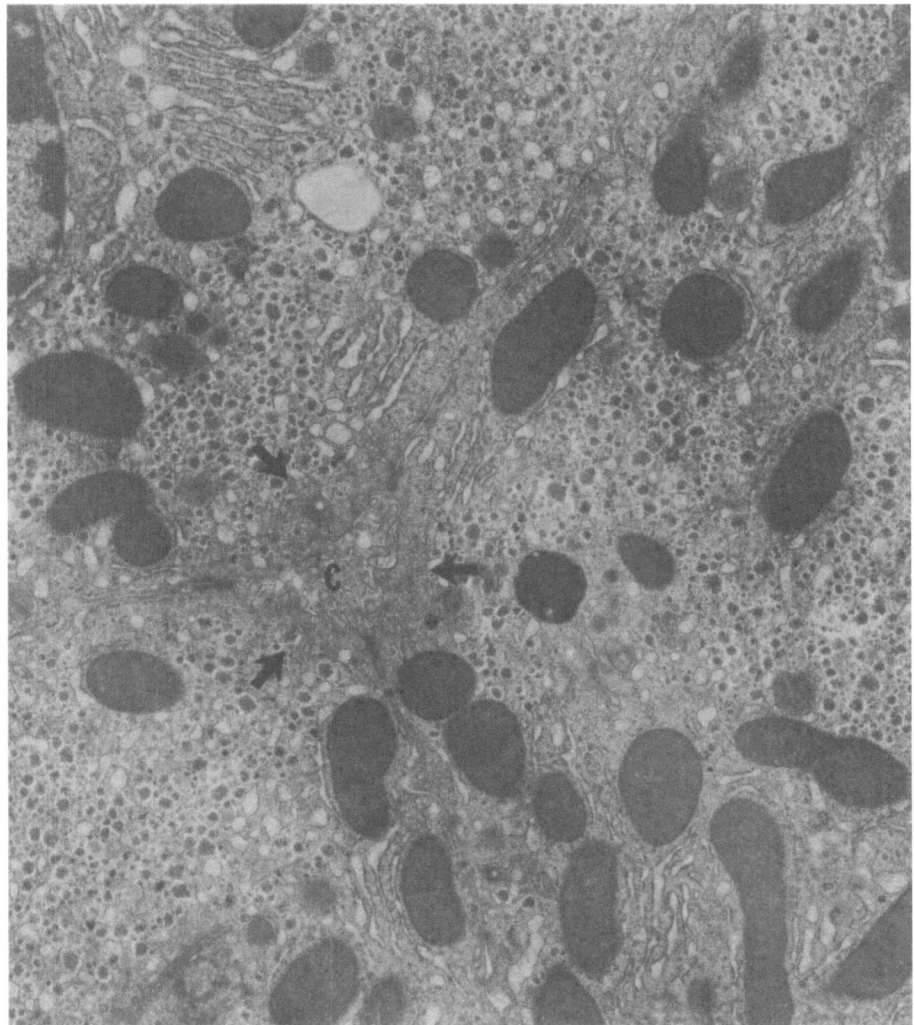

Fig. 10   Control mouse liver.   The triangular-shaped canaliculus (arrows) is
collapsed and filled with microvilli.   The ectoplasmic zone is
narrow.   Uranyl acetate and lead citrate X18,4000.

gizzard smooth muscle (13).   We have demonstrated morphological differences between the MF hyperplasia seen with Phalloidin and MBs.   The MB
protein was antigenically distinguishable from actin using SMA and antisera
to MBs.   Taken together, this evidence supports the conclusion the MBs are
composed primarily of IF protein and not actin.

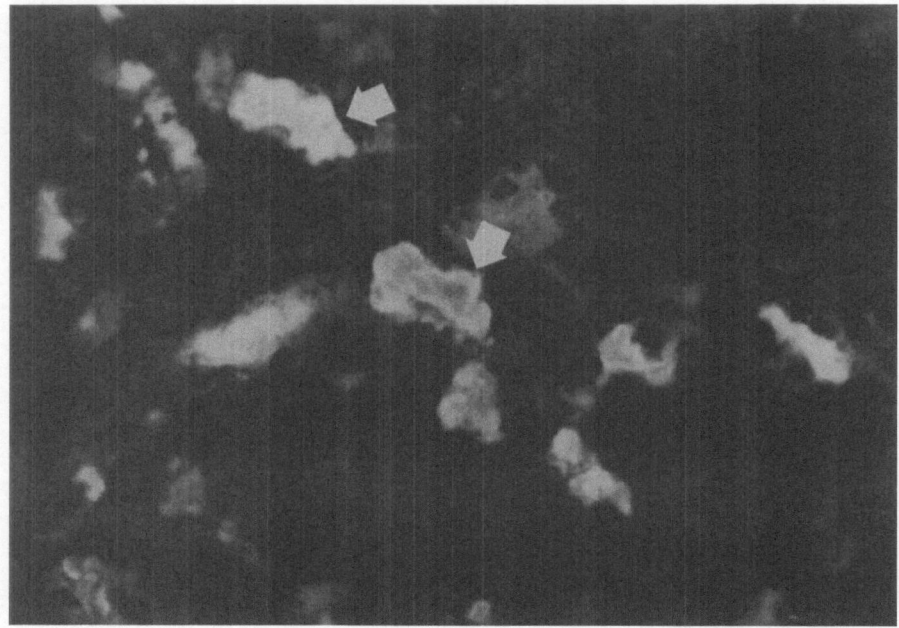

Fig. 11   *Frozen section of liver from a patient with AH. The MBs were stained by the indirect immunofluorescent staining technique using rat anti-MB antibody.   Note the central core of the MB sometimes appears less dense than the rim.   X700*

Given that MBs represent abnormal accumulation of IFs it is then possible to relate MB formation to microtubular failure. IFs increase in number and aggregate in large clusters in cells exposed to antitubulins such as colchicine and colcemide. Colchicine induces the proliferation of 10 nm neurofilaments (IFs) in neurons (28).   De Brabander et al (29) showed in in vitro studies that C3H mouse embryonal cells develop bundles and whirls of IFs five hours after exposure to antitubulins. Over a 24-48 hour period the IF aggregation continued to grow in size. When the antitubulin was removed the filament whirls were slow to diminish and large aggregates persisted more than 48 hours. The antitubulin-induced increase in IFs was blocked by the protein synthesis inhibitor, cycloheximide. These studies suggested that antitubulins induce an excessive synthesis of IF protein. Similar massive accumulations of IFs have been induced in muscle cells in cultures treated with cytochalasin-B followed by colcemide (30). Thus, MB-like aggregates of IFs have been induced in a variety of cells using antitubulin agents.

If antitubulins induce MB-like aggregation of IFs and chronic ethanol feeding has a similar effect on liver cells in AH, what is the evidence that

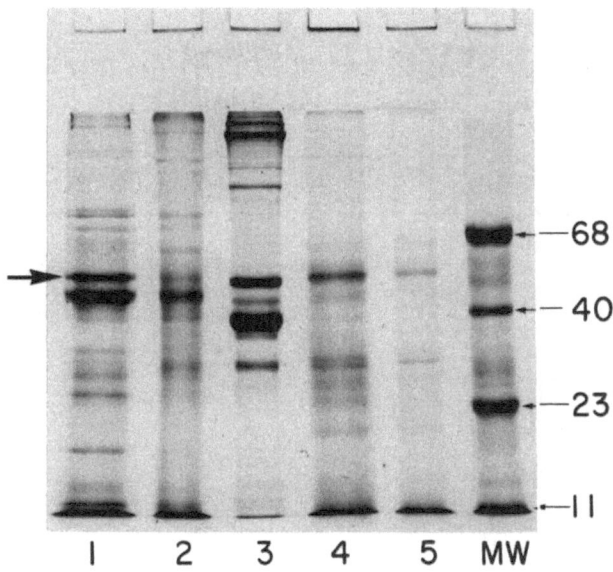

Fig. 12   Slab gel electrophoresis of MB protein (purified and semi-pure), extracts of griseofulvin and control livers, extracts of chicken gizzard smooth muscle and protein standards (MW). Protein standards used were BSA 68,000, actin 40,000, chymotrypsin-A 23,300 and cytochrome-C 11,700. Note that the MB protein band from the AH purified fraction (5) and semi-purified fraction (4) is also present in the griseofulvin-fed (2) and control mouse livers (1). (See solid arrow.). This protein has the same electrophoretic mobility as the IF protein band of the chicken gizzard extract (3).

ethanol may have its effect due to an antitubulin action? It has been shown that colchicine interferes with the secretion of low-density lipoprotein by the liver cell presumably through its antitubulin action (31). Colchicine also inhibits protein secretion (32, 33) and leads to the accumulation of small lipid droplets within the liver cells (34). Le Marchand et al have shown that colchicine inhibits secretion of albumin by the liver (35). Similarly, it has been shown by Annable and Cooper that acute ethanol inhibits the secretion of triglycerides by the liver cell and increases hepatotriglycerides concomitantly (58). Madsen has shown that acute ethanol reduced the serum very low density lipoprotein levels suggesting that hepatic lipoprotein secretion is inhibited by ethanol (36). Baraona et al have shown that the livers of rats fed ethanol for prolonged periods accumulate protein (2). They showed that export proteins increased in the livers of the ethanol-fed rats whereas colchicine-binding protein decreased. This important observation would seem to link the loss of functioning tubulin with the accumulation of protein and lipids and give substance to the hypothesis that MB accumulation in AH

TABLE II

T AND B LYMPHOCTYE* POPULATIONS IN PERIPHERAL
BLOOD (PB), HEPATIC VEIN BLOOD (HV) AND THE LIVER (L)

DX	PB-T	PB-B	L-T&B	L-T	L-B	HV-T	HV-B
	%	%	No./mg	%	%	%	%
AH	80	15	-	73	12	-	
AH+C[†]	58	19	1040	77	14	-	
	73	18	2300	89	-	75	19
	50	24	840	70	17		
CHF [¶]	52	22	5000	46	12	83	25

* *Viability 95-100% tested with 0.1% Trypan blue.*

[†] *Alcohol hepatitis with cirrhosis.*

[¶] *Congestive heart failure.*

is due to an ethanol-induced decrease in microtubular function. This may explain the hypoalbuminemia found in alcoholic patients with normal liver histology (37). Caution must be exercised in interpreting these results since the inhibition of protein secretion by colchicine may not be a result of antitubulin action (38).

The maldistribution of cytoplasmic organelles seen in hepatocytes bearing MBs could also be a reflection of the loss of microtubular function (1). Using antitubulins applied to a variety of cells it has been shown that microtubules are important in maintaining cell shape, the distribution of lysosomal and Golgi elements within the cytoplasm and the direction of saltatory movements of endocytic vacuoles towards the terminal hepatic veins(39). For instance Chang, using liver cells in tissue culture, showed inhibition of the movement of formed endocytic vacuoles to the cytocenter with the concomitant disappearance of cytoplasmic microtubules when the cells are treated with colcemide (40). Elongated mitochondria arranged in orderly parallel radiations become disoriented and intertwined after colcemide treatment. Similar organelle disarray is prominent in liver cells containing MBs in cases of AH (1). In rats treated with colchicine over prolonged periods, skeletal muscle myofilament disorientation becomes prominent so that bundles of myofilaments cross perpendicular or oblique to the long axis of muscle fibers (41). Developing skeletal muscle of embryos treated with antitubulin developed conspicuous aggregates of branching IFs which resembled MBs morphologically (39). Using smooth muscle cell preparations, Cooke has shown that the IFs function as a cytoskeleton, determining cell shape and defining cytoplasmic channels (13). The filaments connect with the plasma membrane of the smooth muscle cells in a way that determines cell polarity. Jimbow and Fitzpatrick reported evidence that the IFs in human melanocytes participate in the elongation of dendritic processes of the cell and in the transfer of melanosomes (42). Moellmann et al showed that microtubules were involved in melanosome aggregation and IFs were involved in dispersion of melanosomes (43). These two processes were under hormonal and cyclic nucleotide control. Colchicine stimulated the dispersion of the melanosomes in melanocytes. These observations indicate a dynamic interrelationship of microtubules and IF function which controls intracytoplasmic movement of organelles and cell shape. This complex of changes seen with antitubulins resembles closely the cellular features seen in liver cells in AH including MB formation. It is, therefore, considered likely that the occurrence of MBs in AH is the result of an antitubulin effect of chronic ethanol ingestion.

It is apparent that the colchicine–like action of chronic ethanol feeding cannot by itself account for the distribution of the cellular injury around the terminal hepatic veins in AH. The griseofulvin–induction of MBs occurs diffusely throughout the hepatic lobule. In an effort to bring together the many factors which could explain the focal nature of the liver damage we have diagramed the mechanisms which could, in combination, explain the AH lesion (Fig. 13). The hypoxia caused by the hypermetabolic state (44) resulting from the ATP deficiency due to an increase in ATPase activity could cause the decrease in microtubular function in the region of the terminal hepatic veins. The ethanol–induced increase in ATPase may result from K^+ efflux secondary to the stimulation of the α adrenergic receptor by epinephrine (45). Alternatively, the decrease in ATP could result from the acetaldehyde–induced mitochrondrial dysfunction (46) or the decrease in mitochondrial adenine translocase activity (47) observed in the ethanol-fed rats.

The failure of the microtubular dependent secretory process could also result from changes in intracellular cAMP and Ca^{2+}. It has been shown that chronic ethanol feeding does induce a β noradrenergic subsensitivity (48) which could reduce the hepatocellular processes that are modulated by cAMP and Ca^{2+}. Liver cell β receptors stimulate cAMP synthesis (48). Cyclic AMP does stimulate the efflux of Ca^{2+} from the mitochondria into the cytosol (49). A decrease in Ca^{2+} efflux could lead to a reduction in hepatocellular secretion of export protein and lipoprotein since hormone stimulated Ca^{2+} efflux triggers microtubular dependent secretory processes in a variety of cells (50). Cyclic AMP could also control cell shape by promoting phosphorylation of tubulin and associated proteins (51-52). By the same mechanism cAMP and Ca^{2+} could modulate intracellular locomotion of organelles (53). However, the possible role played by the hormone-induced changes in Ca^{2+} and cAMP in the control of the secretory functions of hepatocytes has not yet been investigated.

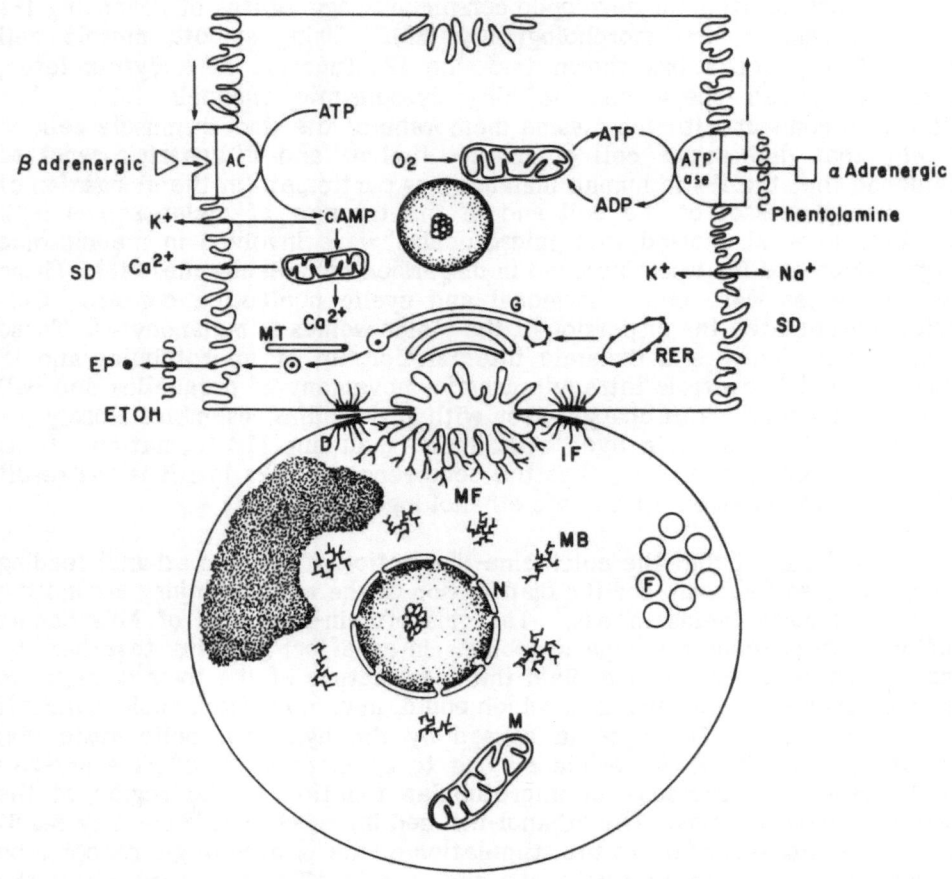

Fig. 13 *Diagramatic representation of the hypothetical role that various factors play in the pathogenesis of the hepatocellular changes seen in AH. SD=space of Disse, BC=bile canaliculus, RER=rough endoplasmic reticulum, G=Golgi, MT=microtubule, AC=adenylyl cyclase, D=desmosome, MF=microfilaments, IF=intermediate filaments, F=fat, MB=Mallory bodies, EP=export protein and N=nucleus.*

The possible importance of lymphocytes in AH was investigated. Piecemeal necrosis and focal lymphocytic infiltrates in the liver parenchyma were noted in 44% of the cases with AH. Lymphocytes were shown to be present between liver cells and to invade liver cells. Similar changes have been noted by light and electron microscopic examination of orthotopic liver homograph rejection (54). This finding suggested a possible role for T-cell "killing" in the propagation of hepatocellular injury in AH.

Brunt et al (3) found a similar frequency of piecemeal necrosis (40%) in AH. Christoffersen and Juhl (55) found lymphocytic infiltrates in 87% of patients with fatty liver and MBs, and in 27% of patients with fatty liver without MBs. This association of MBs with lymphocytic infiltrate correlates with the clinical observation that T-lymphocytes are sensitized to MBs in AH (56). Galambos (57) reported that the proportion of lymphocytes, plasma cells and macrophages increased in the inflammatory exudate in patients with AH who had serial liver biopsies during abstention from alcohol. It is for this reason that we have begun to study the T and B cell population in the peripheral blood, hepatic vein blood and in the liver. If T and B cells are sequestered in the liver this would suggest an autoimmune role for the lymphocyte to explain why AH progresses even after alcohol has been withdrawn from the diet.

SUMMARY

The morphologic findings in 27 consecutive cases of AH were reviewed for clues regarding the pathogenesis of cell injury. Two separate mechanisms were suggested by this study.

1. The swelling of hepatocytes containing MBs in the region of the terminal hepatic veins was postulated to result from the failure of the microtubular system to disperse IFs, maintain cell shape and intracellular organization as well as secrete export proteins. Review of the literature indicated that these changes could be reproduced in a variety of cell types with antitubulins such as colchicine. It was confirmed that the antitubulin griseofulvin induced MB formation and cellular enlargement in mice. It was also shown by immunopathologic, chemical and electron microscopy techniques that both the human and the experimental MBs were composed, in part, of IFs and not MFs. These findings supported the microtubular failure hypothesis of hepatocellular injury in AH.

2. The frequency of parenchymal lymphocytic infiltrate and piecemeal necrosis suggested a cytotoxic role for lymphocytes in AH especially in the later course of the disease. A study of the T and B cell population in the peripheral blood and liver was initiated to find out if T or B cells are sequestered in the liver in AH.

ACKNOWLEDGEMENTS

This research was supported by a VA-supported Grant MRS 612-293. The authors wish to thank Mrs. Mary Castle and Mrs. Virginia Smith for their excellent technical assistance.

REFERENCES

1. FRENCH SW, and DAVIES PL: The Mallory body in the pathogenesis of alcoholic liver disease. In Alcoholic Liver Pathology. JM Khanna, Y Israel, A Kalant, (eds.). Addiction Research Foundation of Ontario, 1975. pp. 113-143

2. BARAONA B, LEO MA, BOROWSKI SA, LIEBER CS: Alcoholic hepatomegaly: Accumulation of protein in the liver. Science 190: 794-795, 1975

3. BRUNT PW, KEW MC, SCHEUER PJ, SHERLOCK S: Studies in alcoholic liver disease in Britain. I. Clinical and pathological patterns related to natural history. Gut 15: 52-58, 1974

4. DENK H, GSCHNAIT F, WOLFF K: Hepatocellular hyalin (Mallory bodies) in long term griseofulvin-treated mice: A new experimental model for the study of hyalin formation. Lab Inv 32: 773-776, 1975

5. FRENCH SW: Effect of chronic ethanol ingestion on liver enzyme changes induced by thiamine, riboflavin, pyridoxine or choline deficiency. J Nutr 88: 291-302, 1966

6. GABBIANI G, MONTESANO R, TUCHWEBER B, SALAS M, ORCI L: Phalloidin-induced hyperplasia of actin filaments in rat hepatocytes. Lab Inv 33: 562-569, 1975

7. SIM J, FRENCH SW: Binding of peroxidase-antiperoxidase complex (PAP) by Mallory bodies in unfixed tissue. Arch Path (in press).

8. WIGGERS KD, FRENCH SW, FRENCH BA, CARR BN: The ultrastructure of Mallory body filaments. Lab Inv 29: 652-658, 1973

9. OUCHTERLONY O: Diffusion-in-gels. Methods for immunological analysis. Prog Allergy 5: 1-78, 1958

10. KYRIAZIS AP, WISSLER RW: Demonstration and purification of a specific antigen in Morris hepatoma 5123. Lab Inv 26: 178-183, 1972

11. ORTEGA LG, MELLORS RC: Analytical pathology: IV. The role of localized antibodies in the pathogenesis of nephrotoxic nephritis in the rat. J Exp Med: 104-151, 1956

12. LAEMMLI UK: Cleavage of structural proteins during the assembly of the head of bacteriophage T_4. Nature 227: 680-685, 1970

13. COOKE P: A filamentous cytoskeleton in vertebrate smooth muscle fibers. J Cell Biol 68: 539-556, 1976

14. OKAMURA K, HARWOOD TR, YOKOO H: Isolation and electrophoretic study of Mallory bodies from the livers of alcoholic cirrhosis. Lab Inv 33: 193-199, 1975

15. FAIRBANKS G, STECK TL, WALLACH DF: Electrophoretic analysis of the major polypeptides of the human erythrocyte membrane. Biochem 10: 2606-2617, 1971

16. AMES GF: Resolution of bacterial proteins by polyacrylamide gel electrophoresis on slabs. J Biol Chem 249: 634-644, 1974

17. WYBRAN J, FUDENBERG HH: Thymus-derived rosette-forming cells in various human disease states: cancer, lymphoma, bacterial and viral infections, and other diseases. J Clin Invest 52: 1026-1032, 1973

18. GIULIANO VJ, JASIN HE, HURD ER, ZIFF M: Enumeration of B-lymphocytes in human peripheral blood by a rosette method for the detection of surface-bound immunoglobulin. J Immunol 112: 1494-1499, 1974

19. VAN BOXEL JA, PAGET SA: Predominantly T-cell infiltrate in rheumatoid synovial membranes. N Eng J Med 293: 517-520, 1975

20. FRENCH SW, DAVIES PL: Ultrastructural localization of actin-like filaments in rat hepatocytes. Gastroenterology 68: 765-774, 1975

21. NENCI K: Identification of actin-like proteins in alcoholic hyalin by immunofluorescence. Lab Inv 32: 257-260, 1975

22. EDMONDSON HA, PETERS RL, FRANKEL HH, BOROWSKY S: The early stage of liver injury in the alcoholic. Medicine 46: 119-129, 1967

23. BIAVA C: Mallory alcoholic hyalin: A heretofore unique lesion of hepatocellular ergastoplasm. Lab Inv 13: 301-320, 1964

24. YOKOO H, MINICK OT, BATTI F, KENT, G: Morphologic variants of alcoholic hyalin. Am J Path 69: 25-40, 1972

25. HORVATH E, KOVACS K, ROSS RC: Subcellular features of alcoholic liver lesion: Alcoholic hyalin. J Path 110: 245-150, 1973

26. MARGULIS L: Colchicine-sensitive microtubules. Intern Rev Cytol 34: 333-361, 1973

27. BANDMANN U, NORBERT B, SIMMINGSKOLD G: Griseofulvin inhibition of polymorphonuclear leukocyte chemotaxis in Boyden Chambers. Scand J Haematol 15: 81-87, 1975

28. SHELANSKI ML, FEIT H: Filaments and tubules in the nervous system. In The Structure and Function of Nervous Tissue. GH Bourne (ed.). Academic Press, N.Y. 1972. pp. 47-80

29. DE BRABANDER M, AERTS F, VAN DE VEIRE R, BORGERGS M: Evidence against interconversion of microtubules and filaments. Nature 253: 119-120, 1975

30. HOLTZER H, CROOP J, DIENSTMAN S, ISHIKAWA H, SOMLYO AP: Effects of cytochalasin B and colcemide on myogenic cultures. Proc Nat Acad Sci 72: 513-517, 1975

31. STEIN O, STEIN Y: Colchicine-induced inhibition of very low density lipoprotein release by rat liver in vivo. Biochem Biophys Acta 306: 142-147, 1973

32. STEIN O, SANGER L, STEIN Y: Colchicine-induced inhibition of lipoprotein and protein secretion into the serum and lack of interference with secretion of biliary phospholipids and cholesterol by rat liver in vivo. J Cell Biol 62: 90-103, 1974

33. FELDMANN G, MAURICE M, SAPN C, BENHAMOU J-P: Inhibition by colchicine of fibrinogen translocation in hepatocytes. J Cell Biol 67: 237-243, 1975

34. SINGH A, LEMARCHAND Y, ORCI L, JEANRENAUD B: Colchicine administration to mice: A metabolic and ultrastructural study. Europ J Clin Invest 5: 495-505, 1975

35. LEMARCHAND Y, PATZELT C, ASSIMACOPOULOS-JEANNET F, LOTEN EG, JEANRENAUD B: Evidence for a role of the microtubular system in the section of newly synthesized albumin and other proteins by the liver. J Clin Invest 53: 1512-1517, 1974

36. MADSEN NP: Reduced serum very low-density lipoprotein levels after acute ethanol administration. Biochem Pharmacol 18: 261-262, 1969

37. KYOSOLA K, SALORINNE Y: Liver biopsy and liver function tests in 28 consecutive long-term alcoholics. Ann Clin Chem Res 7: 80-84, 1975

38. REDMAN CM, BANERJEE D, HOWELL K, PALADE GE: The step at which colchicine blocks the secretion of plasma protein by rat liver. Ann N Y Acad Sci 253: 780-788, 1975

39. ISHIKAWA H, BISCHOFF R, HOLTZER H: Mitosis and intermediate-sized filaments in developing skeletal muscle. J Cell Biol 38: 538-555, 1968

40. WAGNER RC, ROSENBERG MD: Endocytosis in Chang liver cells: the role of microtubules in vacuole orientation and movement. Cytobiologie 7: 20-27, 1973

41. SEIDEN D: Effects of colchicine on myofilament arrangement and the lysosomal system in skeletal muscle. Z Zellforsch 144: 467-473, 1973

42. JIMBOW K, FITZPATRICK TB: Changes in distribution pattern of cytoplasmic filaments in human melanocytes during ultraviolet-mediated melanin pigmentation. J Cell Biol 5: 481-488, 1975

43. MOELLMAN G, MCGUIRE J, LERNER AB: Intracellular dynamics and the fine structure of melanocytes with special references to the effects of MSH and cyclic AMP on microtubules and 10-nm filaments. Yale J Biol Med 46: 337-360, 1973

44. ISRAEL Y, KALANT H, ORREGO H, KHANNA JM, VIDELA L, PHILLIPS MJ: Experimental alcohol-induced hepatic necrosis. Suppression by propylthiouracil. Proc Nat Acad Sci 72: 1137-1141, 1975

45. BERNSTEIN J, VIDELA L, ISRAEL Y: Hormonal influences in the development of the hypermetabolic state of the liver produced by chronic administration of ethanol. J Pharmacol Exp Ther 192: 583-591, 1975

46. CEDERBAUM AI, LIEBER CS, RUBIN E: The effect of acetaldehyde on mitochondrial function. Arch Biochem Biophys 161: 26-39, 1974

47. GORDON ER: Mitochondrial functions in an ethanol-induced fatty liver. J Biol Chem 248: 8271-8280, 1973

48. FRENCH SW, PALMER DS, NAROD ME: Noradrenergic subsensitivity of rat liver homogenates during chronic ethanol ingestion. Res Commun Chem Path Pharmacol 13: 283-295, 1976

49. BORLE AB: Cyclic AMP stimulation of calcium efflux from kidney, liver and heart mitochondria. J Membrane Biol 16: 221-236, 1974

50. BERRIDGE MJ: The interaction of cyclic nucleotides and calcium in the control of cellular activity. Adv Cyclic Nucleotide Res 6: 1-98, 1975

51. OSTLUND R, PASTAN I: Fibroblast tubulin. Biochemistry 14: 4064-4068, 1975

52. SLOBODA RD, RUDOLPH SA, ROSENBAUM JL, GREENBARD P: Cyclic AMP-dependent endogenous phosphorylation of a micro-tubule-associated protein. Proc Nat Acad Sci 72: 177-181, 1975

53. MAGUN B: Two actions of cyclic AMP in melanosome movement in frog skin. J Cell Biol 47: 845-858, 1973

54. COSSEL L, MAHNKE PF, SCHWARZER R: "Killer"-lymphocytes in action? Light and electron microscopical findings in orthotopic liver homografts. Virch Arch Path Anat Histol 364: 179-190, 1974

55. CHRISTOFFERSEN P, JUHL E: Mallory bodies in liver biopsies with fatty changes but no cirrhosis. Acta Pathol Microbiol Scand Section A 79: 201-207, 1971

56. LEEVY CM, ZETTERMAN R: Alcoholic hepatitis and corticosteroids. Ann Intern Med 79: 739-740, 1973

57. GALAMBOS JT: Natural history of alcoholic hepatitis, III. Histologic changes. Gastroenterology 63: 1026-1035, 1972

58. ANNABLE W, COOPER C: Inhibition of release of hepatic triglyceride by ethanol — A reappraisal. Biochem Pharmacol 23: 2063-2068, 1974

DISCUSSION

CHAIRMAN: K.J. ISSELBACHER

ISSELBACHER: Do you think that the presence of more T-cells in the liver and less in the serum is a normal response of the liver to injury, whether it be virus or alcohol or anything else?

FRENCH: Yes, I think that the T-cells may be perpetuating the disease process. They are sequestered in the liver because they bind to sites on the liver cell plasma membrane. In vitro studies indicate that liver cells can turn on circulating T-cells and that these lymphocytes can be cytotoxic to liver cells. There seems to be pretty good correlation between liver cell injury and T-cell sensitization.

FOX: The identification of T and B lymphocytes is a real problem. In a limited number of alcoholics we have found normal circulating levels of T-lymphocytes using conventional rosetting techniques. If the normal population in the blood is 60-70% then you would expect 60-70% of a lymphocyte infiltrate in the liver to be T-lymphocytes.

What does enzyme digestion of the liver do to lymphocyte characteristics in terms of their capabilities of rosetting and such?

FRENCH: Well, since we measured the rosetting simultaneously in the peripheral blood and liver and found the rosetting to be the same or sometimes lower in the peripheral blood, we didn't think there was interference with the rosetting. We studied the lymphocytes from the liver using vital stain techniques and found the great majority to be viable.

FOX: I think there is good evidence now that the lymphocytes of patients with acute damage of the liver regardless of the etiologic agent can be cytotoxic to liver cells in vitro. This would appear to be a nonspecific phenomenon.   Acute liver damage turns on the circulating lymphocytes.

FRENCH: It may be a non-specific reaction to liver injury. But it still might be important in the pathogenesis or progression of the disease.

THE PATHOGENESIS OF ALCOHOLIC CIRRHOSIS

Hans Popper

The Stratton Laboratory for the Study of Liver Diseases
Mount Sinai School of Medicine of the City University of New
York, New York, New York

A discussion of the pathogenesis of alcoholic cirrhosis must 1) define cirrhosis to identify the lesion, 2) describe the forms in ethanol abusers, 3) most important, trace the developmental pathways, of possible significance in rational management, 4) enumerate diagnostic criteria, important in management since alcohol withdrawal can arrest the disorder, and 5) indicate the relation to carcinoma.

Cirrhosis is defined (1) as a scar stage characterized by regenerative parenchymal nodules and connective tissue septa linking terminal hepatic veins and portal tracts. The septa contain vascular anastomoses between the afferent branches of the portal vein and hepatic artery and the efferent tributaries of the hepatic veins. Functionally, cirrhosis is reflected in 1) disturbed hepatic circulation mirrored by a) portal hypertension from compression of efferent vessels by nodules and fibrosis and from anastomoses between hepatic artery and portal vein branches, and b) reduced effective parenchymal blood flow (2, 3), and 2) diminished functional hepatic mass (4). Cirrhosis differs from chronic hepatitis, the usually accepted precursor stage, which may 1) be absent in the presence of cirrhosis, 2) be present with it, 3) have disappeared or 4) never have been conspicuous.

The morphologic classification of alcoholic cirrhosis, confusing despite many proposals (5, 6, 7, 8), is of little clinical significance. A uniform micronodular form with small septa, often designated as Laennec's type, is usually distinguished from a variform macronodular type often associated with broad and irregular scars sometimes resulting in a deformed organ and previously called postnecrotic cirrhosis (9). Supposedly, continued alcohol abuse is associated with the micronodular form, while discontinuation is associated with the macronodular form with broad septa (10, 11). More meaningful is separation into a large hyper-regeneratory liver, and a shrunken, hypo-regeneratory one, although histologically, regeneration is not less conspicuous in the latter (1). The clinically most useful separation distinguishes cirrhosis with active alcoholic hepatitis from that without it.

It is conventionally assumed that alcoholic hepatitis with approximation of terminal hepatic veins and portal tracts is the essential precursor stage of cirrhosis (12). But the histologic analysis to be presented raises the possibility of a creeping development of cirrhosis without conspicuous inflammatory reaction. In the histogenesis the formation of the regenerative nodules and of the connective tissue septa requires analysis. The former is not specific for alcoholic cirrhosis and is either passive or active (13). The parenchyma is dissected by septa and the liver cell plates subsequently rearrange themselves around newly formed efferent vessels. Hepatocellular hypertrophy and hyperplasia may set in subsequently. Active regeneration is more frequent and it starts usually but not necessarily in zone 1 of the acinus. Such foci are distinguished by formation of plates two and even more cells thick (14). In these regeneratory areas, rearrangement of the liver cell plates produces formidable nodules. Secondary degeneration of the regenerates results in destruction of the nodules. This may be caused by the alcoholic liver injury, but also may occur independently by local disturbance of the microcirculation induced by the cirrhosis, or by focal cholestasis. During this destruction, segmented leukocytes and Mallory's hyalin may accumulate, which need not point to an alcoholic etiology since it is seen in nodular destruction of any cirrhosis (15). Therefore in this setting, hyalin is not of diagnostic significance. This secondary collapse differs from primary collapse by the lack of the normal spacing of the terminal hepatic veins and portal tracts, otherwise preserved after disappearance of the liver cells, and by the frequent persistence of small hepatocytic islands.

In contrast to the parenchymal regeneration, the fibrosis culminating in septa is more specific for alcoholic liver injury, and deserves therefore more detailed discussion. As in any fibrosis, fiber excess may be passive or active (16). Following necrosis of hepatocytes, the preexisting connective tissue framework collapses in alcoholic liver injury 1) around the efferent veins and 2) along parenchymal planes linking the area around the efferent veins with the portal tracts, seemingly in the oxygen-poor zone 3 of the acinus (17, 18) (Fig. 1), and 3) with massive necrosis of hepatocytes the connective tissue framework of contiguous acini sometimes collapses, (Fig. 2). Thus, primary massive collapse in severe alcoholic hepatitis explains the rare alcoholic cirrhosis with a conspicuously deformed liver (9).

In any type of collapse, experimental and clinical, new fibers rapidly form, as has been established by chemical analysis in experimental cirrhosis (19). Active fibrogenesis has recently attracted considerable interest because of improved knowledge of the cellular and molecular processes in collagen synthesis including the distinction of forms of collagen which differ in amino-acid composition of the characteristic alpha chains and in immuno-fluorescence visualization (20, 21, 22, 23). Type I collagen, characteristic of

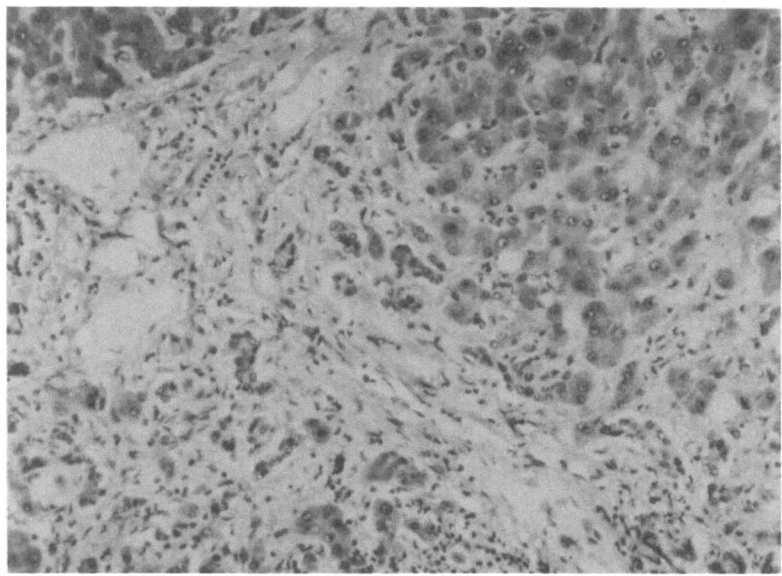

Fig. 1   *Subacute alcoholic hepatitis. Note close approximation between terminal hepatic veins and portal canals with bile ductules and vessels and hard (type I) collagen in the area of connection. Hematoxylin eosin. 100x.*

bone, tendon and skin, is found in the liver as dense double–refractive collagen bundles in portal tracts and around hepatic veins but sparsely in the hepatic parenchyma (24). Type II is in hyaline cartilage and so far not found in the liver. Type III, characteristic of embryonal tissue and blood vessels, corresponds to the hepatic reticulum, and type IV, being rich in cysteine and 3–hydroxyproline, to basement membranes. The main responsible cell is the fibroblast, well defined by its electronmicroscopic features of a rough endoplasmic reticulum with fluffy material in dilated cisternae (25). However, other cells have a repressed potential for fibroplasia (26). This agrees with the observation that at least the embryonal chicken liver is particularly rich in messenger RNA for collagen (27). Fibroblasts are readily demonstrable in the portal tracts but barely found in the parenchyma. Here, a common perisinusoidal cell, the lipocyte (28) or Ito cell (29), is identified. It contains many small fat droplets with strong vitamin A fluorescence (30, 31), but in contrast to the macrophagic Kupffer cells and endothelial cells is free of any phagosomes, even in human or experimental iron overload. The previous suggestion that lipocytes are resting fibroblasts (32, 33) has recently been confirmed by Kent and co-workers (34), who made these cells more conspicuous by vitamin A supplements, which increase and enlarge the fat droplets. In prolonged hepatic necrosis produced by carbon tetra-chloride, lipocytes accumulate and in later stages one can see many forms transitional between these cells and fibroblasts. These transitional cells

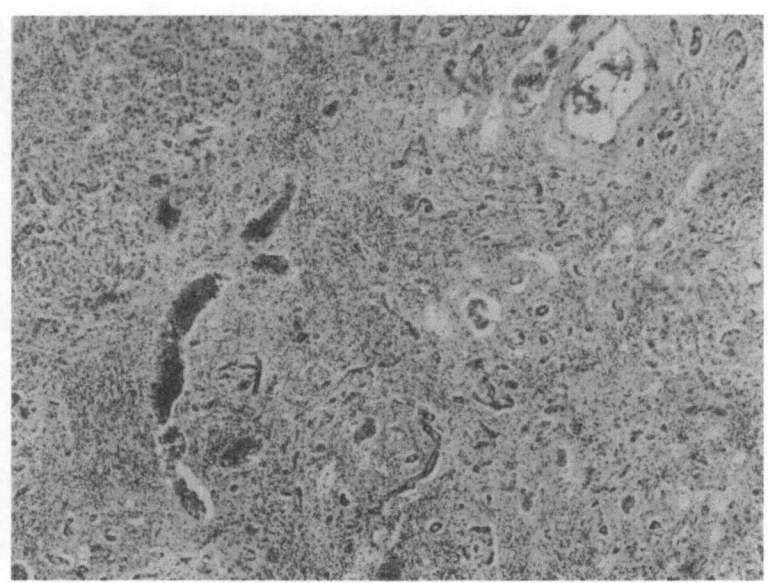

Fig. 2   Alcoholic hepatitis with massive necrosis. Note approximation
            of portal tracts and terminal hepatic veins.   Hepatocytes
            preserved only in left upper corner. Hematoxylin eosin. 40x.

contain fat droplets, have the endoplasmic reticulum characteristic of
fibroblasts, are surrounded by collagen fibrils and may be seen to be
undergoing mitoses. This suggests that liver cell injury, often associated
with macrophages, stimulates accumulation of lipocytes and their transition
to fibroblasts. The fibers formed have initially the character of reticulum
or type III collagen, as demonstrated with immunofluorescence by Gay (35,
36) and supported by chemical analysis (37). This process might become the
target of specific antifibroblastic therapy.

    Fibers form in alcoholic liver injury at the same sites as in liver disease
in general (16), namely around:

    1)   altered hepatocytes, seen particularly well in the region of the
terminal hepatic veins, around cells with hydropic cytoplasm, some of them
containing alcoholic hyalin;

    2) basement membranes of proliferating bile ductules, usually preceded
by periductular inflammation;

    3)   macrophages loaded with phagocytosed material, especially in fat

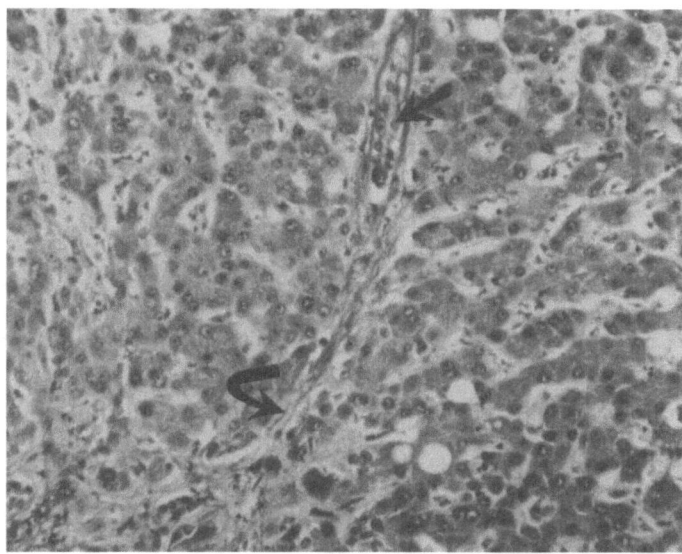

*Fig. 3   Arrested alcoholic cirrhosis.   Septum extending from portal
              tracts containing bile ductules (straight arrow) and vessels
              (curved arrow). Aniline blue. 100x.*

granulomas, that means when the amount of fat exceeds the metabolic
ability of the hepatocytes;

    4) basement membranes of capillaries and venules.

    All these locations have reduced fluid exchange in common, as on the
surface of damaged hepatocytes, where the cell membrane is devoid of
microvilli, at basement membrane of ductules and blood vessels, or with
prolonged life span of macrophages containing phagocytic material.
Reduced oxygen tension, probably inhibiting collagen breakdown on the
border of the acinus, is a localizing factor.

    Three different processes of septa formation occur in alcoholic liver
injury. The first, in active alcoholic hepatitis (38), is the extension of the
initial perivenous necrotizing and subsequently fibrosing process to other
perivenous areas and, more important, to the portal tracts with subsequent
approximation of the terminal hepatic veins and portal tracts (12) (Fig. 1).
Arteries and bile ductules grow out of the portal tracts and, surrounded by
inflammatory exudate and fibrous tissue, extend into the perivenous zones.
Bile ductules observed in the originally perivenous zone were responsible for
the wrong assumption of an initial portal site of alcoholic liver injury (12).

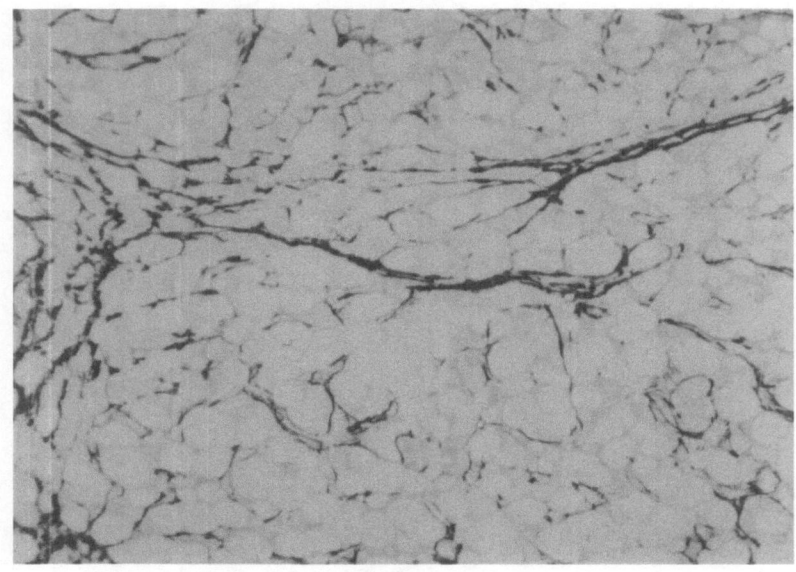

Fig. 4   *Alcoholic steatosis with intralobular fibrosis from newly formed*
              reticulum fibers around fat-loaded hepatocytes and fat
              granulomas. Approximation of connective tissue septa. Silver
              impregnation. 100x.

Deposition of type I collagen in these bridges may account for the pull,
which seems to explain the often rapid transition from alcoholic hepatitis to
cirrhosis.

A second, more insidious fibrogenesis around bile ductules causes
extension of septa from otherwise only slightly inflamed portal tracts (Fig.
3) and produces their stellate shape. This stellate fibrosis seems to be
stimulated by portal fat granulomas. Its functional consequence seems to be
small because without connections between the terminal hepatic veins and
portal tracts it does not disturb the hepatic circulation.

A third process entails the development of septa within the lobular
parenchyma from the merging of reticulum fibers newly formed around
hepatocytes engorged with fat (Fig. 4). These hepatocytes often form fatty
cysts, and are accompanied by fat granulomas (Fig. 5) with macrophages
containing PAS-positive diastase-resistant granules (Fig. 6) and by frequent
lipocytes. These septa often end blindly within the parenchyma (Fig. 4),
while in other instances they link with septa extending from either the
terminal hepatic vein or the portal tracts to result in a dissection of the
parenchyma into nodules (14). This process was demonstrated by three-
dimensional reconstruction 25 years ago (39) (Fig. 7) and the actual

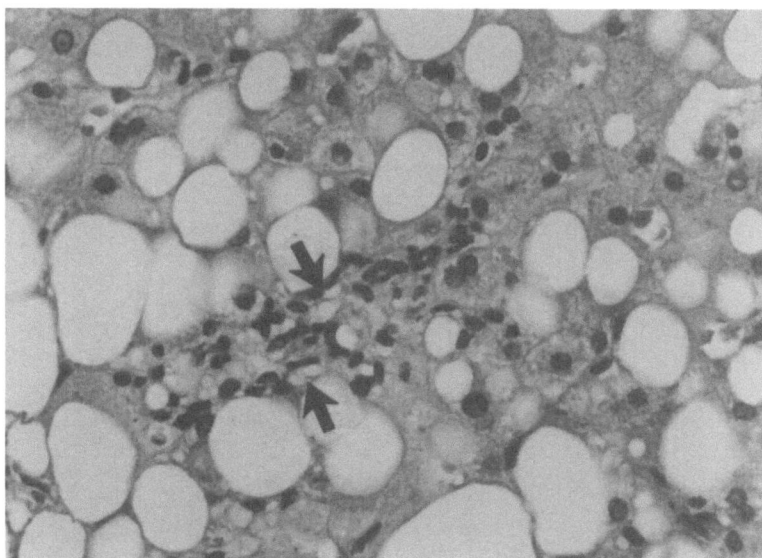

Fig. 5   *Diffuse alcoholic steatosis with intraparenchymal focal fibrosis and fat granulomas.   Note Ito cells (lipocytes) (arrows). Hematoxylin eosin. 240x.*

localization of the septa may be explained on the basis of Rappaport's acinus (17, 18) wherein collagen deposition is favored in the relative oxygen–poor zone 3. This concept that an insidious process of septa connections without conspicuous inflammation may also terminate in cirrhosis contradicts the widely held opinion that alcoholic hepatitis is the sole precursor stage of alcoholic cirrhosis but is in keeping with clinical observations of alcoholic cirrhosis without clinically apparent alcoholic hepatitis.   The described pericellular fibrosis in rare instances is accentuated to produce so–called florid cirrhosis (40), a diffuse interstitial fiber deposition associated with abundant lipocytes and resulting in hepatic failure before cirrhosis develops (Fig. 8).

Creeping septa formation associated with numerous lipocytes agrees with the increased hepatic activity of prolyl hydroxylase, demonstrated in rats after ethanol administration (41) and with other observations of a fibrosis–stimulating effect of ethanol (42, 43, 44).   It seems to be also characterized by early development of hard type I collagen (gray in silver impregnations) (Fig. 9), reflected also in the term 'central hyaline sclerosis'.

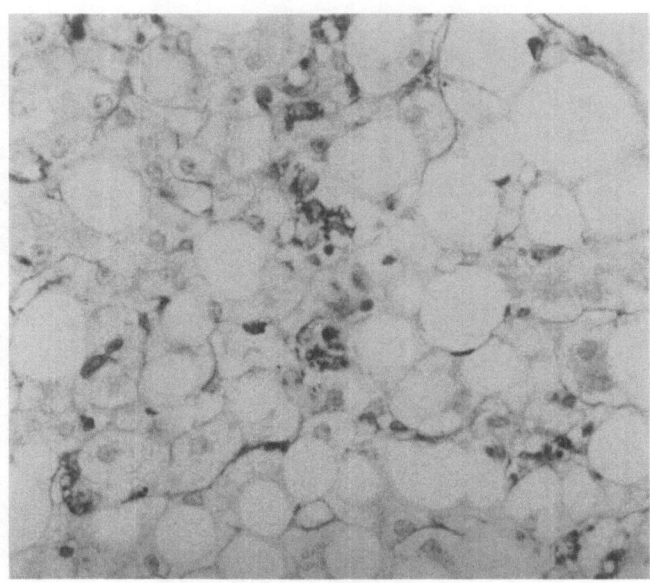

Fig. 6   *Diffuse alcoholic steatosis with fat granulomas around fat-loaded hepatocytes containing macrophages with PAS-positive granules. PAS reaction after diastase treatment. 250x.*

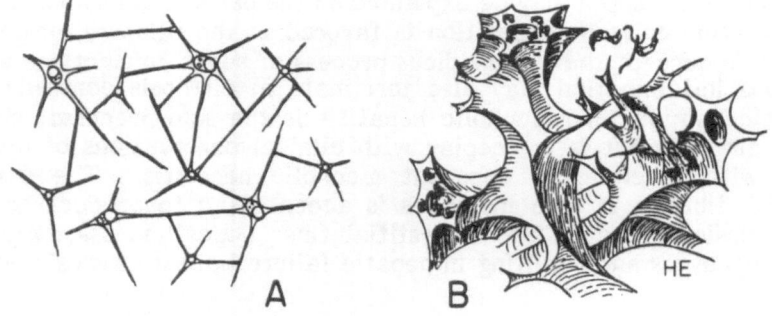

Fig. 7   *Formation of junction of septa   with subdivision of the lobule. A: Two-dimensional diagram. B: Three-dimensional visualization. Reproduced with permission from Popper H, Szanto PB, and Elias H: Transition of fatty liver into cirrhosis. Gastroenterology 28: 183, 1955.*

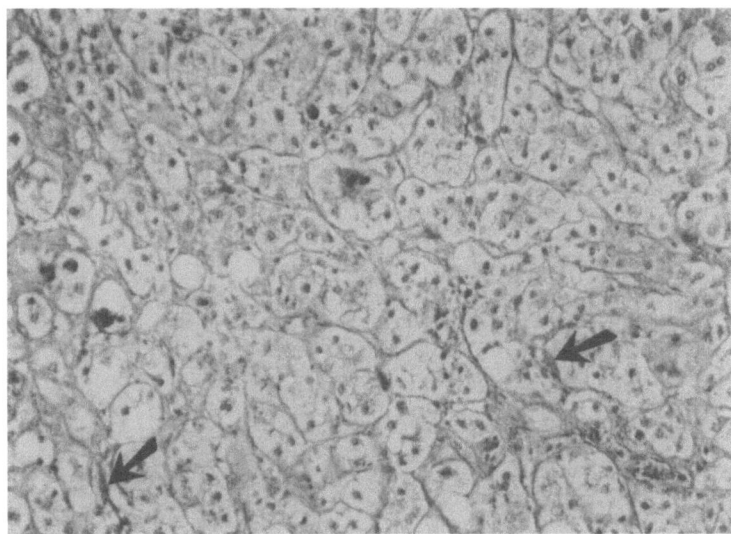

Fig. 8   Florid cirrhosis. Hepatocytic plates, mostly more than one cell
          thick, are uniformly surrounded by a dense reticulum frame-
          work. In places, hard collagen bundles (arrows) are seen. Silver
          impregnation. 100x.

This collagen is double-refractive in polarized light (Fig. 10). In the septa,
vessels form by transformation of sinusoids into venules by acquisition of a
basement membrane and subsequently of a collagen coat (Fig 11). These
vessels, if linking afferent with efferent blood supply, produce the
intrahepatic shunts in cirrhosis (14, 2, 3). The slow septa connection as well
as the pull in alcoholic hepatitis may be arrested and this accounts for the
incomplete irregular types of cirrhosis sometimes designated as posthepatitic cirrhosis in alcoholics (7). However, the described processes do not
include the primary or secondary immunologic processes stimulated either
by release of membrane isoantigens from damaged hepatocytes, or by
neoantigens in the form of alcoholic hyalin, as discussed elsewhere in this
book. They might explain the infrequent self-perpetuation of alcoholic
cirrhosis after alcohol withdrawal.

    In general, the architectural processes, namely, bridging and, exception-
ally, massive collapse as well as septa connections do not differ in principle
from those in viral-induced or cryptogenic cirrhosis although the cytologic
features are different except for the occasional lymphocytic immune
reaction. This explains the difficulty in establishing the alcoholic etiology in
the advanced stages which represent a common terminal pathway. However

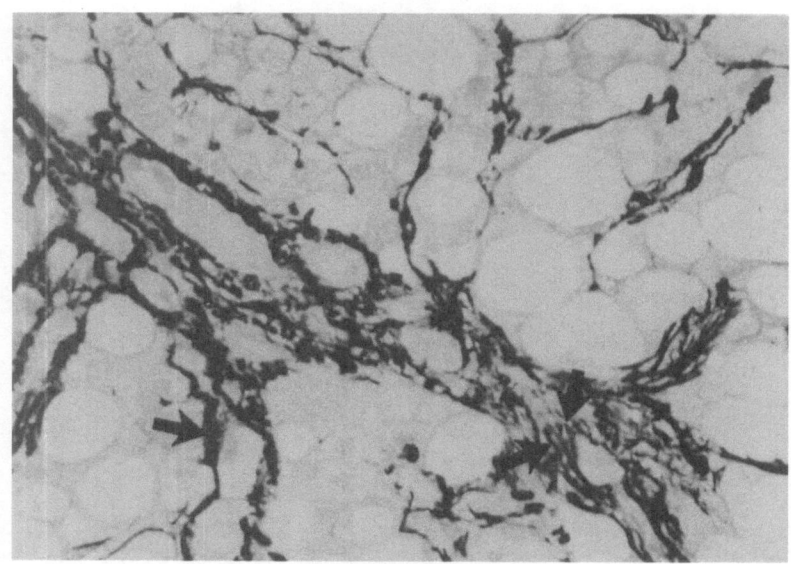

Fig. 9   *Diffuse alcoholic steatosis with intraparenchymal creeping
              fibrosis.   Note increased reticulum and focal hard (type I)
              collagen (arrows) giving gray instead of black reaction.   Silver
              impregnation. 250x.*

Fig. 10   *Diffuse steatosis with creeping fibrosis. Note double-refractive
              hard collagen bundles.   Hematoxylin eosin.   Polarized light,
              100x.*

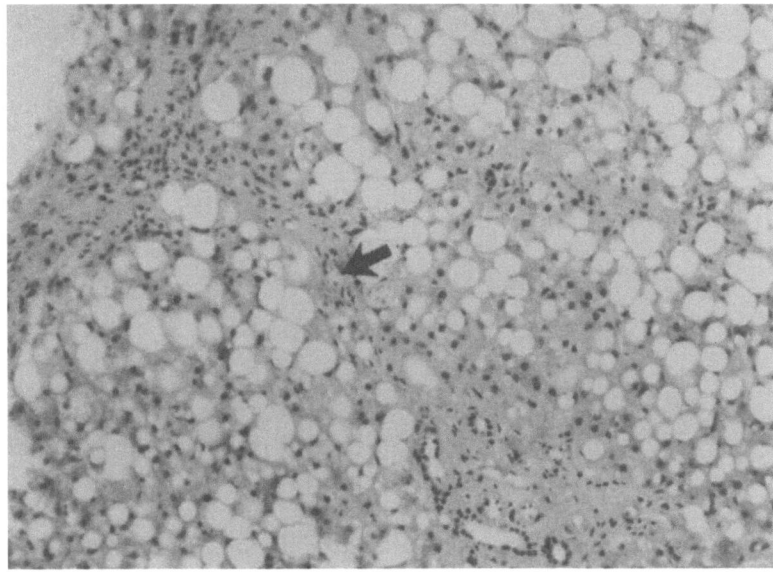

Fig. 11   Alcoholic fatty cirrhosis with multiple septa containing bile ductules and arteries, particularly in the one connecting terminal hepatic vein and portal tract (arrow). Hematoxylin eosin. 100x.

the following features at least raise the suspicion of an alcoholic etiology (45):

1) Alcoholic hepatitis with intraparenchymal accumulation of segmented leukocytes and alcoholic hyalin, predominantly around the terminal hepatic veins. Hyalin can be subsequently seen in the portal zone I but it then has less diagnostic significance because it can be found there also in primary biliary cirrhosis, in prolonged cholestasis, in chronic active hepatitis, and in Wilson's disease (15).

2) Relative integrity of the portal tracts when not connected with bridges. This can also be seen in aflatoxin-induced liver cell injury, in the exceptional cirrhosis from hypervitaminosis A (46), in the cirrhosis following intestinal bypass operations (47) and in the rare cirrhosis following so-called fatty-liver hepatitis (48).

3) Iron overload of hepatocytes is more frequent in alcoholic than in other types of liver injury.

4) Hypocellular dense collagenous septa.

5) Secondary, irregularly limited collapse on gross inspection. Primary collapse with characteristic ghost lobules and involving many lobules is rare.

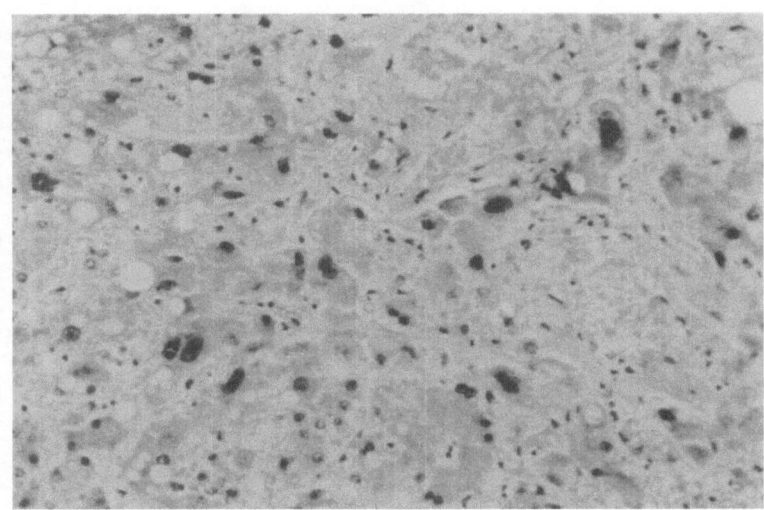

Fig. 12   *Alcoholic cirrhosis with hepatocellular carcinoma. Dysplastic
            hepatocytes in noncarcinomatous part.   Hematoxylin eosin.
            120x.*

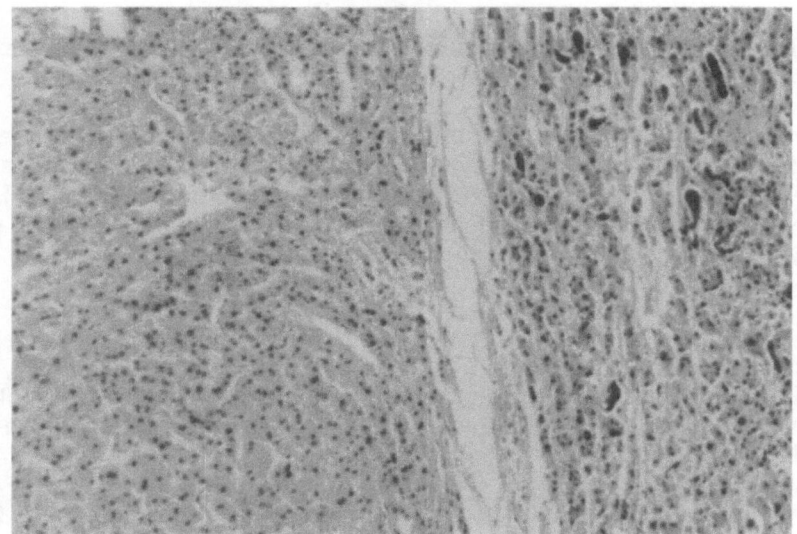

Fig. 13   *Part of hyperplastic nodule in alcoholic cirrhosis with hepato-
            cellular carcinoma.   Note variations in cell populations and
            cholestasis in right part. Hematoxylin eosin. 40x.*

Hepatocellular carcinoma is now observed with greater frequency in alcoholic cirrhosis, presumably because improved management prolongs survival (11, 49, 50). The question arises whether ethanol or its metabolites are carcinogenic, or whether the hepatocellular regeneration in cirrhosis leads to autonomous growth, possibly enhanced by higher susceptibility to additional ubiquitous carcinogens. The second possibility is favored by the seemingly equal incidence of about 15 percent in alcoholic (51) and cryptogenic cirrhosis, by the lack of carcinomas in noncirrhotic livers of alcoholics, and by the fact that the morphogenesis of the carcinoma is similar in other forms of cirrhosis. Dysplastic hepatocytes (52) may be noted outside the tumor (Fig. 12). In the center of regenerative, hyperplastic appearing nodules multiple types of hepatocellular populations develop usually in multicentric fashion, (Fig. 13) (53, 54). These evolve to cancer cells which are first usually smaller, contain small fat droplets, are more homogenous, and form multiple cell plates with reduced reticulum framework. Characteristically, transitions in the same cell plate are seen in many places as indication of a multicentric origin. There is no predilection of malignant degeneration for any of the morphologic types of alcoholic cirrhosis, as has been claimed (11).

SUMMARY

While there are no distinctive features of gross appearance or of formation or degeneration of regenerative nodules in alcoholic cirrhosis, the fibrosis resulting in septa formation has some characteristics. The abundance of lipocytes as precursors of fibroblasts associated with formation of type III collagen or reticulum and the early appearance of hard type I collagen favoring portal hypertension are both in agreement with the described stimulation of hepatic fibrogenesis by ethanol intake. Cirrhosis results from 1) approximation between the terminal hepatic veins and portal tracts in active alcoholic hepatitis, 2) fibrosis around proliferated ductules, and 3) septa formation within the parenchyma around fat-loaded hepatocytes and fat granulomas, with connection of these septa in a creeping process slowly distorting the architecture. Analysis of these processes has provided tentative criteria for the recognition of alcoholic cirrhosis even in late stages although in principle the architectural if not the cytologic features are the same as in other forms of cirrhosis. Carcinomatous degeneration appears to result from the cirrhotic process per se rather than from a carcinogenic action of ethanol or its metabolites.

ACKNOWLEDGEMENTS

Supported by NIOSH Contract 210-75-0044.

REFERENCES

1. POPPER H, ORR W: Current concepts in cirrhosis. Scand J Gastroenterol 6: 203-222, 1970

2. GROSS G, BABEL JF, RITSCHARD J, MEGEVAND R, ROHNER A, DONATH A, PERRIER CV: Quantification of intrahepatic porta-systemic shunting in cirrhotic patients: Possible relevance to the problem of indication for surgical procedure. In The Liver, Quantitative Aspects of Structure and Function. R Preisig, J Bircher, G Paumgartner, (eds.). Aulendorf, Editio Cantor, 1976. pp. 159-166

3. SHALDON S, CHIANDUSSI L, GUEVARA L, CAESAR J, SHERLOCK S: The estimation of hepatic blood flow and intrahepatic shunted blood flow by colloidal heat-denatured human serum albumin labeled with I^{131}. J Clin Invest 40: 1346-1354, 1961

4. PREISIG R, BIRCHER J, PAUMGARTNER G: Physiologic and patho-physiologic aspects of the hepatic hemodynamics. In Progress in Liver Diseases, vol IV. H Popper, F Schaffner (eds.). New York, Grune & Stratton, 1972. pp. 201-216

5. GALAMBOS JT: Classification of cirrhosis. Am J Gastroenterol 64: 437-451, 1975

6. MEISTER HP, SZANTO PB, SCHOOLMAN H: Quantitative-morphologic evaluation of postnecrotic cirrhosis. Virchows Arch Pathol Anat 336: 447-464, 1963

7. GALL EA: Posthepatitic, postnecrotic and nutritional cirrhosis: a pathological analysis. Am J Pathol 36: 241-259, 1960

8. STEINER PE: Precision in the classification of cirrhosis of the liver. Am J Pathol 37: 21-47, 1960

9. RUBIN E, KRUS S, POPPER H: Pathogenesis of postnecrotic cirrhosis in alcoholics. Arch Pathol 73: 288-298, 1962

10. POPPER H, RUBIN E, KRUS S, SCHAFFNER F: Postnecrotic cirrhosis in alcoholics. Gastroenterol 39: 669-685, 1960

11. LEE FI: Cirrhosis and hepatoma in alcoholics. Gut 7: 77-85, 1966

12. GERBER MA, POPPER H: Relation between central canals and portal tracts in alcoholic hepatitis. A contribution to the pathogenesis of cirrhosis in alcoholics. Human Pathol 3: 199-107, 1972

13. RUBIN E, POPPER H: The evolution of human cirrhosis deduced from observations in experimental animals. Medicine 46: 163-183, 1967

14. POPPER H, ELIAS H: Histogenesis of hepatic cirrhosis studied by the three-dimensional approach. Am J Pathol 31: 405-441, 1955

15. GERBER MA, ORR W, DENK H, SCHAFFNER F, POPPER H: Hepatocellular hyalin in cholestasis and cirrhosis: Its diagnostic significance. Gastroenterol 64: 89-98, 1973

16. POPPER J, UDENFRIEND S: Hepatic fibrosis - correlation of biochemical and morphologic investigations. Am J Med 49: 707-721, 1970

17. RAPPAPORT AM: The microcirculatory hepatic unit. In Drugs and the Liver. W Gerok, K Sickinger, (eds.). Stuttgart, FK Schattauer Verlag, 1975. pp. 425-434

18. RAPPAPORT AM: The microcirculatory hepatic unit. Microvasc Res 6: 212-228, 1973

19. KENT G, FELS IG, DUBIN A, POPPER H: Collagen content based on hydroxyproline determinations in human and rat livers. Its relation to morphologically demonstrable reticulum and collagen fibers. Lab Invest 8: 48-56, 1959

20. Collagen Metabolism in the Liver. H Popper, K Becker, (eds.). New York, Stratton Intercontinental Medical Book Corporation, 1975

21. MILLER EJ, MATUKAS VJ: Biosynthesis of collagen. The biochemist's view. Fed Proc 33: 1197-1204, 1974

22. HAHN E, TIMPL R, MILLER EJ: Demonstration of a unique antigenic specificity for the collagen alpha-1 (II) chain from cartilaginous tissue. Immunology 28: 1-8, 1975

23. HAHN E, TIMPL R, MILLER EJ: The production of specific antibodies to native collagens with the chain composition (alpha-1(I)$_3$), (alpha-1(II)$_3$) and (alpha-1(I)$_2$). J Immunol 113: 421-423, 1974

24. WOLMAN M: Polarized light microscopy as a tool of diagnostic pathology. J Histochem Cytochem 23: 21-50, 1975

25. ROSS R: The connective tissue fiber forming cell. In Treatise on Collagen vol. 2. GN Ramachandran, BS Gould, (eds). New York, Academic Press, 1968

26. LANGNESS U, UDENFRIEND S: Collagen biosynthesis of nonfibroblastic cell lines. Proc Nat Acad Sci 71: 50-51, 1974

27. STERN R. Personal communication.

28. BRONFENMAJOR S, SCHAFFNER F, POPPER H: Fat-storing cells (lipocytes) in human liver. Arch Pathol 82: 447-453, 1966

29. ITO T: Recent advances in the study on the fine structure of the hepatic sinusoidal wall; A review. Gunma Rep Med Sci 6: 119-163, 1973

30. POPPER H: Distribution of vitamin A in tissue as visualized by fluorescence microscopy. Physiol Rev 24: 205-224, 1944

31. KOBAYASHI K, TAKAHASHI Y, SHIBASAKI S: Cytological studies of fat-storing cells in the liver of rats given large doses of vitamin A. Nature New Biol 243: 186-188, 1973

32. SCHNACK H, STOCKINGER L, WEWALKA F: Adventitious connective tissue cells in the space of Disse and their relation to fiber formation. Rev Int Hepat 17: 855-860, 1967

33. TANIKAWA K: Ultrastructure of hepatic fibrosis and fat-storing cells. In Collagen Metabolism in the Liver. H Popper, K Becker, (eds.). New York, Stratton Intercontinental Medical Book Corporation, 1975. pp. 93-99

34. KENT G, BAHU R, INOUYE T, MINICK T, POPPER H: The role of the Ito cell (lipocyte) in hepatic injury. Gastroenterol 69: A35/835, 1975

35. GAY S, FIETZEK PP, REMBERGER K, EDER M, KUHN K: Liver cirrhosis: Immunofluorescence and biochemical studies demonstrate two types of collagen. Klin Wschr 53: 205-208, 1975

36. REMBERGER K, GAY S, FIETZEK PP: Immunhistochemische Untersuchungen zur Kollagencharakterisierung in Lebercirrhosen. Virchows Arch A Pathol Anat Histol 367: 231-240, 1975

37. ROJKIND M, MARTINEZ- PALOMO A: Increase in type I and type III collagens in human alcoholic liver cirrhosis. Proc Nat Acad Sci USA 73: 539-543, 1976

38. EDMONDSON HA, PETERS RL, REYNOLDS TB, KUZMA OT: Sclerosing hyaline necrosis of the liver in the chronic alcoholic: a recognizable syndrome. Ann Int Med 59: 646-673, 1963

39. POPPER H, SZANTO PB, ELIAS H: Transition of fatty liver into cirrhosis. Gastroenterol 28: 183-192, 1955

40. POPPER H, SZANTO PB, PARTHASARATHY M: Florid cirrhosis. Am J Clin Pathol 15: 889-901, 1955

41. FEINMAN L, LIEBER CS: Fibrogenic effect of alcohol in rat liver: Role of diet. Science 179: 406-407, 1973

42. GALAMBOS JT: Collagen metabolism in chronic alcoholic liver injury. In Alcohol and the Liver. W Gerok, K Sickinger, HH Hennekeuser, (eds). Stuttgart, FK Schattauer Verlag, 1971. pp. 321-331

43. CHEN TS, LEEVY CM: Collagen biosynthesis in liver disease of the alcoholic. J Lab Clin Med 85: 103-112, 1975

44. MEZEY E, POTTER JJ, MADDREY WC: Collagen turnover in alcoholic liver disease. Gastroenterol 65: A-36/560, 1973

45. POPPER H, SCHAFFNER F: Hepatic cirrhosis, a problem in communications. Israel J Med Sci 4: 1-7, 1968

46. LEITNER ZA, MOORE T, SHARMAN IM: Fatal self-medication with retinol and carrot juice. Proc Nutr Soc 34: 44A, 1975

47. POPPER H, SCHAFFNER F: Nutritional cirrhosis in man? New Eng J Med 285: 577-578, 1971

48. THALER H: Relation of steatosis to cirrhosis. In Clinics in Gastroenterology. H Popper, (ed.). London, WB Saunders Company Ltd, 1975. pp. 273-280

49. McDONALD RA: Primary carcinoma of the liver. Arch Intern Med 99: 266-279, 1975

50. FISHER RL, SCHEUER PJ, SHERLOCK S: Primary liver cell carcinoma: Alcohol and chronic liver disease. Gastroenterol 67: A-14/791, 1974

51. HALLEN H, LINNE I: Cirrhosis of the liver in one community. A study of 768 cases of liver cirrhosis from a city with one hospital: incidence, etiology and prognosis. In Alcoholic Cirrhosis and Other Toxic Hepatopathias. Skandia International Symposia. A Engel, T Larsson, (eds.). Stockholm, Nordiska Bokhandelns Forlag, 1970. pp. 336-352

52. ANTHONY PP, VOGEL CL, BARKER LF: Liver cell dysplasia; a premalignant condition. J Clin Pathol 26: 217-223, 1973

53. FARBER E: Pathogenesis of liver cancer. Arch Pathol 98: 145-148, 1974

54. POPPER H, STERNBERG SS, OSER BL, OSER M: The carcinogenic effect of Aramite in rats. A study of hepatic nodules. Cancer 13: 1035-1045, 1960

DISCUSSION

FRENCH: What is the relative frequency of alcoholic hepatitis versus the non-inflammatory fibrosis in the pathogenesis of cirrhosis?

POPPER: I wish I knew. I believe that there is no complete separation between them. There probably are patients with cirrhosis who never had alcoholic hepatitis but the majority probably had.

PHILLIPS: Do you think that central hyaline sclerosis is a stage in the development of cirrhosis or completely unrelated to cirrhosis?

POPPER: I don't know. We see in man a fibrotic lesion around the terminal hepatic venules. It is hard collagen and it may not be inflammatory. I believe right now that there can be cirrhosis with or without central hyaline sclerosis and that the latter can develop with or without necrosis.

ISSELBACHER: Dr. Rojkind has recently demonstrated that in the rat liver alcohol can lead to a stimulation of collagen synthesis predominantly types 1 and 3. This collagen increase can occur without any morphologic changes. Can you clarify this for me?

POPPER: Perhaps if we refine our morphologic techniques we can come to see it.

307

IMMUNE MECHANISMS IN ALCOHOLIC LIVER DISEASE

Roy A. Fox

Department of Medicine, Dalhousie University

Halifax, Nova Scotia

INTRODUCTION

It is clear that there are many ways in which the liver can be damaged, and these various processes can be manifested as acute or chronic disease. One question that is fundamental in the study of liver disease, as well as many other situations, is what causes the perpetuation of injury following an acute insult. More specifically, why does acute hepatitis become chronic hepatitis or cirrhosis? Many mechanisms have been invoked and a number of hypotheses put forward. A unifying hypothesis may not be possible, if one considers the multiplicity of injurious agents currently extant, but a classification of the hypothesis is possible and might help in understanding. In Table I, a simple classification is outlined, and the examples given are by no means exhaustive. I wish to present the possibility that although extrinsic agents and intrinsic mechanisms might appear to account for most liver diseases, a combination of such events is more likely.

Immune Processes in the Pathogenesis of Liver Disease

The immune response which may be genetically determined has been implicated as one of the intrinsic mechanisms in the progression from alcoholic hepatitis to cirrhosis, even after cessation of alcohol. There are a variety of immune responses and a number of ways by which tissue can be damaged. The two main pathways through which damage can occur are through the production of antibody or by cellular immune mechanisms. The mechanisms are summarized and a classification of these mechanisms given in Table II. The terminology that currently exists in immunological circles with regard to mechanisms of tissue damage can be complicated, and there are in existence at least three classifications. This classification presented in Table II is a simplification, and each mechanism will be referred to by

TABLE I

FACTORS INVOKED AS RESPONSIBLE FOR THE
PERPETUATION OF LIVER INJURY

1. Extrinsic Agents   – repeated ingestion of alcohol
                                        – chronic drug ingestion
                                        – bacterial toxins from diseased bowel

2. Intrinsic Mechanisms   – autoimmune mechanisms
                                        – deranged vascular architecture
                                        – persisting virus infection

3. Extrinsic Agents +
    Intrinsic Mechanisms   – e.g. Alcohol ingestion + immune
                                           mechanisms

TABLE II

MECHANISM OF TISSUE DAMAGE BY IMMUNE MECHANISMS

1. Immediate Hypersensitivity – IgE dependent

2. Cytotoxic Antibody – direct damage with complement
    involved

3. Antigen/antibody complex formation – complement activation

4. Cell mediated immunity (delayed hypersensitivity)

5. Lymphocyte mediated antibody dependent cytotoxicity

title rather than by number so as to prevent confusion with other existing
terminologies.

No convincing evidence has been presented that immediate hypersensitivity reactions might be involved in chronic liver disease. Multiplicity
of autoantibodies has been described in chronic liver disease (1), but despite
this, no evidence has been presented that these antibodies might be
cytotoxic to liver cells. It is, therefore, unlikely that they can be implicated
in disease processes (2). Immune complexes have been detected in blood
vessels in various parts of the body, rarely in the liver, and have been
implicated in the pathogenesis of some extrahepatic manifestations of liver
disease (3, 4). It does not appear likely that immune complexes can be
implicated in the pathogenesis of liver disease itself. Cell mediated
immunity to liver antigen, or viral antigen, has been suggested as being

responsible for damage to the liver in various types of liver disease (5). Direct evidence for these potentially damaging tissue responses has been sought and identified in some situations. There are a number of ways in which cell mediated immunity can be detected in vitro or in vivo. The simplest technique is by a delayed hypersensitivity skin test, and the main limitation in this situation is the preparation of suitable antigen. Obviously, the antigens that one is interested in are related to liver cells, and therefore tissue extracts are required. The drawbacks of this type of approach are obvious, and transmission of disease is a potential risk. Researchers have, therefore, turned to in vitro techniques, and a serious drawback so far has been the inadequacy or inappropriateness of antigens and controls. One is looking for evidence of a reaction initiated by liver specific antigen and mounted against liver cells. In this type of a reaction, the initial interaction is between a T lymphocyte with memory and the antigen. This interaction results in the lymphocytes being turned on, and the population of lymphocytes undergoes transformation which can be measured, for example, by the incorporation of tritiated thymidine.

If we refer to Figure 1, we can see the various ways in which cell mediated mechanisms can be studied. Early work in alcoholic liver disease was concerned with the use of nonspecific mitogens such as phytohemagglutinin (PHA). The use of these tests is limited, and the ability of PHA to turn on T lymphocytes is a simple way of investigating overall immune competence. In patients with alcoholic liver disease, it appears that the circulating T lymphocytes do not respond to PHA normally (6). This is related both to a decrease in numbers of circulating T lymphocytes and blocking factors present in the serum.

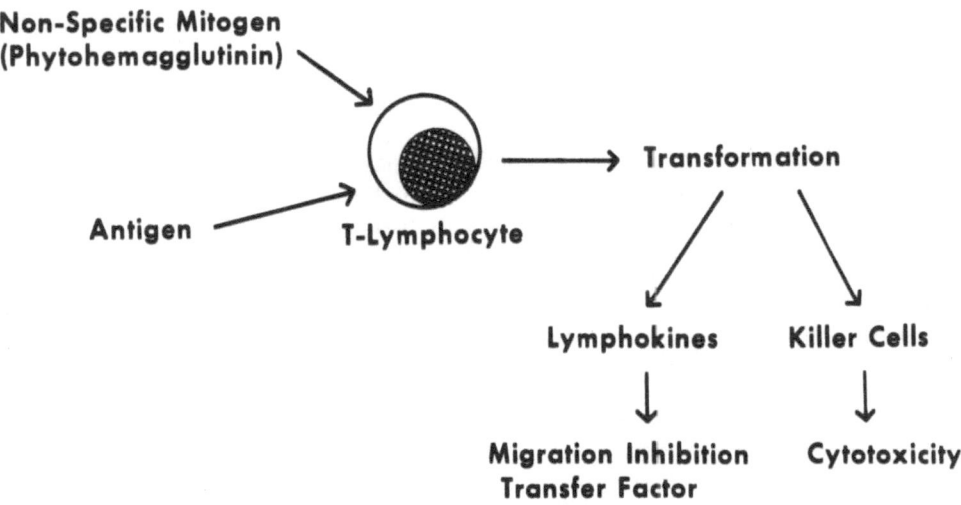

Fig. 1 Cell Mediated Immunity

The ability to turn on lymphocytes in other ways is dependent upon the recognition of the appropriate antigen and the presentation of this antigen in vitro to the lymphocytes. With progress there has been refining of antigen but initially crude antigens were used. Leevy and his associates (7) have used autologous liver homogenate as antigen. They have shown that in vitro lymphocyte transformation occurs in patients with schistosomiasis, chronic active hepatitis and alcoholic hepatitis, but not in normal subjects with normal liver nor in patients with viral hepatitis, alcoholic cirrhosis or alcoholic fatty liver. The specificity of this phenomenon is difficult to define, since other tissue homogenates with comparable protein composition were not used. Furthermore, autologous liver homogenate will turn on the cells from patients with a variety of liver diseases. This suggests that the circulating lymphocyte might well be altered in these diseases, and the effect on them is a nonspecific effect from some intracellular component released by homogenization. Support is given to this concept by the observation that acetaldehyde and ethanol are capable of turning on lymphocytes from patients with both chronic active hepatitis and alcoholic hepatitis (8). Therefore limitations in this work are related to the nature of the antigen. This same antigen has been used in another test system, and if we refer to Figure 1, we see that during transformation, lymphokines are released. We can measure the effect of these lymphokines on such activities as the in vitro migration of peripheral blood leukocytes. It has been shown, using peripheral blood leukocytes, that in vitro migration inhibition is specific and with most antigens, this parallels the development of skin delayed hypersensitivity (9, 10). Much of this work, however, suffers from the limitation of crude antigens. With regard specifically to alcoholic liver disease, some inhibition of in vitro leukocyte migration was seen in a proportion of patients with alcoholic hepatitis, fewer with alcoholic cirrhosis (11). There have been other studies in a variety of liver diseases and Miller et al have demonstrated leukocyte migration inhibition to a liver specific lipoprotein in patients with chronic active hepatitis and primary biliary cirrhosis (12).

From Figure 1, it can be seen that another way to demonstrate cell mediated immunity is via in vitro cytotoxicity. In most studies reported, the cells which act as targets also act as antigens. The principle of the assay is simple. Hepatocytes are separated from liver specimens; the isolated hepatocytes are allowed to grow in microcytotoxicity chambers. These cells adhere to the wells. The potential killer cell population is added in great excess, a ratio of 200-400:1, and the two cell populations are incubated for 48-72 hours. At the end of this time, killed and nonattached cells are separated by gentle washing, and the adherent cells are then counted. Work with this assay has demonstrated direct cytotoxicity against rabbit liver cells with the leukocytes of patients with chronic active hepatitis (13). Human embryonic liver cells (Chang) have also been used as targets and lymphocytes from patients with alcoholic hepatitis were shown to result in killing (14). The specificity of the phenomenon is in some doubt, and this probably rests with the target. Using a slightly different system and measuring killing by specific radioactive chromium release, it has been shown that lymphocytes from patients with various types of chronic liver disease, as well as some healthy controls, will kill Chang liver cells and EL-4 tumor cells (15). This finding, therefore, suggests a certain lack of specificity and inappropriate target in this system.

One group has tried to overcome the problem of specificity by the use of liver cells obtained at liver biopsy. Using autologous liver cells grown in culture, and a technique similar to the one of Thompson et al (13), Paronetto and Vernace found significant killing of autologous liver cells in eight of ten patients with chronic active hepatitis, two patients with chronic persistent hepatitis, one with primary biliary cirrhosis, one with alcoholic hepatitis and three of five with acute viral hepatitis (14). Those individuals with normal livers did not show any cytotoxicity. Thus it can be concluded that almost any liver damage results in in vitro evidence of cell mediated immunity against self. The problem in these findings is the lack of specificity, not only with regard to the disease process, but also with respect to the antigen.

Evidence for Immune Mechanisms in Alcoholic Hepatitis

We should now examine the evidence for involvement of more specific immunological processes in the pathogenesis of alcoholic liver disease. There have been reports of an increased incidence of various autoantibodies, such as antiglobulins, cold agglutinins and antinuclear antibodies in alcoholic cirrhosis (17, 18, 19, 20, 21). But such findings are difficult to interpret in view of other studies where no autoantibodies are found (22, 23, 24), or where the incidence parallels the control population (1). Nevertheless, these observations have led some workers to study immune mechanisms in alcoholic liver disease. Zinneman and Levi, using tissue slices and a sandwich technique with fluorescein tagged immunoglobulin, have shown that the serum of alcoholic cirrhotics possesses antinuclear and anti-Mallory's hyalin activity (25). The former appeared to rest in the serum IgM, the latter in the serum IgA and IgG fractions. This work has been extended, and Zinneman (26) has found that IgM from four noncirrhotic patients possessed no antinuclear activity, whereas eight cirrhotic sera did. With purified IgA from one cirrhotic, and seven pooled cirrhotic IgA, there was fluorescence of alcoholic hyalin. Furthermore, incubation of a liver slice containing alcoholic hyalin with rhodamine tagged anti-IgA, revealed positive staining. These results suggested the presence of antibodies to alcoholic hyalin of the IgA class in patients with alcoholic liver disease. These antibodies would appear to bind in vivo. Another interesting observation in this work, was the finding that the IgG fractions from the cirrhotic sera blocked this fluorescence. It was suggested that this might indicate the presence of blocking antibodies which could serve a regulatory function. Zinneman believes that there are autoantibodies in alcoholic cirrhosis and that they are associated in some way with the elevated immunoglobulins found in this disease.

Leevy and his associates have approached this problem in a slightly different way. These workers have isolated and purified Mallory's hyalin by a standard technique and have used it as antigen in a number of situations

(27).   First of all, the finding of autoantibodies was confirmed (28).   One hundred percent of patients with severe alcoholic hepatitis had antibodies to purified hyalin, 42% with less severe disease had antibodies, and no antibodies were found in eight normal subjects, or in ten patients with acute viral hepatitis, five with fatty liver and five with alcoholic cirrhosis. It is not known which immunoglobulin type possessed the antibody activity.

Circulating lymphocytes from patients with acute alcoholic hepatitis will transform in vitro in response to purified alcoholic hyalin (7, 11). The transformation is most marked in patients with acute alcoholic hepatitis, but can be potentiated by the addition of acetaldehyde or ethanol. Furthermore, the supernatants from these turned on lymphocytes appear to contain lymphokines (see Figure 1), as one would predict. For example, specific transfer factor has been found only from the lymphocytes of patients with acute alcoholic hepatitis (28). Macrophage or leukocyte migration inhibition factor is elaborated and peripheral blood leukocyte migration is inhibited (29). The supernatants also contain activity which promotes the incorporation of tritiated hydroxyproline into liver collagen (7).

It can be concluded from these data that specific immunological processes are taking place within the liver. There is evidence of immune reactivity, both humoral and cellular, to liver antigens and more specifically, to alcoholic hyalin.   This reactivity is enhanced by ethanol and acetaldehyde.   It is of interest that as the damage progresses and with transformation to cirrhosis, the reactivity is found less frequently.

Mechanism of Immunization

The end result of alcoholic cirrhosis in any individual is due to a complex interplay of many factors. For the development of alcoholic liver disease, we know that the ingestion of alcohol is essential. The nature of the other factors which interact is less apparent, and we must rely on circumstantial evidence. It has been suggested that immune processes might play a critical role, and I propose to consider the possible mechanism of immunization to self.

The nature of the immune response is genetically determined, and we have some evidence for a predisposed or susceptible population. Wilson et al (31) detected a variation in the elevation of gamma G-3, related to genetic differences in the G_m system, which has suggested a predisposed alteration of the normal regulatory mechanism for immunoglobulin synthesis.   This might be extrapolated to cellular immune mechanisms. Thus, one might envisage a population of individuals programmed to respond in a certain way. There is ample testimony in the literature and from this symposium that ethanol and its metabolites are damaging. This damage might consist of the disruption of hepatocytes and release of intracellular contents (see Figure 2), and this event can be considered as an immunization event. Certainly, in other situations where there is extensive liver necrosis, there is evidence of release of antigens into the circulation (33).   These materials then act as

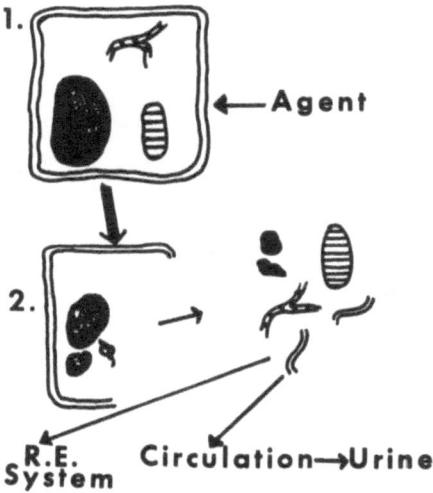

Fig. 2   Immunization

immunogens, either in their natural state, or much more likely, in an altered form. From the work of Meyer zum Buschenfelde, it is clear that a disease akin to chronic active hepatitis can be produced in rabbits by the injection of liver specific protein - but only with repeated injections and the addition of an adjuvant or binding chemical like sulfanilic acid (33). The work of Leevy has revealed the adjuvant action of ethanol and its metabolites by the increased in vitro lymphocyte reactivity (7, 11). Therefore in alcoholic liver disease we have tissue damage, release of potential immunogens, presence of adjuvant, and chronic exposure in a susceptible population.   Thus, immunization results in some perpetuation of liver damage. This is also a probable consequence if one considers the chronic active hepatitis model of Meyer zum Buschenfelde, where the immunogen was altered liver specific protein, and the immune response was against unaltered self.

The possible chain of events is depicted in Table III. I have so far reviewed the experimental evidence for each step and indicated the evidence that presently exists which supports the hypothesis of immuniz- ation to self components. The first event would, therefore, appear to be alcohol ingestion which results in tissue damage. The determinant of tissue damage is presumably related to amount of alcohol ingested and the nutritional status of the individual. The event of tissue damage leads to the release of cell contents and the possibility of prolonged exposure to the immune system. An important determinant here will be the efficiency of clearing by the reticuloendothelial system. The event of exposure to the cellular contents, plus the presence of alcohol and its metabolites, results in either immunization or tolerance. What determines this is presumably the genetic programming of the individual. The final event to consider is the

TABLE III

EXPLANATORY CHART FOR THE PERPETUATION OF LIVER INJURY

EVENT	RESULT	DETERMINANT
Alcohol ingestion	Tissue damage	Amount, nutrition, etc.
Tissue damage	Release of cell contents + prolonged exposure	Efficiency of RE system
Exposure to cell contents + alcohol acetaldehyde	Immunization or Tolerance	Genetic programming
Rechallenge	Perpetuation of liver injury damage to self (unaltered components)	Immunization or Tolerance

rechallenge of the individual with the alcohol and the intracellular contents. I postulate that the result is perpetuation of liver injury and damage to self, the unaltered components of self, and what determines this is whether immunization has taken place or whether the individual is tolerant. The antigen or the immunogen is yet to be completely clarified. Undoubtedly, Mallory's alcoholic hyalin is antigenic, certainly in vitro and possibly in vivo. Whether this antigen is available for immunological attack because of its location (34) is open to debate.

Further dispute might centre around the type of immune mechanism responsible for the tissue damage. This is obviously of importance to determine if one is to plan a logical approach to the abrogation of such responses. We have looked at humoral immunity and examined the evidence for cell mediated immunity. We have not examined the evidence for a Type V response, that is to say, a combination of antibody and cells - lymphocyte mediated antibody dependent cytotoxicity. I am not aware of a specific study to demonstrate this phenomenon in alcoholic liver disease, but this type of reaction is obviously important in other types of liver disease. Hopf, Arnold, Meyer zum Buschenfelde et al have demonstrated the presence of membrane fixed IgG on isolated hepatocytes from patients with chronic active hepatitis (35). This immunoglobulin is unlikely to be cytotoxic, since it has never been found in the serum of patients with liver disease (21). Direct evidence for Type V cytotoxicity has recently been forthcoming. Kawanishi, measuring LDH release, has demonstrated cytotoxicity against Chang liver cells with the sera from patients with chronic active hepatitis (36). This has also been shown for 12 of 17 patients with chronic active hepatitis, using rabbit liver cells as targets (37). It would be logical to look for this in alcoholic liver disease.

Sequelae

The end result of repeated alcohol abuse and repeated immunization is end stage liver disease, alcoholic cirrhosis, and it is of interest that the immune responsiveness of acute alcoholic hepatitis is thereby lost. This is probably not due to simple anergy, although this has been described in a number of liver diseases (38, 39). I suggest that one reason for the disordered growth in cirrhosis, the nodules and twin cells plates, for example, might be an immune reaction. It is conceivable that the immune reactions directed against self select out a cell type that does not possess the same antigens. This selection could truly be a phenomenon of selection or alternatively could arise by a process akin to antigenic modulation or allotypic suppression. The cells which lack or have covered an integral membrane protein (antigen) might well possess different behavioural characteristics and "prefer" different conditions in which to grow. A model might well be set up to test this hypothesis.

There are many well recognized sequelae of cirrhosis which will not be discussed here. One, however, bears mention. That is the phenomenon of apparent increased immune responsiveness. This phenomenon was described by Havens who demonstrated a supernormal response to tetanus toxoid injection in patients with alcoholic liver disease (39). This was not borne out by other studies (40, 41). In fact, in some liver disease, such as primary biliary cirrhosis, the production of antibodies is, if anything, decreased which might relate to impaired T cell function (42). Impaired T cell function has been described in alcoholic liver disease and this also makes supernormal immune responses unlikely (6). There is evidence, however, that the abnormal circulation which exists in cirrhosis allows the Kupffer cells to be bypassed. Therefore, instead of sequestration of antigens absorbed from the bowel, one gets circulating antigens and immunization. Therefore, if one looks for antibodies to the appropriate antigen such as E. coli, an increased incidence of such antibodies is found (42, 43).

CONCLUSIONS

Although the main etiological agent in alcoholic liver disease is unquestionably alcohol, it is likely that immune processes are involved in perpetuation of the disease. Immunization against self might be one of the factors responsible for continuation of the disease process once the extrinsic agent has been removed.

REFERENCES

1. DONIACH D, ROITT IM, WALKER JG, SHERLOCK S: Clin Exp Immunol 1: 237, 1966

2. PARONETTO F, GERBER MA, VERNACE SJ: Proc Soc Exp Biol (N.Y.) 143: 756, 1973

3. POPPER H, PARONETTO F, SCHAFFNER F: Ann N.Y. Acad Sci 124:
    781, 1965

4. NOWOSLAWSKI A, KRAWCZYNSKI K, BRZOSKO WJ, MADALINSKI K:
    Amer J Pathol 68: 31, 1972

5. DUDLEY FJ, FOX RA, SHERLOCK S: Lancet i: 723, 1972

6. HSU CC, LEEVY CM: Clin Exp Immunol 8: 749, 1971

7. LEEVY CM, CHEN T, ZETTERMAN R: Ann N.Y. Acad Sci 252: 106,
    1975

8. SORRELL MF, LEEVY C.M: Gastroenterol 63: 1020, 1972

9. SØBORG M, BENDIXEN G: Acta Med Scand 181: 247, 1967

10. SØBORG M: In Immunology of Liver Disease. Wm Heinenmann Medical
    Books Ltd., 1971. pp. 125

11. ZETTERMAN RK, LEEVY CM: Bull N.Y. Acad Med. 51: 533, 1975

12. MILLER J, SMITH MGM, MITCHELL CG, REED WD, EDDLESTON AL,
    WILLIAMS R: Lancet ii: 296, 1972

13. THOMPSON AD, COCHRANE AMG, MACFARLANE IG, EDDLESTON
    AL, WILLIAMS R: Nature New Biol 252: 271, 1974

14. KAKUMU S, LEEVY CM: Gastroenterol 69: A33/833, 1975

15. VIERLING JM, NELSON DL, STROBER W, BUNDY BM, JONES EA:
    Gastroenterology 69: A75/875, 1975

16. PARONETTO F, VERNACE S: Clin Exp Immunol 19: 99, 1975

17. HARTMANN L, BURTIN P, GRABAR P, FAUVERT R: C.R. Acad Sci
    (D) 243: 1937, 1956

18. PARONETTO F, RUBIN E, POPPER H: Lab Invest 11: 150, 1962

19. SCHNEIDERBAUR A, SCHUSTEN F: Wien Khiu Wochenschr 85: 288,
    1973

20. HOWELL DS, MALCOLM JM, PIKE R: Amer J Med 29: 662, 1960

21. NAKACHE JP, SALMON D, GREMY F, et al . Rev Eur Etud Clin Biol
    15: 71, 1970

22. GÖKCEN M: J Lab Clin Med 59: 533, 1962

23. DONIACH D, WALKER JG: Lancet i: 813, 1969

24. BIANCHINI E, ZANACCHI G: Minerva Med 62: 1715, 1971

25. ZINNEMAN HH, LEVI DF: Arch Int Med 124: 153, 1969

26. ZINNEMAN HH: Amer J Dig Dis 20: 337, 1975

27. FRENCH SW, IHRIG JT, NORVUM ML: Lab Invest 26: 240, 1972

28. CHEN T, KANAGASUNDARAM N, KAKAMU S, LUISADA-OPPER A,
    LEEVY CM: Gastroenterol 69: A13/813, 1975

29. KANAGASUNDARAM N, LEEVY CM: Gastroenterol 69: A33/833,
    1975

30. ZETTERMAN RK, LUISADA-OPPER A, LEEVY CM: Gastroenterol 70:
    382, 1976

31. WILSON D, OUSTAD G, WILLIAMS RC, Jr.: Gastroenterol 57: 59,
    1969

32. FOX RA: Progress in Immunology II Vol 5: American Elsevier
    Publishing Co. Inc., N.Y. 1976. pp. 318

33. MEYER ZUM BUSCHENFELDE KH, KOSSLING FK: Immunology of
    Liver Disease: Wm. Heinemann Medical Book Ltd., 1971 pp. 169

34. YOKOO H, MINICK OT, BATTI F, KEUT G: Amer J Path 69: 25, 1972

35. HOPF U, ARNOLD K, MEYER ZUM BUSCHENFELDE KH, FORSTER
    E, BOLTE JA: Clin Exp Immunol 22: 1, 1975

36. KAWANISHI H: Gastroenterol 69: A34/834, 1975

37. COCHRANE AM, MOSSOUROS A, THOMSON AD, EDDLESTON, AL,
    WILLIAMS R: Lancet i: 441, 1976

38. FOX RA, JAMES DG, SCHEUER PJ, SHARMA O, SHERLOCK S: Proc
    Roy Soc Med 63: 357, 1970

39. HAVENS WP Jr.: Int Arch Allergy 14: 75, 1959

40. CHERRICK GR, POTHIER L, DUFOUR JJ, SHERLOCK S: New
    England J Med 261: 340, 1959

41. BJØRNEBOE M, JENSEN KB, SCHEIKEL L, et al: Acta Med Scand
    188: 541, 1970

42. FOX RA, DUDLEY FJ, SHERLOCK S: Clin Exp Immunol 14: 473, 1973

43. TRIGER DR, KUNTZ JB, WRIGHT R: Gut 15: 94, 1974

44. TRIGER DR, WRIGHT R: Immunology 25: 951, 1973

DISCUSSION

CHAIRMAN: K.J. ISSELBACHER

KISILEVSKY: How does antibody lead to damage of normal cells when the stimulating antigen is sequestered by the cell membrane? Are we perhaps not dealing with the response of a membrane antigen? Perhaps the phenomenon that we actually see is a red herring.

FOX: That's a very good point. I think that alcoholic hyaline often is not accessible to the immune mechanism. Perhaps we are not looking at the appropriate antigen. Someone raised the point earlier that where you get hyaline you don't necessarily get hepatitis. So there must be a number of antigens involved.

FRENCH: Studies of orthotopic homograph rejection of the liver in pigs have demonstrated that lymphocytes can infiltrate liver cells and can actually migrate within them towards certain organelles as if there were a chemotaxic action involved. Do you interpret this as a morphological indication of an immunological phenomenon?

FOX: Yes. It is well recognized that lymphocytes do go into a variety of cells. They go in and out of macrophages for instance. But into what sort of hepatocyte they go, and how they do what they do when they get in there is open to conjecture.

POPPER: What is the evidence for an immune attack directed against alcoholic hyaline? Do we not have an initial attack by alcohol or one of its metabolites against membrane antigens and then secondary antigen-antibody reactions thereafter as in viral hepatitis? Alcoholic hyaline is probably an immune marker for one of these but not of the initial reaction.

FOX: I think that is absolutely right. Whatever the initial event is, you may well end up with sensitization. In my diagram you can substitute virus or toxin for agent. Even if we cure alcoholism by stopping everyone from drinking, I think it is likely that this plan of things will still be applicable with the increasing number of chemicals to which we are exposed.

It is of interest that the evidence of immunization to hyaline disappears when the patient develops an inactive cirrhosis. I wonder if the immunity itself doesn't lead to the development of cirrhotic nodules and twin-cell plates by encouraging preferential growth of cells with different surface antigenic characteristics which are not seen by the immune system.

ISRAEL: Do you think that some of our difficulty in reproducing alcoholic hepatitis and cirrhosis in experimental animals is not only the alcohol dose but also the species' immune system?

FOX: Yes. I think that is a very distinct possibility. For example there is tremendous variation amongst different strains of mice in terms of their tolerance to ethanol.

ISSELBACHER: Most people think of autoimmunity as a self-perpetuating situation. How do you fit alcoholic hepatitis which stops with the discontinuance of alcohol into this concept of a self-perpetuating process?

FOX: This concept of autoimmunity fails to recognize the object of the exercise. Many of the diseases that we have are characterized by immune reactions against self. In tuberculosis or viral hepatitis B it is the immune response in its attempt to eradicate the agent that leads to the tissue damage. Alcoholic liver disease is just another example of this phenomenon.

ALCOHOL INDUCED SUSCEPTIBILITY TO HYPOXIC LIVER DAMAGE:

POSSIBLE ROLE IN THE PATHOGENESIS OF ALCOHOLIC LIVER DISEASE?

Y. Israel, H. Orrego, J.M. Khanna, D.J. Stewart, M.J. Phillips, and H. Kalant

Departments of Pharmacology, Physiology and Pathology
University of Toronto and Addiction Research Foundation
Ontario, Canada

Previous studies in our laboratory (1-3), have indicated that the major rate limiting factor in ethanol metabolism in the intact liver cell is the rate of mitochondrial reoxidation to NAD^+ of NADH produced in the oxidation of ethanol. This has now been confirmed in several laboratories (4-8). In this process oxygen is utilized and water is formed. The capacity of mitochondria to oxidize reducing equivalents is related to the relative availability of phosphate acceptor (ADP), or more generally to the phosphorylation potential (ATP/ADP x Pi) (9-12). Mitochondrial uncouplers such as dinitrophenol (DNP), carbonyl cyanide p-trifluoromethoxyphenyl-hydrazone (FCCP) and arsenate allow the mitochondria to oxidize reducing equivalents independently of phosphate acceptor availability and thus they increase the rate of oxygen consumption (13). Accordingly, the rate of ethanol metabolism has been shown to be increased by uncoupling agents both in vivo (2,4) and in vitro in liver slices (1, 14), perfused liver (3,5) and isolated hepatocytes (8). Figure 1 shows the effect of DNP on the rate of ethanol metabolism by perfused rat liver.

In agreement with the concept that under normal conditions the rate of oxygen consumption limits the rate of ethanol metabolism, is the finding (15) that in different animal species the basal metabolic rate (BMR) correlates remarkably well with the in vivo rate of ethanol metabolism (Figure 2). These data are also in line with reports by Lester and Keokosky (16) who found that ethanol metabolism in vivo is related to (body weight) 0.75 which is, in turn, known to be related to basal metabolic rate. Assuming a proportionality factor between basal metabolic rate and liver oxygen consumption for each species, a correlation between ethanol metabolism and basal metabolic rate is to be expected on the basis that in man and in other species the liver utilizes a very large proportion (60-80%) of its total oxygen consumption to transform alcohol into acetate (17,18). This is done at the

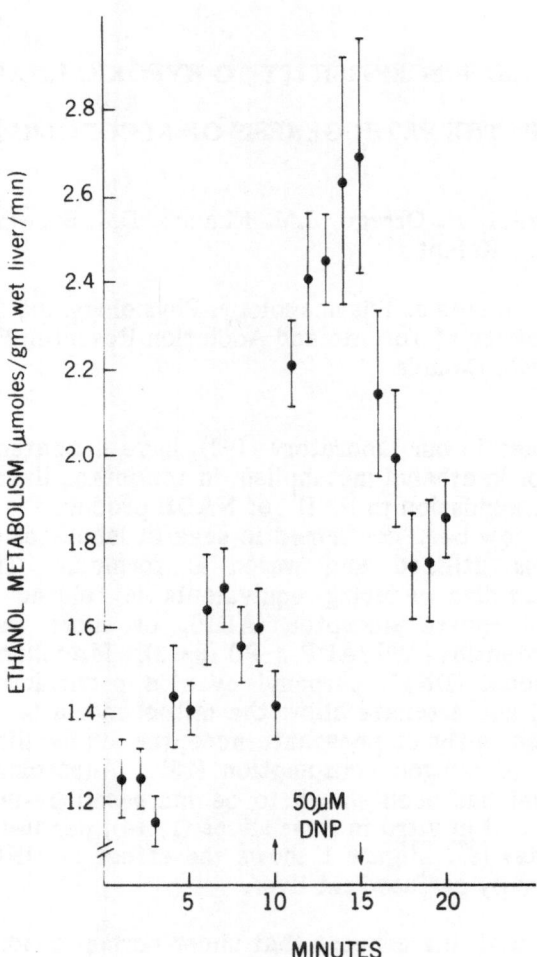

Fig. 1   Effect of 2.4 dinitrophenol on the rate of ethanol metabolism by
          isolated perfused rat liver.
          The arrows show the time at which 2.4 dinitrophenol (DNP) was
          added to and removed from the perfusion fluid (from ref. 3).

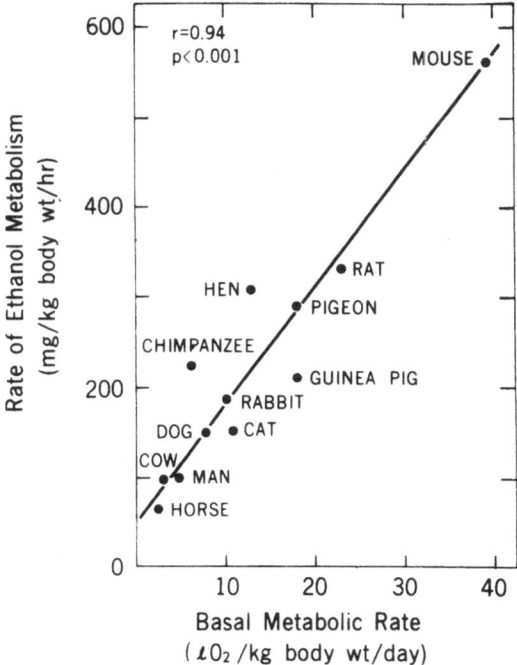

Fig. 2   *Relationship between in vivo rate of ethanol metabolism and basal metabolic rate in several animal species, including man (from ref. 15).*

expense of other physiological substrates, the oxidation of which is greatly inhibited (19,20).

It is known that chronic alcohol ingestion leads to an increase in the rate of ethanol metabolism both in man and in experimental animals (21-29). Increases of up to 100% over control values have been reported in human alcoholics and in Rhesus monkeys following chronic ethanol administration (25,26). Standard laboratory rat strains increase their rates of ethanol metabolism by 30-70% (21,23,27-29). Liver slices prepared from animals chronically treated with ethanol show a hypermetabolic state as evidenced by increases of 20-60% in the rates of ethanol metabolism and of oxygen consumption (QO_2) (14,27,30) (Figure 3). Thurman et al. (6) have shown that perfused livers of rats which have been chronically fed ethanol also utilize oxygen and metabolize ethanol at rates which are 40-70% higher than those of their respective controls (Table I).

In human alcoholic hepatitis, hepatocellular necrosis is most commonly seen in the periphery of the acinus (centrilobular area) (31-35). This is the

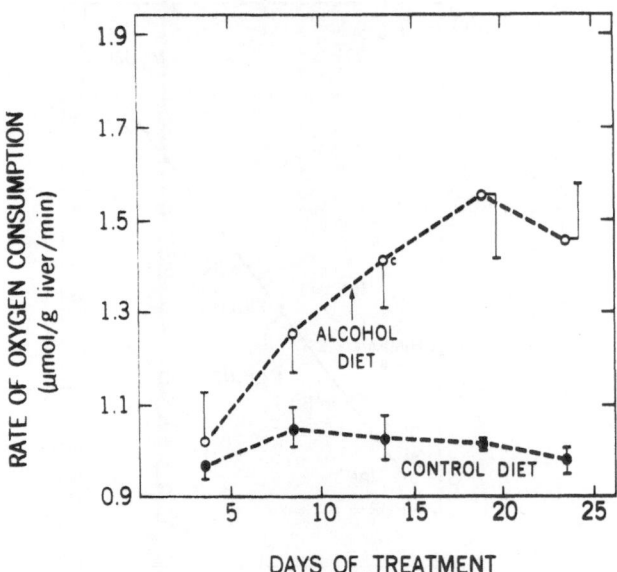

Fig. 3   *Effect of chronic ethanol feeding on the rate of oxygen*
consumption by rat liver slices (data from ref. 14).

zone of the acinus most distant from the points of entry of blood and
therefore the zone in which the oxygen tensions are lowest (36). Since the
livers of ethanol treated animals consume oxygen at higher rates, the
possibility exists that the gradient of decreasing oxygen tension from the
portal vein to the terminal hepatic vein (central vein) is accentuated. We
have proposed (37) that when the availability of oxygen is reduced below
normal by any physiological, pharmacological or pathological condition, this
accentuation of periacinar hypoxia leads to hypoxic damage and necrosis. In
order to test this hypothesis, rats were chronically treated with ethanol and
then subjected to two conditions that are likely to occur in the life of human
alcoholics, that tend to reduce the availability of oxygen to the liver. The
first condition was the exposure of the animals to low oxygen tensions (37),
as this would replicate conditions in which hypoxemia is likely to exist. In
man this can occur in conditions such as respiratory depression due to heavy
alcohol intoxication or in disease states such as pneumonia, emphysema or
pulmonary insufficiency. The second condition was the production of an
experimental anemia by bleeding with simultaneous replacement of serum so
that the hematocrit value was reduced but maximal changes in intravascular
volume did not exceed 5-6% at any time.

TABLE I

EFFECT OF CHRONIC ETHANOL TREATMENT ON
THE RATE OF OXYGEN CONSUMPTION AND
ETHANOL METABOLISM BY PERFUSED RAT LIVER

	Ethanol Metabolism	Oxygen Consumption
	(μmoles/g/hr)	
Control	58 ± 4	127 ± 14
Ethanol-treated	80 ± 5	205 ± 18

n = 5 - 8.   Data from Thurman et al, Ref 6.   With permission of the authors.

In order to determine the severity of liver lesions, samples of the livers were fixed in buffered 10% formalin solution and sections were stained with hematoxylin-eosin for light microscopy. Liver necrosis and other abnormalities were assessed in slides coded to avoid bias. Liver necrosis was scored as follows: 0, no necrosis; 1+ focal necrosis of one or two cells per lesion; 2+ focal necrosis of more than two cells per lesion; 3+ massive confluent necrosis and 4+ zonal massive necrosis plus necrotic bridging between terminal hepatic veins (central veins). Before exposure to low oxygen tensions or bleeding, the rats were fed for 30 days with liquid diets containing 35% of the calories as ethanol (38). Control animals were pair fed with diets containing isocaloric sucrose in place of ethanol. Animal weights at the end of this period ranged between 160 and 260 g in different experiments. All the animals were fasted overnight before the experiments. Rat chow and water were given ad libitum for the 24-hour period following hemorrhage.

In the experiments in which hypoxia was used, the animals were placed individually in cylindrical glass chambers (40 x 20 cm) and were exposed for 6 hours to oxygen at selected concentrations (11%, 7.5% or 5%; the remainder being pure nitrogen). After this time the animals were sacrificed for liver histology studies. In some experimental series the activities of serum glutamic-oxalacetic transaminase (SGOT) and ornithine carbamyl-transferase (SOCT) were determined in each animal before and after hypoxia or bleeding (37). In the experiments in which the experimental anemia was produced, the animals were lightly anesthetized with ether and blood was removed through one femoral vein while the other femoral was used for simultaneous infusion of rat serum prepared freshly from normal rats. This was done with a variable rate infusion pump. The bleeding procedure lasted about 3-4 minutes, while the whole operation did not exceed 12-16 min.

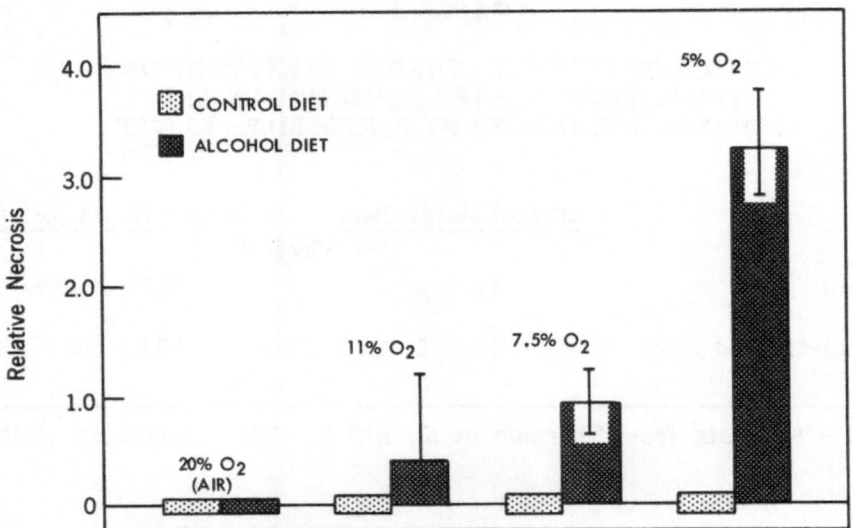

Fig. 4   *Effect of chronic ethanol feeding and exposure to reduced oxygen tensions on liver histology.*
Rats were fed liquid diets containing 35% of total calories as ethanol or as isocaloric sucrose controls for 30 days before exposing them for 6 hours to atmospheres at the oxygen tensions indicated. See text for explanation of lesion scores (data from ref. 37).

Plate 1   a)   *Sucrose control, 5% anoxia 6 hours.   The histology is normal.*
                  Hematoxylin and eosin x 320.

            b)   *Ethanol treated animal, 7.5% anoxia 6 hours.   Note the periacinar (centrilobular) hepatocytes show condensation of their cytoplasm, mild fatty change and occasional focal necrosis and leukocytes (+ - ++ lesion).*
                  Hematoxylin and eosin x 320.

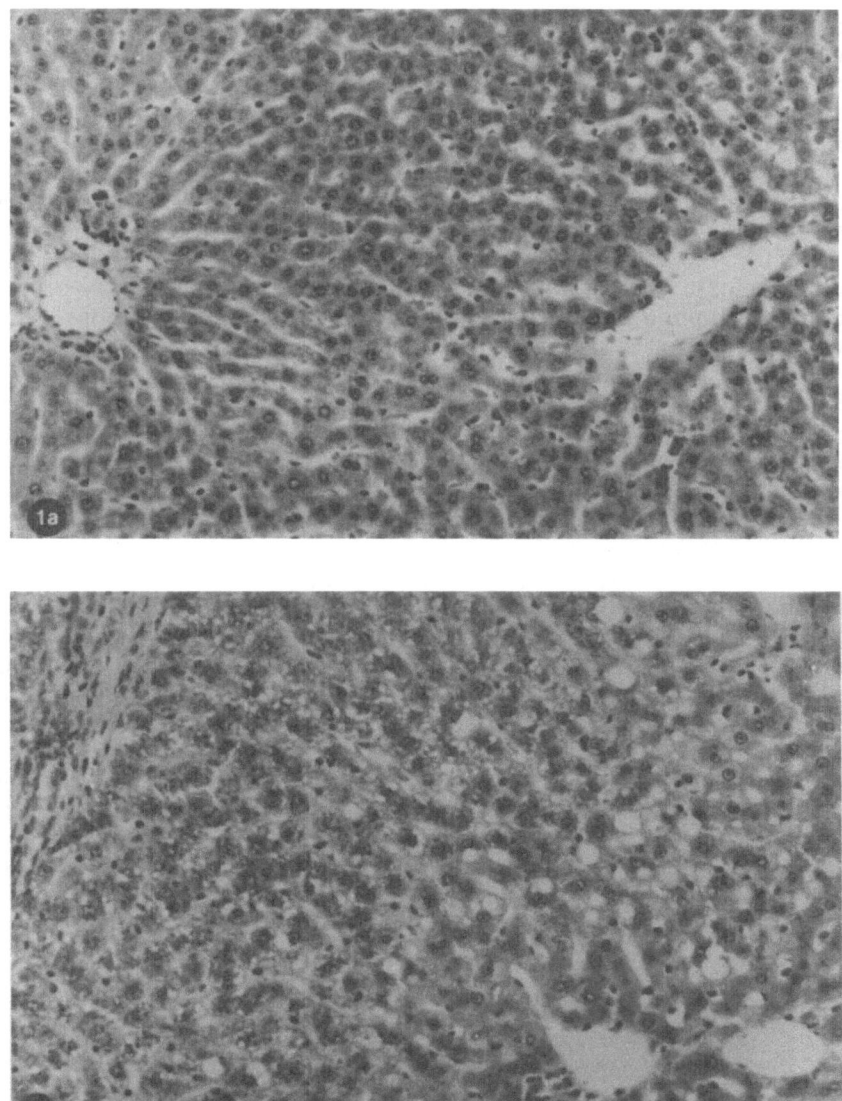

Twenty-four hours after bleeding the hematocrit values were 25.5 ± 1.7 (12) and 25.8 ± 1.1 (12) respectively for ethanol treated and control animals. At this time the animals were sacrificed and a portion of the liver was fixed for light microscopy.

Figure 4 shows the effect of low oxygen tension on animals chronically treated with ethanol and controls. Only the animals chronically treated with alcohol showed liver lesions. Furthermore, the severity of the lesions was proportional to the degree of hypoxia. The alterations were, in all cases, localized in the periacinar (centrilobular) zone and were characterized by necrosis, degeneration and mild leukocytic infiltration. Periacinar (centri-lobular) fat was always present in the ethanol treated animals independently of the presence or absence of necrosis or other alterations. The lesions seen with 11% O_2 and 7.5% O_2 were focal but these became massive at 5% O_2 (Plates 1 and 2). Thus, while the latter resemble the pattern classically ascribed to ischemic liver lesions, the focal lesions correspond more closely to the lesions that are observed in the human alcoholic.

Some aspects of the microscopic appearance of these lesions deserve further consideration. It whould be noted that alcoholic hyaline (Mallory bodies) was (were) not observed in these experiments. Nevertheless Mallory bodies are now believed not to be specific for alcoholic liver disease and they are not considered an essential condition for the diagnosis of alcoholic hepatitis (33,39-42).

Since the above experiments suggest that the liver of alcohol treated animals is very sensitive to a reduction in the availability of oxygen, it was conceivable that pretreatment with a drug such as propylthiouracil, which is known to reduce tissue oxygen consumption through its well known antithyroidal effects (43), would reduce the degree of periacinar ischemia. Thus, propylthiouracil might afford a protective effect in the livers of ethanol treated animals. In order to test this hypothesis rats were pair-fed the ethanol or equicaloric sucrose diets for 30 days. During the last 10 days half of each group received a solution of prophylthiouracil at a dose of 5 mg/100g/day by gastric intubation, while the other half received water (37).

Plate 2   a)   *Ethanol treated animal, 7.5% anoxia 6 hours. Note more advanced fatty change andcellular necrosis (++   -   +++ lesion).*
            Hematoxylin and eosin x 320.

            b)   *Ethanol treated animal, 5% anoxia 6 hours. Massive periacinar (centrilobular) hepatocellular necrosis is present (++++ lesion).*
            Hematoxylin and eosin x 320.

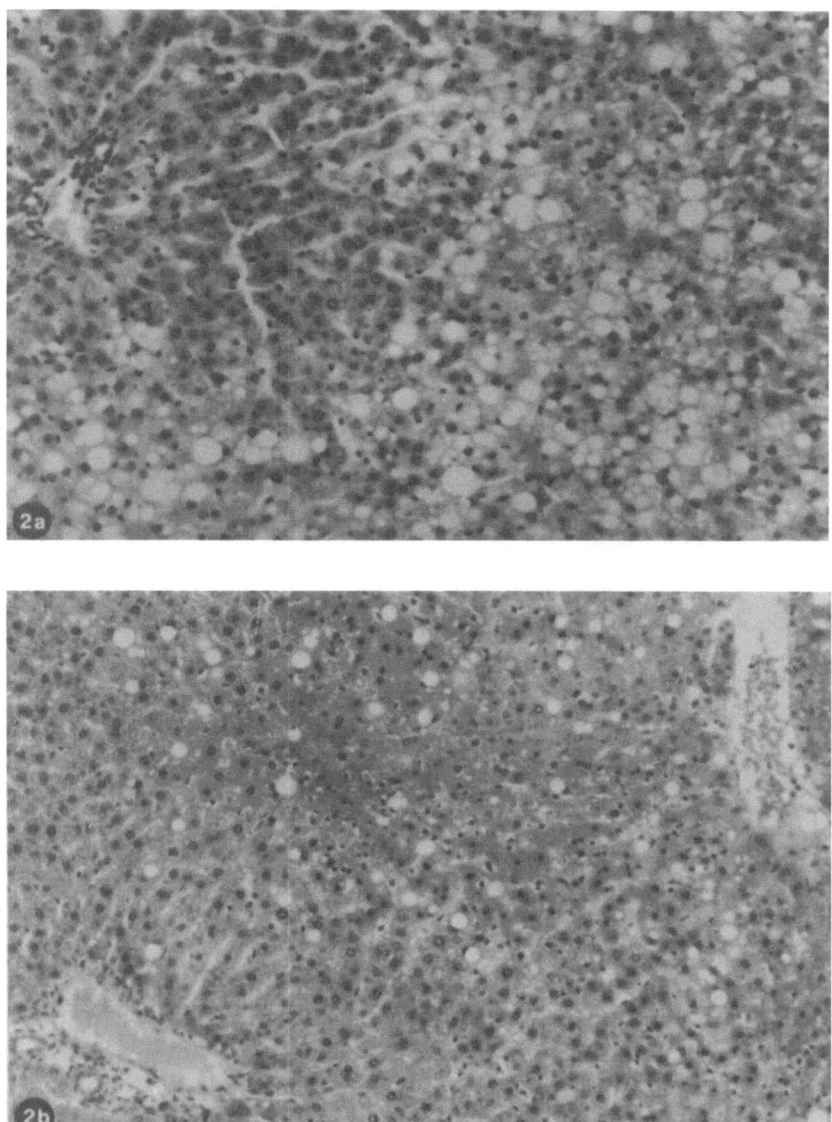

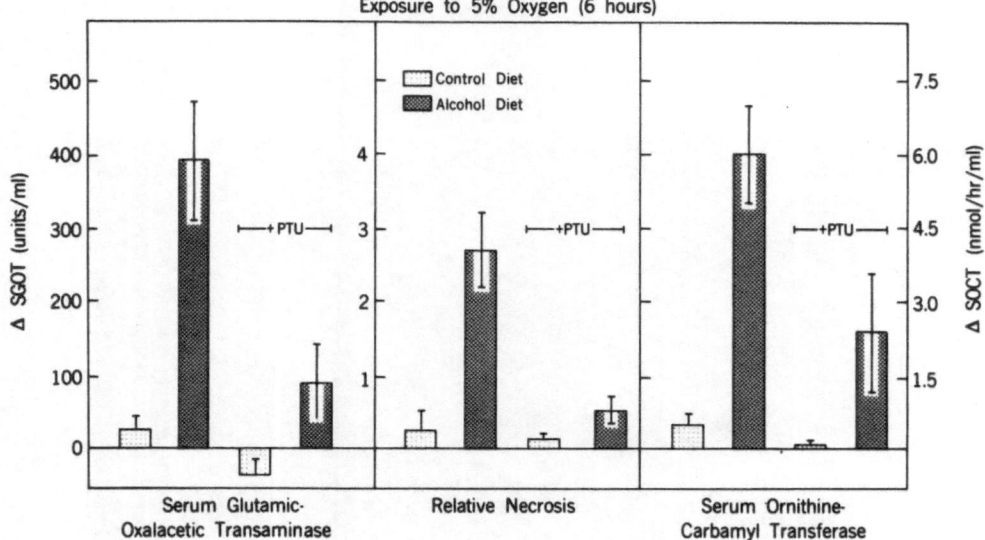

Fig. 5   *Protective effect of propylthiouracil on hypoxic liver damage in*
             ethanol treated rats.
             Conditions as in Fig. 4. Animals were exposed for 6 hours to an
             atmosphere containing 5% O₂. Prophylthiouracil (5 mg/100g/
             day) was administered for last 10 days. Changes in serum
             enzyme activities are expressed as differences (Δ) = Activity
             after hypoxia minus Activity before hypoxia (data from ref. 37).

Propylthiouracil treatment markedly protected against liver damage induced
by hypoxia in ethanol treated animals, as shown by a marked reduction in the
liver necrosis scores, and reductions in SGOT and SOCT (Figure 5).

Table II shows the effect of bleeding and serum replacement on SGOT
and liver necrosis in ethanol treated and control animals. Significant
increases in SGOT were found as early as 6 hours after bleeding. These
changes were accentuated at 24 hours. Liver histology done at this time
showed liver lesions in all the ethanol treated animals. No abnormalities
were observed in the liver of control animals. In the ethanol treated animals
the lesions were always periacinar (centrilobular) and sharply zonal. In all
instances fatty infiltration and hepatocellular degeneration were found. The
necrosis was predominantly focal (1+ to 2+) necrosis and leucocytic
infiltration, and in a few cases, more extensive confluent or early bridging
necrosis were also observed (Plate 3). As in the hypoxia series, no alcoholic
hyaline was observed in the liver of animals fed ethanol and bled.

TABLE II

EFFECT OF BLEEDING WITH SERUM REPLACEMENT
ON SERUM GLUTAMIC-OXALACETIC TRANSAMINASE
(SGOT) AND LIVER HISTOLOGY IN RATS
CHRONICALLY FED ETHANOL

Hours	Controls	Necrosis Scores	Ethanol Treated
24	0.0 (7)		1.56±0.5 (8)
		SGOT (Units/ml)	
0	69.6±9.4 (9)		84.9±10.3 (9)
3	74.0±5.3 (12)		112.5±15.3 (12)
6	89.2±4.7 (12)		173.6±29.0 (12)
24	80.3±11.2 (12)		344.8±110 (12)

At time = 0 hrs animals had been treated for 30 days with ethanol or sucrose
(control) diets and had been fasted for 16 hours. Bleeding with simultaneous
serum replacement was done at time zero. At 24 hours the hematocrits
were: Ethanol treated = 25.5 ± 1.7 (12); Controls 25.8 ± 1.1 (12).

Recent studies in our laboratory have concentrated on the production of
alcohol induced liver damage in strains of rats in which the lesions would
occur spontaneously (i.e. without exposing the animals to low oxygen
tensions or inducing an experimental anemia).

A large body of literature has accumulated on a stressable strain of
rats, namely the Okamoto-Aoki Spontaneously Hypertensive (SH) Rat (see
ref. 44). These animals are essentially normotensive up to about 30–60
days. However, between the ages of 60 and 120 days they develop marked
hypertension reaching systolic blood pressures of 180–200 mm Hg (44,45).
These changes are abolished by thyroidectomy, adrenalectomy or hypo-
physectomy (46). Falkow and co-workers have shown that an increased
stressability in these animals precedes the development of the hypertenion
(47,48). Since we have proposed that the hypermetabolic state produced in
the liver following chronic ethanol ingestion may involve hormonal changes
that are normally associated with the stress response (30,49,50), we thought
that SH rats might develop such a state more readily. Furthermore, it has
been reported that as the SH rats become hypertensive there is dramatic
reduction in cardiac output per kg body weight and a significant reduction in
visceral blood flow (45). These changes should result in a decreased

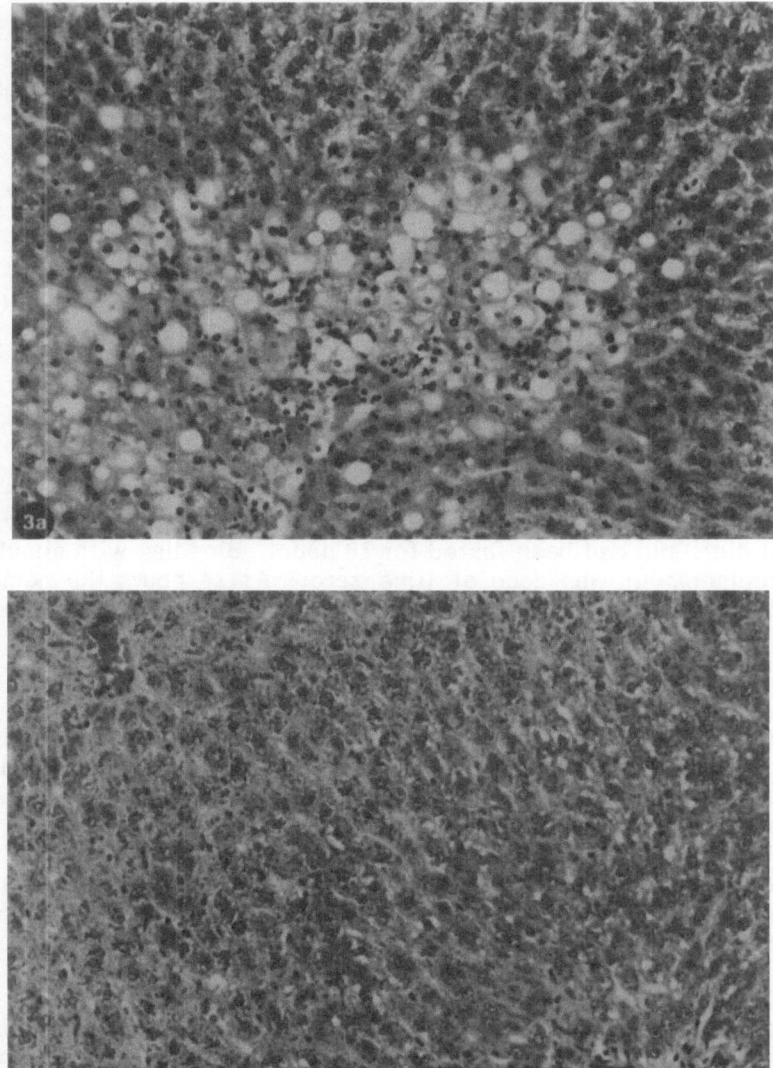

availability of oxygen to the liver of these animals. Thus these animals would conceivably be more sensitive to an ethanol induced ischemic liver damage.

Perfused livers of SH rats chronically fed alcohol in liquid diets metabolize ethanol and consume oxygen at an increased rate with respect to controls. Also, a marked hepatomegaly was induced by the chronic alcohol treatment (Table III). When both the increase in liver mass and the rate of oxygen consumption per unit weight of liver are considered, increases in the rate of oxygen utilization of the order of 80% are found in the livers of ethanol treated SH rats. These animals showed histological evidence of liver damage, seen as cell degeneration and focal necrosis in the periacinar areas (Table IV). In line with these observations, biochemical evidence of cell necrosis was also observed, in the form of increases in SGOT and SOCT in the alcohol treated SH rats (Table V).

Data presented above indicate that different experimental conditions that lead to a reduction in liver oxygenation produce cell necrosis in the periphery of the acinus in the liver of alcohol fed animals. It is also in the area in which collagen is deposited in alcoholic cirrhosis (see Popper, this Symposium). Cell necrosis appears to be a condition sine qua non in the development of experimental cirrhosis by any agent (51). Thus, ischemic necrosis in the periphery of the acinus could conceivably set the conditions for collagen deposition in this area. The question therefore arises as to whether these hypoxic lesions actually occur in the liver of the alcoholic.

Several lines of evidence would indicate that ischemia is more likely to occur in the liver of alcoholics than in the liver of normal individuals. These are listed in Table VI. The first condition refers to the existence of:

(i) A hypermetabolic state in the liver after chronic ethanol. This state most likely exists in man (and also in sub-human primates) as it does in rats since marked increases in the rate of ethanol metabolism, up to 100%, have been reported to occur in alcoholics and in Rhesus monkeys fed ethanol chronically (22,24,25,26). An increased rate of oxygen consumption is required by the liver to transform the massive amounts of alcohol ingested,

---

Plate 3   *Bleeding plus serum replacement*

a)   *Ethanol treated animal. Periacinar (centrilobular) region is shown. Note the hepatocellular necrosis, leukocytic infiltration and the zonal distribution of the lesion. Hematoxylin and eosin x 320.*

b)   *Control animal. The hepatic histology is normal. Hematoxylin and eosin x 320.*

TABLE III

OXYGEN CONSUMPTION AND ETHANOL METABOLISM IN
PERFUSED LIVER AFTER CHRONIC ALCOHOL TREATMENT
IN MALE SPONTANEOUSLY HYPERTENSIVE RATS

PERFUSED LIVER

	Control	Chronic Alcohol	(p)
Ethanol Metabolism (μmoles/g/min)	1.33 ± 0.14 (4)	2.33 ± 0.20 (4)	1.0 ($p < 0.05$)
Oxygen Consumption (μmoles/g/min)	3.02 ± 0.16 (6)	3.63 ± 0.21 (6)	0.61 ($p < 0.01$)
Liver/Body ratio (g liver/100g animal)	3.69 ± 0.15 (6)	5.485 ± 0.16 (6)	($p < 0.01$)
Total Liver Oxygen Consumption (μmol/100g animal/min)	11.2 ± 0.83 (6)	19.8 ± 1.1 (6)	($p < 0.01$)

Animals = Age: 98 – 108 days ; 48 – 58 days on diets.

The recirculation technique of liver perfusion was used. Ethanol was added
to the perfusate to a final concentration of 40 mM.

which in some alcoholics can amount to 50-75% of their total caloric intake.
This should occur independently of the enzymic mechanism invoked to
increase the rate of ethanol metabolism, since all the systems known utilize
oxygen.

(ii) Apart from an increase in the rate of oxygen consumption per unit
mass of liver, total liver mass should also be considered in determining the
total oxygen consumption of this organ.   In this respect it should be
mentioned that the most constant concomitant of alcoholic liver disease
(before the final cirrhosis stage) is hepatomegaly. Data by Lishner et al.
(52) and Fallon (53) indicate that hepatomegaly occurs in 81-92% of
alcoholics with alcoholic hepatitits.   Hepatomegaly has been classically
considered part of the liver damage that has been described in alcoholics
after chronic alcohol intake.   In this regard one can, however, ask if
hepatomegaly could not be regarded as a possible contributory cause rather
than only as a consequence of the liver lesions in the alcoholic. It should be
borne in mind that hepatomegaly per se cannot be regarded as pathogenic, as
it also occurs in a large percentage of alcoholics with fatty liver, in the
absence of cell necrosis (53).

TABLE IV

LIVER NECROSIS IN SPONTANEOUSLY
HYPERTENSIVE RATS AFTER CHRONIC
ALCOHOL TREATMENT

Pair Number	Ethanol	Control
29/30	1+ ; 1.5+	0 ; 0
37/38	0 ; 2+	0 ; 0
39/40	1+ ; 0.5+	0 ; 0
15/16	0.5+ ; 0.5+	0 ; 0
19/20	1+ ; 1+	0 ; 0
23/24	1+ ; 1.5+	0 ; 0
27/28	1.5+ ; 0.5+	0 ; 0
31/32	0 ; 1+	0 ; 0

Animals were fed the alcohol or control diets for
48 - 75 days.

Duplicate samples were examined for each of the
ethanol and control animals in separate blocks of
liver tissue.

(iii) Another condition commonly associated with alcoholism is anemia
(59-61). This can be produced by many alcohol related effects which can
precede alcoholic liver damage such as bleeding due to alcoholic gastritis
(54-56) or nutritional problems (57-59). Studies by Lischner et al. (52)
showed that 43% of patients with alcoholic hepatitis had anemias with
hematocrit values below 30%. This is within the hematocrit range at which
ethanol treated rats showed liver damage after bleeding, in our studies.
Bleeding due to esophageal varices resulting from an increased portal
pressure due to an already injured liver in alcoholics can obviously not be an
etiological factor in the production of the initial lesion. However, anemia
due to this cause could create a vicious circle perpetuating the lesions.

An inefficient oxygen delivery can also occur in alcoholics due to
"functional anemias" i.e. alterations in which the curve of oxygen dissociation of hemoglobin is shifted to the right. One such type of functional
anemia occurs in alkalosis, a condition that occurs in alcoholics upon
discontinuation of drinking (62,63) and that is due to the increased
respiratory activity accompanying the alcohol withdrawal syndrome (respiratory alkalosis) (62). A different type of functional anemia may be related to

TABLE V

SERUM ENZYMES IN
SPONTANEOUSLY HYPERTENSIVE RATS (MALES)
TREATED 75 DAYS (I) OR 34 DAYS (II)
WITH ETOH AND WITHDRAWN 24 HOURS

	SGOT (units/ml)	
	(I)	(II)
CONTROLS	182.8 ± 9.2 (12)	186.8 ± 9.8 (9)
	($p < 0.01$)	($p < 0.02$)
ETHANOL	308.7 ± 26.9 (9)	292.7 ± 29.5 (8)

	SOCT (pmol/hr per ml)	
CONTROLS	64.4 ± 17.1 (7)	-
	($p < 0.01$)	
ETHANOL	673 ± 285 (7)	-

Animals I = Age 125 days; 75 days on liquid diets

Animals II = Age 84 days; 34 days on liquid diets

the fact that abnormally low levels of ATP and 2,3 diphosphoglycerate (2,3 DPG) - both allosteric modifiers of the hemoglobin dissociation curve - have been observed in red cells of malnourished alcoholics, in which plasma phoshate levels are reduced (64).

(iv) Another group of abnormalities found with an increased frequency in the alcoholic population, leading to inadequate tissue oxygen supply relates to problems of blood oxygenation due to abnormal lung function. Alcohol, as many other general depressants, leads to respiratory depression when high enough concentrations are attained in blood (65). It is also known that heavy smoking is very common in alcoholics (66). Carbon monoxide in cigarette smoke is known to bind to hemoglobin, with an affinity that is 200-300 times greater than that of oxygen (67), thus reducing the oxygen carrying capacity of blood. Heavy smoking has been shown to reduce the amount of hemoglobin available for combination with oxygen by as much as 9-10% (68). Emirgil and co-workers (69) have shown that 91% of all alcoholics in a detoxification unit had chronic bronchitis while 60% of them showed dyspnea. Several other parameters of pulmonary function were also found to be consistently altered in the alcoholics (69). It is not clear

TABLE VI

FACTORS THAT PREDISPOSE TO HEPATIC HYPOXIA IN CHRONIC ALCOHOLICS

		References
(i)	Hypermetabolic State	(22) (24) (25) (16)
(ii)	Hepatomegaly	(52) (53)
(iii)	Anemia	
	a) Concomitant Nutritional Problems	(57) (58) (59)
	b) Bleeding, Acute Gastritis	(54) (55) (56)
	c) Functional Anemias	
	(1) Withdrawal Alkalosis	(62) (63)
	(2) ATP and 2, 3 DPG abnormalities	(64)
(iv)	Respiratory Dysfunction and Hemoglobin Saturation	
	a) Respiratory Depression	(65)
	b) Cigarette Smoking	(66) (67) (68)
	c) Pulmonary Dysfunction	(69)
	d) Respiratory Infections	(70) (71) (72) (73)
(v)	Hemodynamic Factors	
	a) Alcoholic Cardiomyopathy	(75) (76)

however, to what extent these might be the result of liver damage. Nevertheless, these abnormalities may be of importance in the perpetuation and progression of the disease.

Another factor leading to hypoxemia in alcoholics is the well established fact that the severity of upper respiratory diseases is greater in these individuals than in controls (70). A study of the autopsy records of those who died of lobar pneumonia over a 10 year period in a large institution showed that 70% of the patients were alcoholics (71). An increased incidence of several types of pneumonia has also been reported to occur in alcoholics (72,73). Baboons fed ethanol chronically appear to show an increased susceptibility to upper respiratory infections. In a recent report (74), four out of nine animals fed ethanol chronically developed upper respiratory infections. The latter two showed cirrhosis on autopsy. No such problems were reported for the control animals.

(v) Finally, hemodynamic alterations known to occur in alcoholics, such as those produced by alcoholic cardiomyopathy (75-76), might also contribute to reducing the availability of oxygen to the liver.

From the above discussion it is clear that many factors tend to accentuate periacinar hypoxia in the liver of alcoholics. Based on our studies in animals, a combination of several such factors could conceivably be of relevance in the development and perpetuation of liver lesions in the alcoholic.

SUMMARY

Chronic ethanol feeding leads to increased rates of ethanol metabolism in man and in animals (metabolic tolerance). This appears to be due to an increased rate of general metabolism of the liver and to an increased liver mass. Both conditions increase the oxygen demand by this organ thus making it more vulnerable to a variety of conditions that reduce oxygen availability. Liver necrosis and leukocytic infiltration in the periacinar region (centrilobular area) occur in chronically ethanol fed animals after exposure to a brief period of hypoxia or after hematocrit reduction by bleeding plus serum replacement. These liver alterations are not seen in similarly treated control animals.

The liver of the Spontaneously Hypertensive strain of rats shows marked increases in the rates of ethanol metabolism and of oxygen consumption following chronic ethanol feeding. These animals, in which cardiac output and liver perfusion rates are known to be reduced by the hypertension, develop liver lesions spontaneously (i.e. without exposure to hypoxia or bleeding), when fed ethanol chronically.

Apart from a general increase in liver metabolic rate and an increase in liver mass, many other conditions reviewed here occur with an increased frequency in alcoholics and increase the risk of producing hepatic ischemia. It is suggested that ischemia, resulting from a combination of metabolic factors and subclinical and clinical conditions, may play a pathogenic role in the production of liver lesions in the alcoholic.

REFERENCES

1. VIDELA L and ISRAEL Y: Factors that modify the metabolism of ethanol in rat liver and adaptive changes produced by its chronic administration. Biochem J 118: 275-281, 1970

2. ISRAEL Y, KHANNA JM and LIN R: Effect of 2.4 - dinitrophenol on the rate of ethanol elimination in the rat in vivo. Biochem J 120: 447-448, 1970

3. SEIDEN H, ISRAEL Y and KALANT H: Activation of ethanol metabolism by 2.4 - dinitrophenol in the isolated perfused rat liver. Biochem Pharmacol 23: 2234-2337, 1974

4. KREBS HA and STUBBS M: Factors controlling the rate of alcohol disposal by the liver. In Alcohol Intoxication and Withdrawal, vol II, MM Gross (ed.). Plenum Press, N.Y. 1975. pp. 149

5. ERIKKSON CJ, LINDROS KO and FORSANDER OA: 2.4 - dinitrophenol-induced increase in ethanol and acetaldehyde oxidation in the perfused liver. Biochem Pharmacol 23: 2193, 1964

6. THURMAN RG, McKENNA WR and McCAFFREY TB: Pathways reponsible for the adaptive increase in ethanol utilization following chronic treatment with ethanol: Inhibitor studies with hemoglobin - free perfused liver. Molec Pharmacol 12: 156, 1976

7. CARTER EA and ISSELBACHER KJ: The effect of ethyl-x-chloro-phenoxisobutyrate. Life Sci 13: 907, 1973

8. MAIJER AJ, VAN WOERKOM GM, WILLIAMSON JR and TAGER JM: Rate-limiting factors in the oxidation of ethanol by isolated rat liver cells. Biochem J 150: 205, 1975

9. CHANCE B and WILLIAMS GR: The respiratory chain and oxidative phosphorylation. Adv Enzymol 17: 65, 1956

10. CHANCE B and MIATRA PK: Determination of the intracellular phosphate potential of ascites cells by reversed electron transfer. In Control Mechanisms in Respiration and Fermentation, B Wright (ed). Ronald Press, N.Y., 1963. pp. 307

11. KLINGENBERG M: The respiratory chain. In Biological Oxidations, TP Singer (ed.). Interscience, N.Y., 1958. pp. 3

12. KLINGENBERG M: Respiratory control as function of the phosphory-lation potential. In The Energy Level and Metabolic Control in Mitochondria, S Papa, JM Tager, E Quagliariello and EC Slater (eds.). Adriatica Editrica Bari, 1969. pp. 189

13. MAHLER HR and CORDES EH: Biological Chemistry, Harper and Row, N.Y., 1966

14. ISRAEL Y, VIDELA L, VIDELA-FERNANDEZ V and BERNSTEIN J: Effects of chronic ethanol treatment and thyroxine administration on ethanol metabolism and liver oxidative capacity. J Pharmacol Exp Ther 192: 565, 1975

15. VIDELA L, FLATTERY KV, SELLERS EA and ISRAEL Y: Ethanol metabolism and liver oxidative capacity in cold acclimation. J Pharmacol Exp Ther 192: 575, 1975

16. LESTER C and KEOKOSKY WZ: Alcohol metabolism in the horse. Life Sci Part I 6: 2313, 1967

17. TYGSTRUP N, WINKLER K and LUNDQUIST F: The mechanism of the fructose effect on the ethanol metabolism of the human liver. J Clin Invest 44: 817, 1965

18. FORSANDER OA: Effects of ethanol on metabolic pathways. In International Encyclopedia of Pharmacology and Therapeutics, J. Tremolieres (ed). Pergamon Press, N.Y., 1970. Section 20, pp. 117

19. WILLIAMSON JR, SCHOLZ R, BROWNING ET, THURMAN RG, and FUKAMI MH: Metabolic effects of ethanol in perfused rat liver. J Biol Chem 244: 5044, 1969

20. FORSANDER OA and HIMBERT JJ: Effect of glucose on liver metabolism during ethanol oxidation. Metabolism 18: 776, 1969

21. HAWKINS RD, KALANT H and KHANNA JM: Effects of chronic intake of ethanol on the rate of ethanol metabolism. Can J Pharmacol 44: 241, 1966

22. KATER RM, CARULLI N and IBER F: Differences in the rate of ethanol metabolism in recently drinking alcoholic and non-drinking subjects. Am J Clin Nutr 22: 1608, 1969

23. MEZEY E: Duration of the enhanced activity of the microsomal ethanol oxidizing system and rate of ethanol degradation in ethanol fed rats after withdrawal. Biochem Pharmacol 21: 137, 1972

24. MISRA PS, LEFEVRE A, ISHII H, RUBIN E and LIEBER CS: Increase of ethanol, meprobamate and pentobarbital metabolism after chronic ethanol administration in man and in rats. Am J Med 51: 346, 1971

25. PIEPER WA and SKEEN MJ: Changes in the rate of ethanol elimination associated wtih chronic administration of ethanol to chimpanzees and Rhesus monkeys. Drug Metabolism and Disposition 1: 634, 1973

26. UGARTE G and VALENZUELA J: Mechanisms of liver and pancreas damage in man. In Biological Basis of Alcoholism, Y Israel and J Mardones (eds). Wiley, N.Y., 1971. Chapter 5

27. VIDELA L, BERNSTEIN J and ISRAEL Y: Metabolic alternations produced in the liver by chronic ethanol administration. Increased oxidative capacity. Biochem J 134: 507, 1973

28. TOBON F and MEZEY E: Effect of ethanol administration on hepatic ethanol and drug-metabolizing enzymes and on rates of ethanol degradation. J Lab Clin Med 77: 110, 1971

29. LIEBER CS and DE CARLI LM: Hepatic microsomal ethanol oxidizing system. In vitro characteristics and adaptive properties in vivo. J Biol Chem 245: 2505, 1970

30. ISRAEL Y, VIDELA L and BERNSTEIN J: Hypermetabolic state after chronic ethanol consumption. Hormonal interrelations and pathogenic implications. Fed Proc 34: 2052, 1975

31. EDMONSON HA, PETERS RL, TELFER BR, REYNOLDS RB and KUZMA OT: Sclerosing hyaline necrosis of the liver in the chronic alcoholic. Ann Inter Med 59: 646, 1963

32. EDMONSON H, PETERS RL, FRANKEL HH and BOROWSKY S: The early stage of liver injury in the alcoholic. Medicine 46: 119, 1967

33. SCHAFFNER F and POPPER H: Alcoholic hepatitis in the spectrum of ethanol – induced liver injury. Scand J Gastroenterol (Suppl 7) 5: 69, 1970

34. JEWELL LD, MEDLINE A and MEDLINE NM: Alcoholic hepatitis. Can Med Assoc J 105: 711, 1971

35. REYNOLDS TB and EDMONSON HA: Alcoholic hepatitis. Ann Int Med 74: 440, 1971

36. RAPPAPORT AM: The microcirculatory hepatic unit. Microvasc Res 6: 212, 1973

37. ISRAEL Y, KALANT H, ORREGO H, KHANNA JM, VIDELA L, and PHILLIPS MJ: Experimental alcohol-induced hepatic necrosis: Suppression by propylthiouracil. Proc Natl Acad Sci (USA) 72: 1137, 1975

38. KHANNA JM, KALANT H and BUSTOS G: Effects of chronic intake of ethanol on rate of ethanol metabolism, II. Can J Physiol Pharmacol 45: 777, 1967

39. BECKETT AG, LIVINGSTONE AV and HILL KR: Acute alcoholic hepatitis. Brit Med J 2: 1113, 1961

40. HARINASUTA U and ZIMMERMAN HJ: Alcoholic steatonecrosis I. Relationship between severity of hepatic disease and presence of Mallory bodies in the liver. Gastroenterology 60: 1031, 1971

41. BIRSCHBACH HR, HARINASUTA U and ZIMMERMAN HJ: Alcoholic Steatonecrosis. II. Prospective study of prevalence of Mallory bodies in biopsy specimens and comparison of severity of hepatic disease in patients with and without this histological feature. Gastroenterol 66: 1195, 1974

42. GREEN J, MISTILIS S and SCHIFF L: Acute alcoholic hepatitis. Arch Int Med 112: 67, 1963

43. HANDBOOK OF PHYSIOLOGY, Section 7, Endocrinology, vol III. Am Physiol Soc. Washington, 1974

44. In Spontaneous Hypertension, its Pathogenesis and Complications, K Okamoto (ed.). Springer-Verlag, N.Y., 1972

45. ALBRECHT I, VIZEK M and KRECEK J: The hemodynamics of the rat during ontogenesis, with special reference to the age factor in the development of hypertension. In Spontaneous Hypertension, its Pathogenesis and Complications, K. Okamoto (ed). SpringerVerlag, N.Y., 1972. pp. 121

46. AOKI K: Experimental studies on the relationship between endocrine organs and hypertension in spontaneously hypertensive rats, III. Role of the endocrine organs and hormones. Jap Heart J 5: 57, 1964

47. FOLKOW B, HALLBACK M, LUNDGREN Y, SILVERTSSON R and WEISS L: The importance of adaptive changes in vascular design for the establishment and maintenance of primary hypertension as studied in man and in spontaneously hypertensive rat. In Spontaneous Hypertension, its Pathogenesis and Complications, K. Okamoto (ed). Springer-Verlag, N.Y., 1972. pp. 103

48. FOLKOW B, HALLBACK M and WEISS L: Cardiovascular responses to acute mental stress in spontaneously hypertensive rats. Clin Sci and Molec Med 45: 1315, 1973

49. BERNSTEIN J, VIDELA L and ISRAEL Y: Hormonal influences in the development of the hypermetabolic state of the liver produced by chronic administration of ethanol. J Pharmacol Exp Ther 192: 583, 1975

50. BERNSTEIN J, VIDELA L and ISRAEL Y: Role of the sodium pump in the regulation of liver metabolism in experimental alcoholism. Ann New York Acad Sci 242: 560, 1974

51. CONN HO: Therapy of alcoholic liver disease. In Alcohol and Abnormal Protein Biosynthesis, M.A. Rothschild, M. Oratz and S.S. Schreiber (eds). Pergamon Press, N.Y., 1975. pp. 509

52. LISHNER MW, ALEXANDER JF and GALAMBOS JT: Natural history of alcoholic hepatitis. I. The acute disease. Am J Digest Dis 16: 481, 1971

53. FALLON HJ: Alcoholic liver disease. In Alcohol and Abnormal Protein Biosynthesis, MA Rothschild, M Oratz and SS Schreiber (eds). Pergamon Press, N.Y., 1975. pp. 473

54. JEFFRIES GH: Gastritis. In Gastrointestinal Disease, Pathophysiology, Diagnosis, Management, MH Sleisenger and JS Fordtran (eds). Saunders, Philadelphia, 1973. pp. 560

55. DAVENPORT HW: Gastric mucosal hemorrhage in dogs. Effects of acid, aspirin and alcohol. Gastroenterol. 56: 439, 1969

56. IVEY KJ: Gastritis. Med Clin North Amer 58: 1289, 1974

57. LEEVY CM and ZETTERMAN RK: Malnutrition and alcoholism - An overview. In Alcohol and Abnormal Protein Biosynthesis, MA Rothschild, M Oratz and S Schreiber (eds). Pergamon Press, N.Y., 1975. pp. 3

58. LEEVY CM, VALDELLON E and SMITH F: Nutritional factors in alcoholism and its complications. In Biological Basis of Alcoholism, Y Israel and J Mardones (eds). Wiley, N.Y., 1971. pp. 365

59. EICHNER ER: The hematologic disorders of alcoholism. Am J Med 54: 621, 1973

60. HINES JD and COWAN DH: Anemia in alcoholism. In Drugs and Hematological Reactions, NV Dimitrov and JH Nodine (eds). Grunne and Stratton, N.Y., 1974. pp. 141

61. HERBERT V and TISMAN G: Hematological effects of alcohol. Ann New York Acad Sci 252: 307, 1975

62. VICTOR M: The role of hypomagnesemia and resiratory alkalosis in the genesis of alcohol withdrawal symptoms. Ann New York Acad Sci 215: 235, 1973

63. SERENY G, RAPOPORT A and HUSDAN H: The effect of ethanol withdrawal on electrolyte and acid-base balance. Metabolism 15: 896, 1966

64. TERRITO MC and TANAKA KR: Hypophosphatemia in chronic alcoholism. Arch Int Med 134: 445, 1974

65. GOODMAN LS and GILMAN A (eds). In The Pharmacological Basis of Therapeutics. MacMillan, N.Y., 1975. pp. 138

66. RANKIN JG and WILKINSON P: Alcohol and tobacco smoking. In The Health of a Metropolis, J. Krupinski and A. Stoller (eds). Heineman Educational Australia, 1971

67. LAMBERTSEN CJ: Effects of excessive pressures of oxygen, nitrogen, carbon dioxide and carbon monoxide: implications in aerospace, undersea and industrial environments. In Medical Physiology 13th Ed., V.B. Mountcasle (ed). Mosby, Saint Louis, 1974. pp. 1563

68. WALD N, HOWARD S, SMITH PG and BAILEY A: Use of carboxy-haemoglobin levels to predict the development of diseases associated with cigarette smoking. Thorax 30: 133, 1975

69. EMIRGIL C, SOBOL BJ, HEYMANN B and SHIBUTANI K: Pulmonary function in alcoholics. Amer J Med 57: 69, 1974

70. SMITH F and PALMER DL: Alcoholism, infection and altered host defenses: A review of clinical and experimental observations. J Chron Dis 29: 35, 1976

71. CHOMET B and GACH BM: Lobar pneumonia and alcoholism: An analysis of thirty seven cases. Amer J Med Sci 253: 300, 1967

72. TILLOTSON JR and LERNER AM: Characteristics of pneumonias caused by Escherichia coli. New Engl J Med 277: 115, 1967

73. JOHNSON WD, KAYE D and HOOK EW: Hemophilus influenzae pneumonia in adults. Amer Rev Resp Dis 97: 1112, 1968

74. LIEBER CS and DE CARLI LM: Animal models of ethanol dependence and liver injury in rats and baboons. Fed Proc 35: 1232, 1976

75. BURCH GE and DE PASCUALE NP: Alcoholic cardiomyopathy. Am J Cardiol 23: 723, 1969

76. ABELMAN WH and RAMIREZ A: Alcoholic cardiovascular disease. In Alcohol and Abnormal Protein Biosynthesis, MA Rothschild, M Oratz and SS Schreiber (eds). Pergamon Press, N.Y., 1975. pp. 459

DISCUSSION

CHAIRMAN: K.J. ISSELBACHER

JOLY: You are chronically feeding ethanol to rats and then you find that hypoxia creates a lesion. What are we looking at?Are we looking at the fact that hypoxia potentiates the liver damage which is already there? Could we create chronic hypoxia and see what the effects of ethanol are? I just don't understand your model.

ISRAEL: There is no doubt that this is the lesion of hypoxia and that it occurs preferentially in the alcohol treated animals. So we are dealing with a liver which alcohol has rendered more susceptible to hypoxia. In man these two types of insults can co-exist. We tried to do your reverse experiments. We kept animals for some time under hypoxic conditions and then tried to give them alcohol. Unfortunately the red cells increased about 60-70% and the blood was so viscous that the experiments couldn't be done.

LUNDQUIST: Have you tested your theory by using some other means of increasing the need of the liver for oxygen?

ISRAEL: We gave animals thyroid hormones and found exactly the same pattern. Dr. Orrego in our Department has infused proteins and has measured the amount of urea formed. He has calculated that the livers are using about 30% more oxygen considering the amount of urea that is formed. These animals are also more susceptible to hypoxic lesions. So these two conditions fit the theory perfectly well.

PHILLIPS: We still have a major problem in studying alcoholic liver disease in experimental animals. I have never seen the lesion of alcoholic hepatitis in a rat. In fact I have not seen in the rat pathology which has looked even close to that which one sees in the human. And this is a big problem when one is trying to decide what is

347

due to alcohol or what is due to ischemia. In these studies of Dr. Israel, the early 1+, 2+ lesions feature fat and focal necrosis of liver cells. These changes are those which one sees in alcohol induced injury in the rat. These changes are not seen in the control animals but only in the group with anoxia. The more severe 3+, 4+ lesions feature bridging necrosis and this to me is predominantly an ischemic lesion. So the morphology is not clear-cut.

FRENCH: We sometimes see massive necrosis of the liver after emergency portacaval anastomosis. Could this represent vulnerability induced by an increased metabolic rate?

ISRAEL: Yes, I think it could.

FRENCH: You haven't actually tried to reproduce this in your animals?

ISRAEL: No we haven't.

FISHER: It is obvious that there should be a pO_2 gradient across the liver acinus from zone 1 to 3 but has such a pO_2 gradient actually been documented? I don't think we can assume that a difference between what arrives in the portal tract and what leaves at the terminal hepatic vein necessarily represents a functionally effective gradient in terms of the hepatocytes in zone 1 versus those in zone 3.

ISRAEL: This is still a problem but Dr. Chance's laboratory in Philadelphia is working on it. Dr. Chance and his associates are exposing rats to a brief period of hypoxia, full nitrogen, zero oxygen for about 30-60 seconds. The animal is then cut in two and the liver frozen within a fraction of a second. They then prepare sections at -70°, examine them microscopically and determine NADH and heme proteins in their oxidized and reduced forms. In the rats exposed to hypoxia one can see areas that are completely reduced around the terminal hepatic vein and areas close to the portal vein that are completely oxidized. This isn't proof of a pO_2 gradient but it is excellent circumstantial evidence.

THE NATURAL HISTORY AND MANAGEMENT OF ALCOHOLIC LIVER DISEASE

Kurt J. Isselbacher and Edward R. Feller

Department of Medicine, Harvard Medical School and
Gastrointestinal Unit, Massachusetts General Hospital,
Boston, Massachusetts 02114

It is evident from the title of this presentation that it is one which could be the topic of an entire symposium rather than the subject of a brief dissertation. Thus, of necessity, this presentation will be a limited review of a series of selected components of this very complex problem.

In assessing the natural history of alcoholic liver disease, one is dealing primarily with the development of cirrhosis and its complications. Alcohol has a variety of morphologic effects on the liver which includes the development of alcoholic hepatitis, the production of fatty liver and also, perhaps separately rather than via hepatitis per se, the development of fibrosis.

Alcoholic liver disease constitutes one of the major challenges of clinical medicine in the Western Hemisphere. Cirrhosis ranks as the fourth most common cause of death in adults in the United States (1). One is called upon to treat the spectrum of complications including alcoholic hepatitis, bleeding varices, hepatic encephalopathy, ascites, hepatorenal syndrome as well as bacterial peritonitis, pancreatitis and the many metabolic derangements that accompany alcoholism and alcoholic liver disease. This presentation will focus on the survival of patients with alcoholic cirrhosis, review the problem of bleeding varices in the natural history of liver disease, and also include some comments about alcoholic hepatitis and certain metabolic derangements.

Factors Influencing Survival

The role of abstinence has elicited considerable interest in assessing and perhaps modifying the natural history of alcoholic liver disease. In a series of 283 histologically documented cases of Laennec's cirrhosis, Powell and

TABLE I

CAUSES OF DEATH IN ALCOHOLIC CIRRHOSIS

	Abstinence	Continued Drinking
	% Survival	
Liver failure	38	51
GI bleeding	22	27
Unrelated	34	18
Renal failure	3	1
Infection	3	3
Unknown	3	4

(From Powell WJ and Klatskin G. <u>Am J Med 44</u>: 406-420, 1968)

Klatskin (2) demonstrated that abstinence appeared to reduce the five-year death rate caused by the two major determinants of mortality, namely, liver failure and gastrointestinal bleeding (Table I). More importantly, these investigators demonstrated that abstinence was associated with a statistically significant increase in 5-year survival in cirrhosis in the presence of ascites, jaundice or hematemesis, as well as in the absence of major complications and in cirrhotics as a group (Table II). A similar series from the Royal Free Hospital in London showed a 5-year survival of 77% in cirrhotics who subsequently abstained compared to a 48% survival in those who continued drinking (3). In contrast to these reports, a study from the Boston Inter-Hospital Liver Group showed no advantage in the 10-year survival of cirrhotics with varices who abstained from drinking (4).

It can be appreciated, that given our current knowledge (and ignorance) concerning the pathogenesis of cirrhosis and its complications, one could entertain certain reasons as to why abstinence might not significantly modify survival. Thus, the presence of esophageal varices may constitute an irreversible injury and adversely influence survival even though alcohol ingestion has stopped. In addition recent observations support the suggestion that continued liver injury may persist as a result of immunologic reactions; under these circumstances, progression of liver disease might be expected even in the absence of alcohol ingestion (5). Nevertheless, it is obvious that abstinence should be stressed, in spite of the fact that certain conditions may modify the degree of expected improvement with cessation of drinking.

TABLE II

5 YEAR SURVIVAL IN ALCOHOLIC CIRRHOSIS

	Abstinence	Continued Drinking
	% Survival	
After diagnosis	63	40.5
After onset of <u>ascites</u>	52.4	32.7
After onset of <u>jaundice</u>	57.5	33.3
After onset of <u>hematemesis</u>	35.3	20.7
No ascites, jaundice or hematemesis	88.9	68.2

(From Powell WJ and Klatskin G. <u>Am J Med 44</u>: 406-420, 1968)

Current Status of Portasystemic Venous Shunts

One of the major questions remaining after more than a quarter of a century of clinical experience with portasystemic shunts relates to the appropriate role and value of these shunts in the management of esophageal varices. In examining this problem, one must consider separately 1) prophylactic shunts, 2) therapeutic shunts, or 3) emergency shunts performed for active variceal hemorrhage.

The impetus to perform <u>prophylactic portacaval anastomoses</u> stemmed from the prohibitive 50-80% mortality of the initial hemorrhage from esophageal varices. Despite early enthusiasm for this procedure based on an apparent increase in survival in shunted patients (6), subsequent controlled investigations (7-9) indicate, in fact, that prophylactic portacaval shunts do not enhance survival. Cumulative data from four controlled studies (Table III) reveal a mortality of 58% in shunted patients versus 44% in the control group during a one to seven year follow-up period. Thus prophylactic shunts are now deemed inadvisable.

The role of <u>therapeutic portacaval shunts</u> in improving survival after variceal hemorrhage remains controversial. In 1971, Jackson et al (10) published the results of a controlled study performed by the VA Cooperative Study Group of 135 cirrhotic patients randomly assigned to a therapeutic shunt or non-surgical control group. This study concluded that survival was

TABLE III

MORTALITY IN CONTROLLED PROPHYLACTIC SHUNT STUDIES

Senior author	Controls		Shunt group		Statistical Significance ($x2$)
	No. of Pts.	Deaths	No. of Pts.	Deaths	
Jackson, 1967	30	19 (63%)	25	23 (97%)	$p < 0.05$
Resnick, 1968	43	19 (44%)	46	22 (48%)	NSS*
Conn (I), 1972	58	16 (28%)	37	19 (51%)	$p < 0.025$
Conn (II), 1972	29	16 (55%)	22	11 (50%)	NSS*
Total	160	70 (44%)	130	75 (58%)	$p < 0.05$

*NSS = Not Statistically Significant

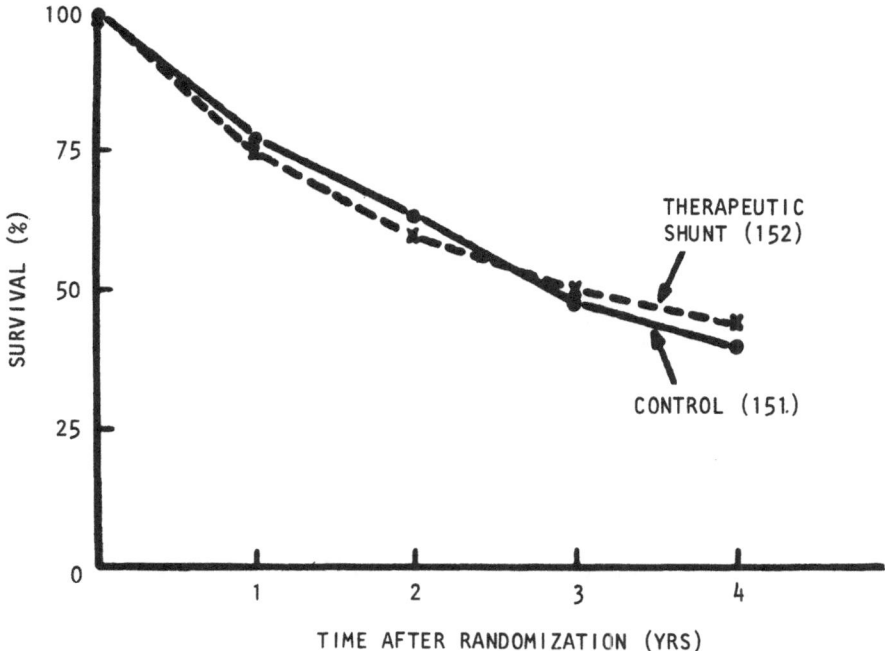

Fig. 1   *Cumulative survival after therapeutic portacaval shunts: combined data from Veterans Administration Cooperative Group, Boston Inter-hospital Liver Group (BILG) and Hôpital Beaujon studies.*
(From Conn H.A.   Gastroenterology 67: 1065-1071, 1974)

enhanced by a therapeutic shunt. Two subsequent controlled trials have been conducted (11, 12). Cumulative data from these studies (Fig. 1) do not reveal a statistically significant difference in survival between the control and shunted groups although the mortality tended to be lower in the surgical group. Shunted patients have a lower incidence of recurrent bleeding, but are more prone to the development of fatal hepatic failure. Current studies in this area include attempts, especially by hemodynamic methods, to improve the preoperative identification of those patients who are prone to develop hepatic encephalopathy. Other efforts are being directed at the design of the surgical procedures such that one could hopefully achieve portal decompression without producing hepatic failure.

In 1963, Warren et al (13) reported that cirrhotics with the greatest decrease in hepatic blood flow after portacaval anastomosis had the greatest risk of developing hepatic failure. More recently, Zimmon and Kessler (14) have presented a hemodynamic classification of cirrhotics with bleeding varices which assesses the response of hepatic sinusoidal pressure to extra-corporeal diversion of portal venous flow. Preliminary data suggest that patients who respond with a marked decrease in hepatic sinusoidal pressure have an increased incidence of encephalopathy since residual hepatic sinusoidal pressure may be inadequate to maintain hepatic blood flow. At the same time, data are being obtained which suggest that, compared to other shunting procedures, the distal splenorenal shunt may result in a reduced incidence of post-operative hepatic failure and subsequent variceal hemorrhage (15, 16); however, whether there is a difference in survival between the spleno-renal and other shunts remains to be determined. Thus, at present, while it seems reasonable to perform therapeutic shunts on patients who have bled from varices on more than one occasion in an attempt to reduce the incidence of recurrent bleeding, there is a "price tag" associated with this benefit and the adverse systemic effects of the surgical procedures in controlling portal hypertension cannot be ignored.

Emergency portasystemic venous shunts are also frequently carried out to control active variceal bleeding. The surgical mortality in this situation ranges from 25-65% in various series (17-20). The mortality rate seems to depend, in part, on how early emergency surgery is performed and how seriously ill the patients are at that time. Although no controlled studies exist comparing emergency shunts with the medical management of bleeding varices, the overall short-term mortality of 50-80% of patients with active variceal hemorrhage strongly suggests that emergency shunts may enhance survival.

Alcoholic Hepatitis

Alcoholic hepatitis, one of the major complications of alcoholism, still poses a significant therapeutic dilemma. In one series of 164 patients (21), the mean 5-year survival rate was 56% after the initial biopsy diagnosis of alcoholic hepatitis. This study also demonstrated a beneficial effect of subsequent abstinence on survival; approximately 80% of abstainers survived five years compared to 50% of those who continued drinking.

Recently a series of investigations has been carried out to evaluate the effectiveness of prednisone on the course of this disease. Corticosteroids have of course multiple effects, including anti-inflammatory actions and a modification of the immune response. In this regard, observations have appeared in recent years, especially from the laboratory of Leevy and associates (5), to suggest that immunologic reactions occur in alcoholic hepatitis and that they may have a pathogenetic role. These investigators (5) have reported that lymphocytes from patients with alcoholic hepatitis respond to the presence of purified alcoholic hyalin by an increased liberation of MIF (migration inhibiting factor). These and other findings support the concept of an immunologic component in the development of alcoholic hepatitis.

The place of corticosteroid treatment in alcoholic hepatitis remains controversial. If one examines all grades of severity of alcoholic hepatitis, the mortality in the control and steroid-treated groups in the published

TABLE IV

STEROID TREATMENT OF ALCOHOLIC HEPATITIS
(ALL GRADES OF SEVERITY)

Authors	Controls		Steroid-treated	
	No. of Pts.	Deaths	No. of Pts.	Deaths
Helman, 1971 (22)	17	6	20	1
Porter, 1971 (23)	9	7	11	6
Campra, 1973 (24)	25	9	20	7
Blitzer, 1973 (25)	16	5	12	6
Resnick, 1973 (26)	9	5	8	6
Maddrey, 1975 (27)	23	5	20	1
Total	99	37 (37%)	91	27 (30%)

reports is not statistically different (22-27). Results from six studies are shown in Table IV and reveal a mortality of 37% in the control group and 30% in the steroid-treated group. However, if one examines the subgroup of severe alcoholic hepatitis (Table V), differences do seem to emerge which suggest that survival may be enhanced in patients treated with steroids. Although the study groups are somewhat heterogeneous, they were all categorized by encephalopathy or a prolonged prothrombin time. Thus, based on an analysis of these data, corticosteroids may yet prove to have some beneficial effects in the management of severe alcoholic hepatitis.

Other studies are being carried out in the management of alcoholic hepatitis and cirrhosis, based on considerations of the possible pathogenetic factors. As mentioned above, corticosteroids may have a salutary effect because of their anti-inflammatory action or because of their suppression of the immune response. However, corticosteroids also act on collagen metabolism by inhibiting proline hydroxylase (28). Several agents that interfere with collagen metabolism are currently being investigated; these include penicillamine, which inhibits collagen fiber cross-linking (29) and cysteine, which interferes with this mechanism, but also acts on collagenase (28). Colchicine has been shown by Rojkind to reduce fibrosis and cirrhosis (30), although the exact mechanism of action of colchicine on collagen metabolism is still not well understood. Rojkind et al have shown that colchicine increases collagenase production and interferes with transcellular movement of collagen (28). Azetidine-2-carboxylic acid, which inhibits proline hydroxylase and collagen synthesis, has been shown to be effective in preventing fibrogenesis in the liver of rats treated with CCl_4 (28). Finally,

TABLE V

CORTICOSTEROIDS AND MORTALITY IN
SEVERE ALCOHOLIC HEPATITIS

Authors	Controls		Steroid Rx	
	No. of Pts.	Mortality %	No. of Pts.	Mortality %
Helman et al* (22) (1971)	6	100	8	12.5
Porter et al[†] (23) (1971)	9	78	11	55
Campra et al* (24) (1973)	10	80	8	50
Maddrey et al** (27) (1975)	10	50	9	11.1

*Encephalopathic patients

[†]Average patient: bilirubin, 24 mg%; albumin, 2.5 gm%; ascites & encephalopathy (75%)

**Coagulation abnormalities precluded liver biopsy

one should comment on the elegant studies of Israel and his associates (31) demonstrating the presence of a hypermetabolic state in chronic alcoholism (especially in experimental animals) and that propylthiouracil has a beneficial effect in blocking this hypermetabolism. It is reasonable to speculate that propylthiouracil may also be of value in the treatment of alcoholic hepatitis.

Some Metabolic Complications

Finally, we would like to comment briefly on some metabolic complications of alcoholism, most of which have already been reviewed in this Symposium. As mentioned above, there is evidence for a hypermetabolic or hyperthyroid-like state, at least in chronic alcoholic rats (31). In addition, one of the important metabolic consequences is an alteration of drug metabolism, especially an increase in metabolism of those drugs metabolized by the smooth endoplasmic reticulum (32). Some of the important potential consequences of alcoholism include 1) elevations of serum triglycerides, 2) a reduction in blood glucose, 3) moderate elevations of serum lactate leading secondarily to increased elevations of uric acid, 4) a reduction in serum magnesium and phosphate levels which may in turn have other sequelae, 5) an increase in serum acetaldehyde, which may have adverse effects on various organ systems, and 6) the occurrence of ketoacidosis.

Ketoacidosis in the alcoholic may be much more common than the available data suggest (34, 35). For some reason this type of ketoacidosis appears to be more common in females and often the same patient may have recurrent episodes. In general, before being hospitalized with this disorder, the patient has evidence of a heavy ethanol intake and vomiting, the latter undoubtedly contributing to the acidosis. Typical laboratory features include a slight elevation of the blood glucose at the time of hospital admission, but these levels rarely are of the magnitude seen in diabetic acidosis. Serum free fatty acid concentrations are usually increased. The serum ketone and lactate levels are only minimally elevated, a finding which is important in view of the fact that these patients have a very large anion gap. The latter observation should alert the physician that agents other than acetone or acetoacetic acid may be accounting for the acidosis. In fact, one of the major substances contributing to the acidosis is beta-hydroxybutyrate and the beta-hydroxybutyrate/acetoacetate ratio is significantly increased (35). The therapeutic approach is relatively straight-forward involving the administration of glucose, saline and minimal amounts of alkali.

The mechanism leading to the production of alcoholic ketoacidosis still remains to be elucidated. It would appear that two pathogenetic factors are important, namely 1) the increased hepatic production of NADH (reduced nicotinamide adenine dinucleotide) and 2) the effect of ethanol on glucose metabolism leading to the production of hypoglycemia. The increased production of NADH will favor the reduction of pyruvate resulting in greater production of lactate; however, as emphasized above, the serum lactate levels tend to be only minimally inceased while the serum beta-hydroxybutyrate levels become significantly elevated. Patients with alcoholic ketoacidosis seem to have increased serum levels of growth hormone, epinephrine, cortisol and glucagon and these elevations may possibly be a consequence of the hypoglycemic effect of ethanol. These hormones and chemical mediators in turn, or course, tend to elevate the blood sugar so that at the time of hospital admission the blood sugar may no longer be low. There are some data to suggest that patients with the greatest degree of hypoglycemia tend to have the greatest degree of ketosis. Agents such as growth hormone and epinephrine also tend to stimulate fatty acid mobilization from peripheral adipose tissues. This results in an increased flux of fatty acids into the liver leading to enhanced fatty acid oxidation and an increase in the generation of beta-hydroxybutyrate. The high beta-hydroxybutyrate-acetoacetate ratio seen in patients with alcoholic ketoacidosis is also influenced by NADH, which favors the conversion of acetoacetate to beta-hydroxybutyrate.

SUMMARY

The effect of chronic alcohol ingestion on the liver results in fatty liver, fibrosis, alcoholic hepatitis and cirrhosis. Since the major complications of alcoholic liver disease cannot be reviewed in detail, we have focused on some aspects of the natural history; i.e. mortality and survival, the role of portacaval shunts, the course and treatment of alcohol hepatitis and some selected metabolic derangements. Liver failure and gastrointestinal bleeding are the major sequelae of alcoholic cirrhosis but their role as a cause of death may be reduced by abstinence. Most studies suggest that abstinence may, to a limited extent, improve survival but enhanced survival may be limited by presence of varices (? irreversible), and possibly by immunologic processes leading to continued cell injury. Survival, as expected, is reduced when patients have ascites, jaundice or have had gastrointestinal bleeding.

Neither prophylactic nor therapeutic shunts seem to alter survival and the exact role of emergency shunts still remains to be determined. Improvement in assessment of pre-operative hemodynamic factors and development of newer methods to control portal hypertension may decrease post-operative morbidity and mortality. Steroid treatment of alcoholic hepatitis has been reviewed and analysis of controlled studies suggests that mortality in severe disease may be reduced by corticosteroids. However, more studies are needed before definite conclusions can be drawn about their overall therapeutic value. It is possible that, in the future, agents that modify collagen synthesis or degradation may have an important role in preventing development or progression of fibrosis or cirrhosis.

Of the metabolic derangements, alcoholic ketoacidosis is probably more common than hitherto recognized. A key finding is a high β-hydroxy-butyrate/acetoacetate ratio in the serum. Increased levels of NADH and hypoglycemia may be important in contributing to the pathogenesis of this entity.

REFERENCES

1.   Viewpoints on Digestive Diseases, Vol 1, No 1, April, 1969

2.   POWELL WJ, KLATSKIN G: Duration of survival in patients with Laennec's cirrhosis. Am J Med 44: 406-420, 1968

3.   BRUNT PW, KEW MC, SCHEUER PJ, SHERLOCK S: Studies in alcoholic liver disease in Britain.   I.   Clinical and pathologic patterns related to natural history. Gut 15: 52-58, 1974

4.   SOTERAKIS J, RESNICK RH, IBER F: Effect of alcohol abstinence on survival in cirrhotic portal hypertension. Lancet 2: 65-67, 1973

5. LEEVY CM, CHEM T, ZETTERMAN RK: Alcoholic hepatitis, cirrhosis. and immunologic reactivity. Ann NY Acad Sci 252: 106-115, 1975

6. PALMER ED, JAHNKE EJ, HUGHES CS: Evaluation of clinical results of portal decompression in cirrhosis. JAMA 164: 746-748, 1957

7. JACKSON FC, PERRIN EB, SMITH AG, DAGRADI AE, NADAL HM: A clinical investigation of the portacaval shunt. II. Survival analysis of the prophylactic operation. Am J Surg 115: 22-42, 1968

8. RESNICK RH, CHALMERS TC, ISHIHARA AM, GARCEAU AJ, CALLOW AD, SCHIMMEL EM, O'HARA ET: A controlled study of the prophylactic portacaval shunt. A final report. Ann Int Med 70: 675-688, 1969

9. CONN HO, LINDERMUTH WW, MAY CJ, RAMSBY GR: Prophylactic portacaval anastomosis. A tale of two studies. Medicine 51: 27-40, 1972

10. JACKSON FC, PERRIN ED, FELIX R, SMITH AG: A clinical investigation of the portacaval shunt. V. Survival analysis of the therapeutic operation. Ann Surg 174: 672-701, 1971

11. RESNICK RH, IBER FL, ISHIHARA AM, CHALMERS T, ZIMMERMAN H: A controlled study of the therapeutic portacaval shunt. Gastroenterology 67: 843-857, 1974

12. RUEFF B, DEGOS F, DEGOS JD, MAILHARD JN, PRANDI D, SICOT J, SICOT C, FAUVERT R, BENHAMOU JP: A controlled study of therapeutic portacaval shunt in alcoholic cirrhosis. Lancet 1: 655-659, 1976

13. WARREN WD, RESTRAPO JE, RESPASS JC, MULLER WH, JR: The importance of hemodynamic studies in the management of portal hypertension. Ann Surg 158: 387-392, 1963

14. ZIMMON DS, KESSLER RE: Hepatic hemodynamic factors reflect prognosis after portacaval shunt. Gastroenterology 64: 166, 1973

15. ZEPPA R, WARREN WD: The distal splenorenal shunt. Am J Surg 122: 300-303, 1971

16. HUTSON DG, PEREVICS R, ZEPPA R, LEVI JU, SCHIFF ER, FINK P: The fate of esophageal varices following selective distal spleno-renal shunt. Ann Surg 183: 496-501, 1976

17. WEINBERGER HA: Emergency portacaval shunt for esophagogastric hemorrhage. Arch Surg 91: 333-337, 1965

18. PRESTON FW, TRIPPEL OH: Emergency portacaval shunt; use in patients with alcoholic cirrhosis. Arch Surg 90: 770-781, 1965

19. CONN HO: The prognosis and management of bleeding esophageal varices. Ann NY Acad Sci 170: 345-357, 1970

20. ORLOFF MJ, CHARTERS AC, CHANDLER JG, CONDON JK, GRAMBORT DE, MODAFFERI TR, LEVIN SE, BROWN NB, SVIOKLA SC, KNOX DG: Portacaval shunt as emergency procedure in unselected patients with alcoholic cirrhosis.   Surg Gynecol Obstet 141: 59-68, 1975

21. ALEXANDER JF, LISCHNER MW, GALAMBOS JT: Natural history of alcoholic hepatitis. Am J Gastroenterology 56: 515-525, 1971

22. HELMAN RA, TEMKO MH, NYE FW, FALLON HJ: Alcoholic hepatitis. Natural history and evaluation of prednisolone therapy. Ann Int Med 74: 311-321, 1971

23. PORTER HP, SIMON FR, POPE CE III, VOLWILER W, FENSTER LF: Corticosteroid therapy in severe alcoholic hepatitis. N Eng J Med 284: 1350-1355, 1971

24. CAMPRA J, HAMLIN EM, JR, KIRSHBAUM RJ, OLEVIER M, REDEKER AG, REYNOLDS TB: Prednisone therapy of acute alcoholic hepatitis. Ann Int Med 79: 625-631, 1973

25. BLITZER BC: Adrenocorticosteroid therapy in alcoholic hepatitis. A prospective, double-blind, randomized study.   Yale M.D. Thesis, 1973

26. RESNICK RH, cited by CONN HO in L. Schiff, Diseases of the Liver, 4th Ed., Philadelphia, Lippincott, 1975. pp.917

27. MADDREY WC, BORTNOTT JK, WEBER FL, JR, BEDINE MS, HARRINGTON DP, WHITE RI, MEZEY E: Corticosteroid therapy of active alcoholic liver disease. A controlled trial.   Gastroenterology 69: 813, 1975

28. ROJKIND M, KERSHENOBICH D: Hepatic fibrosis.   In Progress in Liver Diseases.   H. Popper and F. Schaffner, (Eds.).   New York, Grune and Stratton, 1976. pp. 294-310.

29. NIMNI ED, BAVETTA LH: Collagen defect induced by penicillamine. Science 150: 905-907, 1965

30. ROJKIND M, URIBE M, KERSHENOBICH D: Colchicine and the treatment of liver fibrosis. Lancet 1: 38-39, 1973

31. ISRAEL Y, VIDELA L, BERNSTEIN J: Liver hypermetabolic state after chronic ethanol consumption: Hormonal interrelations and pathogenic implications. Fed Proc 34: 2052-2059, 1975

32. KHANNA JM, KALANT H, YEE Y, CHUNG S, SIEMENS AJ: Effect of chronic ethanol treatment on metabolism of drugs in vitro and in vivo. Biochem Pharmacology 25: 329-335, 1976

33. CEDERBAUM AI, RUBIN E: Molecular injury to mitochondria produced by ethanol and acetaldehyde. Fed Proc 34: 2045-2051, 1975

34. LEVY LJ, DUGA J, GIRGIS M, GORDON EE: Ketoacidosis associated with alcoholism in nondiabetic subjects. Ann Int Med 78: 213-219, 1973

35. COOPERMAN MT, DAVIDOFF F, SPARK R, PALLOTTA J: Clinical studies of alcoholic ketoacidosis. Diabetes 23: 433-439, 1974

DISCUSSION

CHAIRMAN: J.G. JOLY

SENIOR: We have an enormous number of alcoholics in urban Philadelphia and we have seen something alarming which may explain the mystery of sudden death in the alcoholic. We are seeing alcoholic patients with a fulminant metabolic acidosis which is not diabetic and not ketotic but which is characterized by elevation of serum hydroxybutyric acid and an even more marked elevation in serum lactate. We have found blood lactates in the 25-30 millimolar range. This type of alcoholic can walk into the Emergency Room with an arterial pH of less than 7 and not look particularly ill. We have had two such people within the past year. Both died of cardiac arrest and shock despite vigorous treatment. At autopsy we found nothing but fatty liver. This extremely severe metabolic acidosis of the alcoholic may be related to but it is slightly different than alcoholic ketoacidosis which is milder and tends to be recurrent.

Dr. Isselbacher, you have shown that cirrhotics are really a heterogeneous group and I think that this is probably the case also of the patient who has portal hypertension. There are certain patients who can tolerate shunts better than others. Zimmon and Kessler have demonstrated that some people can and others cannot adapt to diversion of portal flow. What do you think arterialization of the portal stump offers those people who cannot adapt to diversion of the portal vein flow?

ISSELBACHER: I know that Dr. Reynolds and others feel that the direction of portal blood flow is the crucial thing, and that if this could be determined effectively it would help determine the appropriateness of a shunt. Until we get such data it will be difficult to be definitive as to which shunt is best for a given patient.

FISHER: Extrapolating from the rat literature, one might be inclined to favour the use of medium chain triglycerides instead of long chain triglycerides in the prevention of fatty liver, and I wondered if you had any information or suggestions along those lines? The other thing that I think has been coming into the pharmacology literature is that SH binders, such as penicillamine, may prevent the development of fatty liver in the rat and have an influence quite apart from their possible influence on collagen. Have you any comments on that?

ISSELBACHER: As far as a medium chain triglyceride is concerned, I guess there could be several responses. First, does fatty liver do any harm? As you know, if the spree drinker stops drinking the fat is going to be dissipated. Obviously you could modify that, but I don't know whether the effort would be worthwhile. It would seem to me that in the case of the alcoholic the main emphasis should be on removing the offending agent.

Obviously penicillamine has effects beyond those involving the cross-linking of collagen. But it remains to be determined whether it has a salutary effect or not. It has been used effectively in patients with Wilson's Disease and to the best of my knowledge, except for allergies, it has not had any deleterious effects. Whether penicillamine would have any greater merit in postnecrotic cirrhosis, primary biliary cirrhosis and Laennec's cirrhosis, I have not been able to determine. The Boston Interhospital Liver Group has decided to use penicillamine in patients with primary biliary cirrhosis. I think that, based on their experience with the heterogeneous alcoholic population, they felt that this would be a better place to start. Therefore I can't answer about effects of penicillamine other than what is known in vitro.

THE NATURAL HISTORY AND MANAGEMENT OF THE PATIENT WITH ALCOHOLIC LIVER DISEASE

James G. Rankin

Addiction Research Foundation

Toronto, Ontario M5S 2S1

INTRODUCTION

The aim of this paper is to examine the natural history of alcoholic liver disease as it is related to the natural history of alcoholism, its prognosis and treatment. Some of the problems of managing liver disease in alcoholic patients and deficiencies in our present care of these individuals will be identified and suggestions made about how they can be resolved.

One of the vivid memories from my days as a medical resident in an Australian teaching hospital is of making a home call in 1955 on a woman aged about 40 who lived alone in a small apartment in Sydney's well-known cosmopolitan area, King's Cross. The purpose of that visit was to perform an abdominal paracentesis on an individual who had a very tense ascites and signs of advanced liver disease. I performed the procedure and left this pitiful creature never expecting to see her again. Many months later I was stopped in the hospital by an attractive, extremely fit-looking woman and had to admit that I had no recollection of meeting her before. As you will have anticipated, it was the same woman whose ascites I had drained. In her view the reason for the difference was that she had stopped drinking alcohol.

I have other memories from the subsequent years of my postgraduate training, of patients suffering from alcoholic liver disease in whom progressively more advanced methods of supportive care were used, but in whom the ultimate factor which determined whether they lived or died from their liver disease was whether they were able to abstain from or drastically reduce their intake of alcohol. Because of these experiences I became progressively more interested in the relationship between alcohol consumption and disease, in how medical care for disease complications could be combined with treatment aimed at helping the individual abstain from alcohol and in the potential changes in morbidity and mortality that might result from a reduction or elimination of alcohol intake. The frustration and the challenge of cirrhosis in the alcoholic patient is the clear association between continued alcohol consumption and the occurrence of and death from the disease, and conversely the knowledge that in alcoholic subjects abstention is associated with both a prevention of cirrhosis as well as a reduction in the morbidity and mortality of those with established hepatic disease.

There is no doubt that hepatologists have learned a great deal more about the nature of alcoholic liver disease and its symptomatic treatment in the years since I first encountered the alcoholic woman in King's Cross. However, unfortunately during that time we have not discovered specific ways in which we can predictably alter the individual's behaviour with alcohol when he or she is living in a natural setting. Even more unfortunately there have been only minimal efforts to combine what we do know about the overall management of the alcoholic behaviour with our knowledge of alcoholic liver disease. This failure to link scientific knowledge is paralleled by a similar failure in clinical practice when it comes to total patient care. Increasingly more intensive methods of medical treatment for the complications of alcoholic liver disease are usually instituted in a vacuum in which there is little or no consideration either of the likely prognosis with regard to the patient's future use of alcohol, or to the provision of ongoing care which considers his total needs and problems.

NATURAL HISTORY OF ALCOHOLIC LIVER DISEASE AND ITS RELATIONSHIP TO CONSUMPTION

Alcoholic Consumption and Occurrence of Liver Disease

It has been known for many years that international differences in the prevalence of cirrhosis are closely related to levels of alcohol consumption. However, it is only in recent years that evidence has been available regarding daily or cumulative levels of individual consumption that increase the risk of developing severe alcoholic liver disease.

Whether there is any safe level of alcohol consumption is still an open question. It could well be that any consumption of alcohol contributes to an increased susceptibility to severe alcoholic liver disease[1]. It was found by Péquignot that the risk of developing alcoholic liver disease occurred when the daily consumption of ethanol exceeded 80 g. per day (1), this level becoming known as the one at or above which consumption was hazardous to health. However, because of observations which apparently demonstrated an increased susceptibility in women to alcoholic liver disease, it has also been

---

[1] In this paper the term severe alcoholic disease refers to both precirrhotic and cirrhotic lesions, while cirrhosis denotes that lesion alone or in combination with fatty infiltration and/or alcoholic hepatitis.

suggested that for women the hazardous level could be substantially lower. The situation became more confused with Péquignot's finding in one French population that the risk of cirrhosis began to rise exponentially when the level of consumption rose above 60 g. per day in men and 20 g. per day in women (2). The work of Lelbach is outstanding in its clear elucidation in one particular population of alcoholic men, of the relationship between total alcohol consumption and the occurrence of severe alcoholic liver disease and cirrhosis (3). Three factors were found to be of importance: the daily level of consumption, the number of years of drinking and individual susceptibility, this last factor being of decreasing importance as the cumulative level of alcohol consumption rose.

Alcohol Consumption and Mortality and Morbidity of Patients with Alcoholic Liver Disease

A number of studies have demonstrated that in patients with severe alcoholic liver disease, continued consumption is associated with increased morbidity and mortality, while conversely abstinence is associated with an improved prognosis. The largest, and probably the best of these studies, is that of Powell and Klatskin of 273 alcoholic patients with histologically proven cirrhosis (4). Ninety-three of this group abstained from alcohol and 185 continued drinking. During the first year after diagnosis the mortality rate was approximately the same in both groups, the one-year survival being 81 and 82% respectively. However, at five years the survival rate was 63.0% in the abstinent group and 40.5% in those who continued drinking. The differences between the groups were dramatic when examined over the last four years of the study, i.e. by excluding those who presented with and died from severe liver disease within the first year after diagnosis. In the last four years the mean survival rates were $86.2 \pm 4.7\%$ in the abstinent and $56.2 \pm 4.7\%$ in the drinking group. The four-year survival in the abstinent group was close to the expected survival for individuals of a similar age in the same country. It was also found that deaths in the abstinent group were less likely to be from hepatic disease and its complications as compared with those who continued drinking.

Interrelationship Between Alcohol Consumption and the Occurrence of and Deaths from Hepatic Disease

If continued hazardous consumption of alcohol is associated separately with the occurrence of severe alcoholic liver disease and deaths from cirrhosis, how may these three variables be interrelated in drinking populations? In an attempt to answer this question I have taken Lelbach's data on the relationship between alcohol consumption and the occurrences of severe alcoholic liver disease (3), and Powell's and Klatskin's data on survival of alcoholic patients with cirrhosis (4), made some simple assumptions and developed speculative data which are presented for consideration. These speculations should be viewed as potentially having qualitative rather than any precise quantitative value.

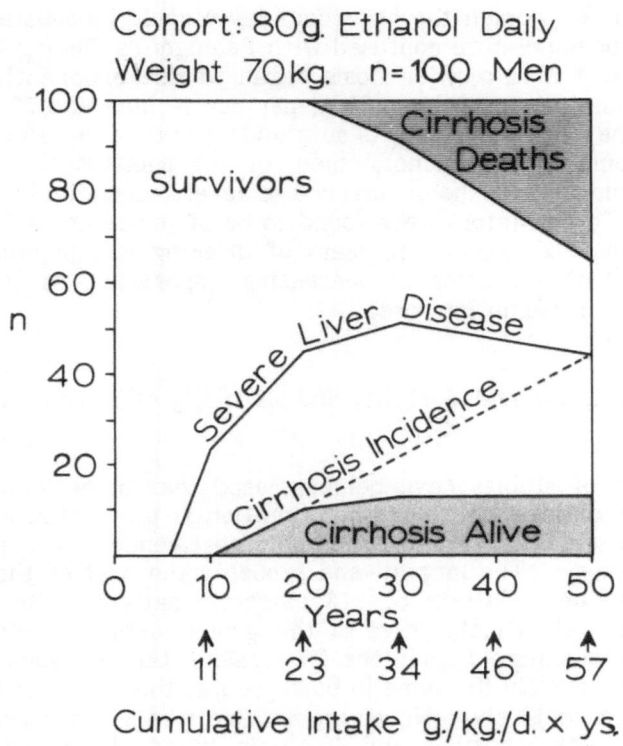

Cohort: 80g. Ethanol Daily
Weight 70kg.   n=100 Men

Fig. 1   *Schematic representation of the development of severe liver*
            disease and death from cirrhosis in a cohort of 100 men, of
            identical age and with identical drinking histories, who drink 80
            g. of alcohol daily.

These speculations on the potential interrelationship between alcohol
consumption, occurrence of severe alcoholic liver disease and deaths from
cirrhosis are illustrated in Figures 1 through 3.   Figure 1 is a schematic
representation of the development of severe liver disease and death from
cirrhosis in a cohort of 100 men, of identical age and with identical drinking
histories, who drink 80 g. of alcohol every day.   On the vertical axis is
represented the number of men and on the horizontal axis the years of
drinking and cumulative intake of alcohol.   In making the calculations on
which this figure was based, it was assumed that there were no deaths from
other causes, and that if a patient developed cirrhosis he had an 85% chance
of dying within the next ten years, the small survival being related to
abstinence.   The composite data suggest that at this level of consumption
severe liver disease occurs after about six years of drinking and is found in
approximately 23% after ten years.   Cirrhosis occurs for the first time after
10 years of drinking and is found in between 10 to 13 of those men who
survive in each subsequent decade.   The number alive with cirrhosis in each

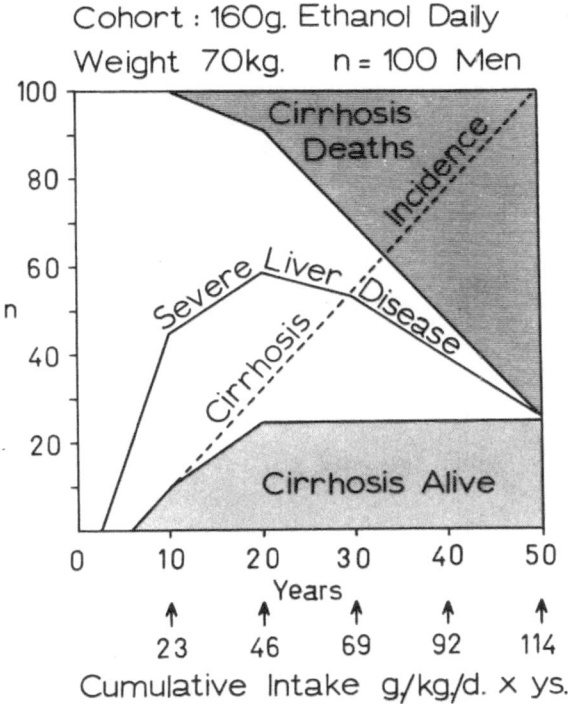

Fig. 2 *Schematic representation of the development of severe liver disease and death from cirrhosis in a cohort of 100 men, of identical age and with identical drinking histories, who drink 160 g. of alcohol daily.*

decade consists of the number of new cases plus the survivors with cirrhosis from the previous decade. After 50 years of drinking in this fashion, it is suggested that the incidence of severe liver disease and cirrhosis in the total group would be 76% and 44% respectively. The data suggest that, at this rate of drinking, alcoholic liver disease becomes a significant problem in terms of progressive morbidity and mortality after about 20 years.

In Figure 2 similar data are presented of a cohort of men consuming 160 g. of ethanol per day, this level being referred to by Péquignot as the cirrhogenic level of consumption (1). It is suggested that, in this group, severe liver disease would occur after about three years and cirrhosis after about six years. After 10 years, approximately 10 men would have cirrhosis and after 20 to 50 years the number of men alive with cirrhosis in each decade would be approximately 25, the difference between new cases and deaths. It is suggested that, in this group, severe liver disease becomes a problem after about 10 years of drinking and that all of those who survive 50 years will have cirrhosis.

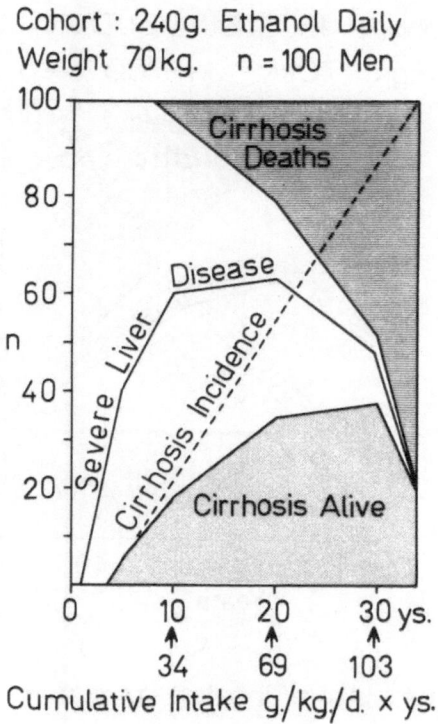

Cohort : 240g. Ethanol Daily
Weight 70 kg.   n = 100 Men

Cumulative Intake g./kg./d. x ys.

Fig. 3   Schematic representation of the development of severe liver
          disease and death from cirrhosis in a cohort of 100 men, of
          identical age and with identical drinking histories, who drink
          240 g. of alcohol daily.

In the last cohort of 100 men, the level of daily consumption is 240 g.
(Figure 3) which is near the mean daily consumption of men at or about the
time of their presentation to special units for the treatment of alcoholism.
At this level of consumption severe liver disease would be predicted to occur
for the first time after about two years and cirrhosis after about four years.
After six years severe liver disease would be a significant clinical problem.
During the period from six to 34 years the number of men alive with
cirrhosis would vary up to a maximum of 38 at 30 years. After 34 years 79
men would have died from cirrhosis and 21 would still be alive with the
disease.

We are unable to speculate in a similar way with women. However, it is
clear that they drink a smaller amount for a shorter period and end up with a
higher incidence of cirrhosis. For example, Wilkinson et al. (5) found an
incidence of cirrhosis of 8.1% in men and 16.8% in women. They also found
that alcoholic women with cirrhosis had consumed less for a shorter period

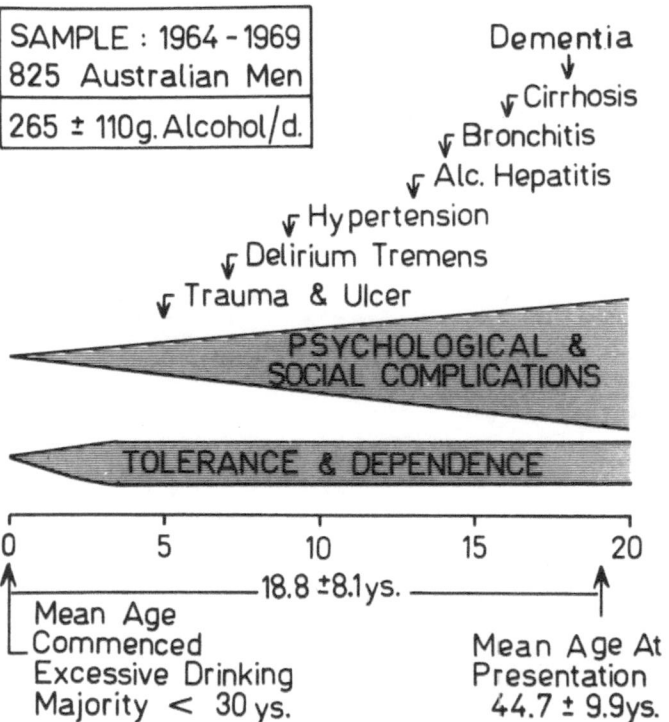

Fig. 4   *Drinking history and development of tolerance, dependence and psychological, social and physical complications in 825 Australian alcoholic men.*

than men.   Although alcoholic women appear to develop cirrhosis more readily than men, Powell and Klatskin found no sex difference in mortality from this disease (4).

Natural History of Alcoholism

The pattern of information presented in this section is derived from Australian alcoholics (6).   However, it resembles data obtained in Canada (7,8) and would probably be representative of general patterns in North America, Western Europe (excluding major wine consuming countries) and New Zealand during the same period.

Figure 4 is a composite of information from 825 Australian alcoholic men who had a mean daily ethanol intake at presentation of 265 g.   Most of

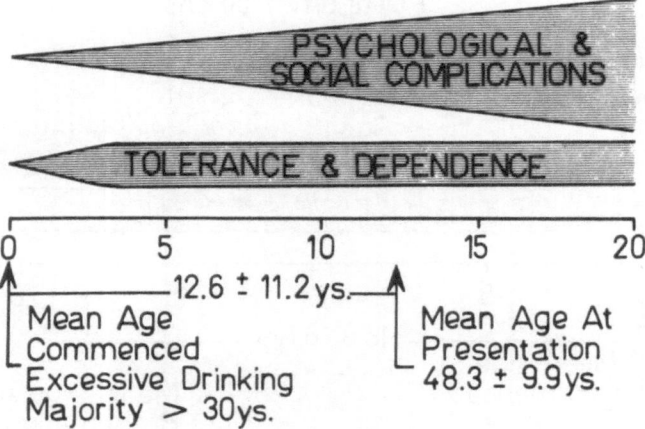

SAMPLE : 1964 - 1969
175 Australian Women
170 ± 65g. Alcohol Day

PHYSICAL DISEASES : Similar Pattern
to Men, Accelerated Course.

PSYCHOLOGICAL &
SOCIAL COMPLICATIONS

TOLERANCE & DEPENDENCE

0   5   10   15   20

————12.6 ± 11.2 ys.————

Mean Age   Mean Age At
Commenced   Presentation
Excessive Drinking   48.3 ± 9.9 ys.
Majority > 30 ys.

Fig. 5   *Drinking history and development of tolerance, dependence and
psychological, social and physical complications in 175
Australian alcoholic women.*

these men had commenced drinking excessively[2] before the age of 30 years,
their mean period of hazardous drinking was 19 years and they presented at
a mean age of 44.7 years. Schematically represented is the development of
tolerance, dependence, and psychological and social complications, and the
age at which the first quartile presented with various physical complications. It can be seen that cirrhosis of the liver was a late complication and
that affected individuals might have been expected to have presented for
medical, social and psychological care numerous times and for many years
before they finally presented with cirrhosis.

Similar information from women is presented in Figure 5. In the case of
women the mean alcohol consumption was 170 g., most commenced drinking
excessively after the age of 30, their mean duration of excessive drinking
before presentation being 12.6 years and age at presentation 48 years.

---

[2]"Excessive" in this study was defined as equal to or more than 100 g. per
day.

Although the pattern of physical diseases was similar to that for men the developmental course in women was accelerated.

General Conclusions Concerning Alcoholic Liver Disease

If the occurrence of alcoholic liver disease is dependent upon daily intake, duration of drinking and individual susceptibility, then several things are apparent:

- Because of the wide variations both in level of consumption and duration of drinking, the risk of developing liver disease varies greatly but is higher the greater the cumulative consumption. Conversely, individual susceptibility to alcohol as an aetiological factor becomes progressively less important as the total consumption increases.

- Alcoholic populations do not drink at high enough levels for long enough periods to achieve the very high incidences of cirrhosis that are theoretically possible. They presumably either die from causes other than liver disease, their alcoholic behaviour remits spontaneously or they respond to treatment.

- Marked fluctuations in total individual consumption readily explain the common occurrence of reversible forms of alcoholic liver disease and the wide variations in the incidence of cirrhosis observed in different alcoholic populations.

MANAGEMENT AND PROGNOSIS OF THE ALCOHOLIC PATIENT WITH LIVER DISEASE

Symptomatic Liver Disease

When the alcoholic patient presents with symptomatic liver disease there are several immediate general problems: the difficulty of establishing an accurate diagnosis on clinical and laboratory grounds alone, the relatively high mortality during the first year after diagnosis in this group and the realization that, in patients presenting for treatment the first time, their ultimate behaviour with alcohol is largely unpredictable.

Although certain patient characteristics provide some guide as to whether or not a patient will recover from his alcoholic liver disease, and beyond that achieve abstinence and the possibility of a life not too shortened by disease, all of this information is of little value in treating the individual patient. Therefore, all efforts should be made to assist each individual to recover from his first clinical episode of liver disease and at the same time to alter his behaviour with alcohol. However, it is usually found that those patients who present with a second or subsequent episode of alcoholic liver disease, and who have not responded to previous attempts to alter their drinking behaviour, usually continue drinking despite all therapeutic efforts.

The cirrhotic patients with jaundice, ascites and/or severe gastrointestinal haemorrhage who were reported by Powell and Klatskin had a mortality rate, during the first year, of approximately 22% whether or not they abstained from alcohol (4). This is a period when progressive hepatic decompensation may be anticipated and continues even after the patient's admission to hospital and withdrawal from alcohol. The benefits of abstinence in patients with symptomatic liver disease are only apparent in those who survive beyond the first year.

Asymptomatic Liver Disease

Knowledge that the patient has subclinical hepatic disease may help the physician in his therapeutic plans concerning both the behaviour with alcohol as well as its physical consequences. It can be argued that in the absence of clinical features, a biopsy-confirmed diagnosis of subclinical alcoholic liver disease by the physician will have little influence on the patient's behaviour with alcohol. On the other hand, knowledge that he has asymptomatic liver disease may help the patient decide that there are serious enough reasons to stop drinking. Certainly it is one piece of potentially available information which the affected individual can consider when deciding whether the adverse consequences outweigh apparent benefits of continued alcohol use.

If a diagnosis of subclinical alcoholic hepatic disease is not confirmed by biopsy evidence then medical mismanagement may occur. It is certainly true that grave prognostications, based on incorrect diagnoses of severe liver disease not backed by histological proof, have frequently gone awry. We probably all can recall the patient who said something like "my doctor warned me ten years ago that I had cirrhosis and that I would die soon if I did not stop drinking. Well I am still alive and still drinking."

Specific Diagnostic Approaches

Percutaneous Liver Biopsy: Because of the significant incidence of severe alcoholic liver disease and our inability clinically to differentiate between patients with cirrhosis, alcoholic hepatitis and fatty liver (9), it is recommended that percutaneous liver biopsy be included in the medical assessment of men and women whose hazardous drinking has lasted more than 10 and five years respectively.

Drinking History: Although comments are frequently made about the unreliability of drinking histories obtained from alcoholics, I have not found them, as a group, to be any less reliable in this regard than other patients. It is usually possible to determine whether or not and when the individual's

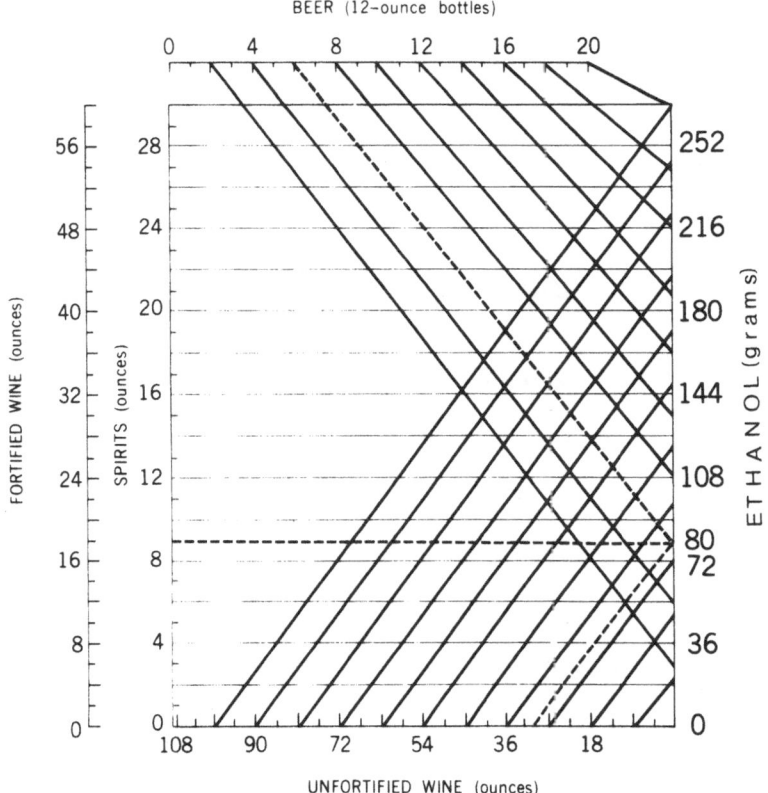

Fig. 6   *Alcoholic beverage conversion nomogram, calculated on the basis of beer, 5% v/v; wine, 12.0% v/v; fortified wine (e.g. sherry), 20% v/v; and spirits, 40% v/v ethanol. Specific gravity of ethanol, 0.78 g./ml.; 1 oz. = 28.5 ml. Dashed lines indicate approximate level of hazardous daily intake (30 oz. of wine, 9 oz. of spirits, 18 oz. of fortified wine or 6 bottles of beer).*

pattern of drinking became hazardous, as well as their pattern of consumption over the last year. The drinking history can usually be cross-checked with family members and others. This information enables us to make some estimate of the cumulative alcohol intake and of the approximate risks of severe alcoholic liver disease and cirrhosis. If we are concerned with the early diagnosis of problems of alcohol use then we should also enquire about alcohol consumption in all patients under our care and in particular those who present with illnesses or other problems commonly associated with hazardous alcohol consumption. Calculations of alcohol intake can be facilitated by the use of nomograms (Figure 6) (10).

TABLE I

PROGNOSTIC FEATURES IN ALCOHOLISM

FEATURE	GOOD PROGNOSIS	POOR PROGNOSIS
SOCIAL STABILITY - MARRIAGE - LIVING ARRANGEMENTS - OCCUPATION	+	-
HIGH SOCIOECONOMIC STATUS	+	-
SOCIOPATHY	-	+
"LAW BREAKING"	-	+
PSYCHOSIS	-	+
BRAIN DAMAGE	-	+
PERSISTENT AETIOLOGICAL FACTOR - HOME - OTHER	-	+
"MOTIVATION"	+	-

+ = FEATURE PRESENT   - = FEATURE ABSENT

Prognosis of Alcoholism (Table I)

After the onset of a hazardous pattern of alcohol consumption it is possible that one may observe in each individual several possible outcomes: continual progression of the drinking behaviour, death from one of the many diseases related to alcohol consumption, spontaneous remission or remission as an apparent result of treatment. Before the age of 60 years the mortality rate of alcoholic individuals is twice that of nonalcoholics, with the majority of deaths occurring between 40 and 60 years (11). Of those patients seeking treatment for their drinking problem, improvement has been found in 32 to 68% of those with favourable prognostic features and in 0 to 18% with unfavourable features (12). Observations by Drew suggest that there must also be significant spontaneous remissions in the drinking behaviour of alcoholic men after the age of 40 (13). It is at this age that the observed prevalence of alcoholism begins to fall well below the expected prevalence, the large difference not being explicable by death or successful treatment.

A favourable prognosis correlates with social stability and high socioeconomic status and an unfavourable one with social instability, psychopathy, psychosis and brain damage. The presence and persistence of aetiological or aggravating factors, in the home or other environment, are also important prognostically, e.g.:

- The presence of others in the home with drinking problems, particularly spouses. In the case of alcoholic married women approximately 50% have husbands who drink hazardously.

- The presence of conflicts between husbands and wives which either precipitate or contribute to the drinking behaviour.

- Engagement in an occupation associated with easy availability and/or high use of alcohol.

One-third of the cirrhotic patients reported by Powell and Klatskin stopped drinking (4). Presumably the percentage of those achieving abstinence would have been much higher if the skid-row and brain damaged members of the group, that is those with little if any chance of achieving prolonged abstinence, had been excluded. In another study of cirrhotic patients by Rankin et al. it was found that 10 of 21 with features suggesting a favourable prognosis stopped drinking, compared with only 4 of 36 where the prognostic features suggested an unfavourable outcome (16).

HOW CAN ALCOHOLIC LIVER DISEASE BE PREVENTED OR MORE EFFECTIVELY TREATED?

In the case of alcoholic liver disease we are confronted with a problem common to medicine generally and that is the degree to which we are able to translate available medical and other knowledge into effective health care resources that are available to the population in need at some reasonable cost. Therefore, some of the deficiencies that are apparent in relation to health care of the patient with alcoholic liver disease are generic to problems of health care generally, but, in addition, are aggravated by factors specifically related to problems of health when they occur in an alcoholic population.

How many physicians endeavour to help the alcoholic patient understand that his physical disease is linked to alcohol intake and try to help him abstain or modify his behaviour with alcohol? There is a marked tendency amongst physicians and other health care personnel to generalize when it comes to alcoholic patients, particularly about the likelihood that they will stop drinking. Such "therapists" are quite likely to exhibit intolerance, frustration or despair toward their alcoholic patients who are not helped and possibly hindered by such emotions, attitudes and related behaviour. The physician's professional vision and perspectives also may be so distorted or obscured by his attitudes and emotions that he is unable to make clinically obvious diagnoses either of drinking problems or of alcohol-related illnesses.

Recommendations

Improvement in Medical Education: A stage has been reached where physicians clearly acknowledge that alcoholism is a common and important medical as well as psychosocial problem and, therefore, that physicians should play a major role in relation to both diagnosis and care of patients with this disorder.   Numerous statements have been issued by medical organizations, calling attention to the fact that alcoholism is a disease and should be accorded appropriate treatment.   Despite all these statements, there is little practical evidence that practising physicians are any more interested in problems of alcoholism.   Meanwhile many students are entering medical schools with an interest in problems of alcohol use, as they have in other areas, where there is a clear relationship between physical illness, behaviour and the environment.   Unfortunately these interests are neither being met nor fostered in most medical schools.   The lack of any real improvement in the medical care for individuals with alcohol problems can be attributed in large part to the failure to develop significant programs on this subject in undergraduate and postgraduate medical programs both in North America and elsewhere.   This failure rests as much with those in charge of policy as it does with teachers.   If all medical schools provided an appropriate curriculum on problems of alcohol use, it seems likely that this would be reflected in major improvements in the attitudes and behaviour to, and care of alcoholic patients by physicians.

Early Recognition and Attempts at Intervention in Hazardous Drinking, Alcoholism and Alcoholic Liver Disease: A reduction in hepatic problems of alcohol use, as with other medical complications, is dependent not only on early diagnosis and effective treatment of the behaviour with alcohol, but also its disease complications.   Recurrently within the community, individuals with alcohol problems are presenting in large numbers to physicians who either are unable to recognize the problem or who are not prepared to deal with the behaviour associated with alcohol use or its complications.   The major locations where alcoholics tend to present with problems are general practice, hospitals and industry.

Development and Availability of Therapeutic Resources: Although a great deal is known about the ways in which therapeutic resources can be set up in existing clinical settings to provide care for alcohol-damaged individuals, these resources are not generally available.   It is important that physicians ask themselves questions, such as: "What do I do if I have an alcoholic patient?" "What does my department or clinic do if it has alcoholic patients who present with various medical problems of alcohol use?" "Why are clinics not available for the care of alcoholic patients within the framework of general hospitals?"   This last question is particularly important when we think of the wide range of specialized clinics which are common in hospital practice.   Not only must the verbal commitment of physicians in this field be reflected by improvements in medical education, they must also accept the responsibility for ensuring that appropriate care is available within existing therapeutic settings.   Such resources often can be developed by redeployment of resources rather than expansion.

Interdisciplinary Cooperation: This last recommendation addresses the problem of the continued general isolation from one another of those therapists who are concerned with the physical health and those who are concerned with the social-behavioural consequences of alcohol use. The need for effective cooperation is obvious.

CONCLUSION

At the time when I was visiting the patient in King's Cross, preventive and social medicine was still mainly concerned, in Australia, with infectious diseases, sanitation and gross forms of industrial pollution. In the 1970s it has become clear that further improvement in health and reductions in morbidity and premature death will require more and more change in the behaviour of nations, governments, industries, corporations and individuals. The maintenance of a healthy lifestyle is more than just an individual concern or responsibility. In the case of alcoholic liver disease we have an important problem resulting largely from lifestyle. In Canada, alcoholic cirrhosis is now the fifth major cause of death for men in the productive years from 25 to 64. This disease is increasing in incidence and mortality so that by the early 1990s it could reach a level of 40/100,000 i.e. similar to France. Efforts to prevent these high levels being reached provide an excellent test of our ability and commitment to preventive and social medicine. Meanwhile the alcoholic patient with liver disease is a test of our ability and commitment to apply the knowledge we have in an effective fashion to ensure adequate patient care.

ACKNOWLEDGEMENTS

Permission is gratefully acknowledged to Dr. E. M. Sellers and the Editor of the Canadian Medical Association Journal for permission to reproduce Figure 6.

REFERENCES

1. PÉQUIGNOT G: Enquête par interrogatoire sur les circonstances diététiques de la cirrhose alcoolique en France. Bull Inst National Hygiene 13: 719-939, 1958

2. PÉQUIGNOT G, CHABERT C, EYDOUX H, COURCOUL MA: Increased risk of liver cirrhosis with intake of alcohol. Rev Alcohol 20: 191-202, 1974

3. LELBACH WK: Cirrhosis in the alcoholic and its relation to the volume of alcohol abuse. Ann NY Acad Sci 252: 85-105, 1975

4. POWELL WJ, KLATSKIN G: Duration of survival in patients with Laennec's cirrhosis. Influence of alcohol withdrawal, and possible effects of recent changes in general management of the disease. Am J Med 44: 406-420, 1968

5. WILKINSON P, SANTAMARIA JN, RANKIN JG: Epidemiology of alcoholic cirrhosis. Aust Ann Med 18: 222-226, 1969

6. WILKINSON P, KORNACZEWSKI A, RANKIN JG, SANTAMARIA JN: Physical disease in alcoholism. Initial survey of 1,000 patients. Med J Aust 1: 1217-1223, 1971

7. ASHLEY MJ, OLIN JS, LE RICHE WH, KORNACZEWSKI A, SCHMIDT W, RANKIN JG: A sociomedical profile of alcoholism. I. Demographic, sociological and drinking characteristics of 1001 alcoholics. Submitted for publication.

8. ASHLEY MJ, OLIN JS, LE RICHE WH, KORNACZEWSKI A, SCHMIDT W, COREY PN, RANKIN JG: A sociomedical profile of alcoholism. II. The physical disease characteristics of 1001 alcoholics. Submitted for publication.

9. RANKIN JG, ORREGO H, MEDLINE A, DESCHENES J, FINDLAY J, ARMSTRONG A: Diagnostic problems in alcoholic liver disease. Submitted for publication.

10. SELLERS EM: Alcohol consumption nomogram. Can Med Assoc J 114: 109-110, 1976

11. DE LINDT J, SCHMIDT W. Mortality from liver cirrhosis and other causes in alcoholics. A follow-up study of patients with and without a history of enlarged fatty liver. Quart J Stud Alc 31: 705-709, 1970

12. BAEKELAND F, LUNDWELL L, KISSIN B: Methods for the Treatment of Chronic Alcoholism: A Critical Appraisal. In Research Advances in Alcohol and Drug Problems Vol 2. R Gibbins, Y Israel, H Kalant, R Popham, W Schmidt, R Smart (eds.). John Wiley and Sons, N.Y., 1975. pp. 247-327

13. DREW LR: Alcoholism as a self-limiting disease. Quart J Stud Alc 29: 956-967, 1968

14. RANKIN JG, WILKINSON P, SANTAMARIA JN: Factors influencing the prognosis of the alcoholic patient with cirrhosis. Aust Ann Med 3: 232-239, 1970

15. SCHMIDT W: The epidemiology of cirrhosis of the liver: A statistical analysis of mortality data with special reference to Canada. In Alcohol and the Liver. JG Rankin, MM Fisher (eds.). Plenum, New York, 1977

16. RANKIN JG, WILKINSON P, SANTAMARIA JN: Factors influencing the prognosis of the alcoholic patient with cirrhosis. Aust Ann Med 3: 232-239, 1970

DISCUSSION

CHAIRMAN: J.G. JOLY

TAMBURRO: We must consider what we are seeing in medical practice. A great number of people have already been lost by the time that they actually get to the hospital or to the doctor. You are absolutely right when you say there is going to have to be a more aggressive approach to the education of those who may get into trouble with alcohol before they reach the age of 25 years. Alcohol consumption in the state of Kentucky is increasing rapidly among the young and it isn't going to change. One should consider that if alcohol was being presented for the first time to the Federal Food and Drug Agency in the United States or to the National Institute of Health and Safety, both agencies would exclude its being used. However, since alcohol was with us before these agencies recommended against it, one should really consider two possibilities: first, having a progressive reduction in the alcohol content of beverages, maybe over a period of the next decade, and secondly, letting the price increase as some people have already suggested. The question is, do you think this is feasible, in two countries like our own in which freedom is such an important thing?

RANKIN: I don't know the answer. However, if we don't keep on raising the issue and re-examining its feasibility then it certainly will never be feasible. I would like to be slightly optimistic on the one hand, but also slightly pessimistic. The reason is because I've lived in Canada just over six years, and I have watched the various educational techniques used to try and persuade the population to wear seat belts. Even if you take something with a clear, beneficial effect, such as seat belt legislation, people will still argue about the hazards of the legislation. There is no doubt that behaviour modification through legislation is an extremely sensitive area. My general view, and that of the Addiction Research Foundation, is that education may not change people's alcohol use, but it may change how people view alcohol and what they are prepared to accept in legislative controls. Surveys were conducted just over a year ago in this Province concerning alcohol control measures. It was interesting that the majority of people who replied in that study were in favour of various forms of control. In summary if you raise the level of community appreciation of the problems of alcohol use, and have enough agitation and concern in the community for change, then control legislation is possible. In this province there has been a lot of controversy over the last six months about the possibility of raising the legal drinking age from 18 to 19.

FISHER: Could we make this a reportable disease? When patients get gonorrhea we rip through their private lives to identify other sources of the problem. Often when one admits a patient to hospital with cirrhosis and then ends up talking to the spouse, one wonders why the spouse isn't in the next bed. It runs in families. Many marriages drink together to stay together. Could this be a reportable disease?

RANKIN: I suppose one could make alcoholism a reportable disease but I wonder to what end. I suggest that it is far more important that physicians recognize alcohol-related problems when they exist, advise their patients accordingly, and actively assist them in seeking help to resolve these problems.

MOORE: I would like to make a comment on Dr. Fisher's remark and question. Don't you think that it would penalize the patient to report on the chart that the patient is suffering from alcoholism? It often happens that pension and invalid plans are cancelled if the word alcoholism appears on the chart. We are often stuck with reporting false information really in order to protect the patient.

RANKIN: Yes, the patient might be penalized under the present rules. It seems there is a need to change the rules of some pension and sickness plans.

MOORE: How could we improve the Canadian scene with regard to using the diagnosis of alcoholism?

RANKIN: I think a large part of the problem is that the word "alcoholism" is like "venereal disease"; it got a bad name a long time ago. I'm not certain it would help to change the name now. Given the right circumstances, the right environment and other appropriate cues, probably anybody in this room might develop an alcohol problem. I think that one should keep on using the diagnosis alcoholism, but reinforce what the diagnosis really means today, and not what it meant 20 years ago.

SANDERS: I wanted to ask if the use of Antabuse is contraindicated in patients with acute alcoholic hepatitis or established cirrhosis. I would like to comment that I've had a number of patients tell me that they have taken 500 mg a day of Antabuse, coupled with a good slug of alcohol, and have had absolutely no reaction whatsoever. Have you found this to be a common or uncommon observation?

RANKIN: Antabuse, or disulfiram, is a drug that we don't commonly use in our hospital. If one looks at the available research information on efficacy in terms of changing behaviour, there is no evidence that the drug improves the rehabilitation rate. For those people that take Antabuse consistently and do well, the taking of Antabuse is a mark of their commitment to wanting to do something about their drinking. One thing that has concerned us over the last year have been comments in the United States and Canada that Antabuse may not be quite as safe as it was thought to be. Certainly it is said to be contraindicated in the presence of liver disease. I think that it is contraindicated in clinically manifest alcoholic hepatitis.

FOX: The Chairman's comments on the social stigma of the term alcoholism reminded me of the data that Dr. Schmidt presented from the U.K. The information from the U.K. should be interpreted with caution because we were warned as interns that if a patient died from cirrhosis we should put down very carefully a non-alcoholic etiology. If one used the term alcoholic, or left the term cirrhosis open, that automatically implied a coroner's inquest. Therefore I think that a lot of the statistical data from the U.K. are questionable.

Have there been any prospective studies on high risk occupations comparing those who do not become alcoholic to those who do? In other words, what stops people from becoming alcoholic?

RANKIN: We certainly can identify some high risk populations but I am not aware of any studies that identified which individual becomes an alcoholic and which one does not in a particular population.

SUMMARY OF THE SYMPOSIUM AND A LOOK AHEAD

Hans Popper

The Stratton Laboratory for the Study of Liver Diseases
Mount Sinai School of Medicine of the City University of
New York, New York, New York

In summarizing this conference on the hepatic effects of alcohol, it is my duty to integrate the past achievements with the new data presented here and to look into the future. In a recent article on futurism in Time magazine I read that "prophecy is the art of selling one's credibility for future delivery." I wonder whether my look into the cloudy crystal ball will enhance my credibility.

The conference we are now closing had several aims. It should benefit the patient. Government officials, increasingly controlling the practice of medicine, hopefully will listen. It should provide new knowledge for physicians and stimulate hepatologists in their research. It should maintain friendship and communication among scientists, since alcohol, and the research on it, is an excellent vehicle with which to travel to conferences in the most beautiful places of this world.

Canada has a specific role. First, alcohol abuse is rampant here. Secondly, excellent research on all its aspects is conducted here in the medical school and particularly in the Addiction Research Foundation. Thirdly, the Canadian Hepatic Foundation is unique; it is the most successful voluntary health agency concerned with problems of the liver anywhere. This Foundation brought us here together, and we want to express our appreciation to its officers and directors.

As the liver injury caused by alcohol abuse is the main concern of this symposium, we might briefly dwell on the history of hepatology (1), a discipline which was organized only in the last 25 years. It developed by the confluence of three main currents of biomedical activity. One was the study of the biology of the liver, emphasized in the Anglo-American, Germanic and Scandinavian countries. The second was the preoccupation with liver disease in the Latin countries, where, already learned from Moliere, many subjective symptoms were explained by a "sick liver". The third current was the concern in developing countries with hepatic cancer, schistosomiasis and cirrhosis, diseases which represent health hazards for young people and are indeed an urgent public health problem. Improved global communications after World War II led to a unified hepatology which was fertilized by four areas of medical endeavors, each surfacing with increasing urgency. One was epidemiology; the second, environmental medicine - important since the liver is not only a target, but also a key organ in the handling of drugs and other enviromental chemical agents. The third was the appreciation of the social aspects of liver diseases, including the role of malnutrition and the greater susceptibility of the poor. The fourth area was the reciprocal relation between liver and brain, including the psychologic aspects of liver disease. Alcoholic liver injury represents the prototype of a disease in which biological, clinical, epidemiologic, sociologic and psychologic factors converge.

The main unresolved problem in liver disease is first and foremost our ignorance about the mechanism of necrosis of the hepatocyte. This explains the absence of a causal therapy of liver cell injury. We do not know how to protect the cell from degeneration and death or how to stimulate regeneration of sick or surviving cells. The second problem is the mechanism of chronicity. Immunologic initiation and perpetuation of alcoholic or other chronic liver diseases is a challenging question, whether one invokes humoral antibodies or immunologically active cells. Another immunologic question is the nature of the target antigen, whether it is a normal, possibly exposed, component of the cell membrane, or a neoantigen. The fate of fibrosis, its stimulation, development and turnover enters into the question of chronicity and we should also point to the role of the macrophages which are conventionally considered scavengers, but which are also important in processing factors influencing immunologic and fibro-blastic reactions. The third problem is the symptomatic management of developed alcoholic liver disease, the role of the shunt operations and of diuretics, the treatment of bleeding varices, and hepatic transplantation. The fourth problem, important in all chronic liver diseases, including the alcoholic variety, is hepatocellular cancer, which was not emphasized at this symposium although the number of these cancers in alcoholics is increasing (2,3). The fifth problem, specific to alcoholic liver injury, is prevention, when social and psychologic modalities are being stressed. Their limited effect indeed is the reason why we met here.

Reviewing the discussions of this conference, the epidemiology was well put into focus, and Canadian researchers deserve great credit for applying the ratio of death rate from cirrhosis to alcohol consumption. One should emphasize the time lag between initiation of alcohol abuse and death, which may explain some minor discrepancies in an excellent presentation. One should also consider other causes of cirrhosis, particularly the recent increase of the one produced by hepatitis, where the hepatitis-associated antigen provides now a diagnostic tool, and the recently more important role of drugs.

   This may be the time to submit the thought that the pattern of alcohol intake in a nation reflects its life style.   Let us not forget that the cultivation of grapes was one of the earliest attempts of agriculture.   Wine made from grapes is one of the oldest horticultural achievements of mankind, already ancient when the Greeks drank their wine.   In our society, alcoholism reflects our freedom, our permissiveness and also our frustration. It is also found in socialized countries like Sweden and is rampant in the Soviet Union.   Its absence in China and in the major parts of the populations of the developing countries might suggest that a complete change of the distribution of wealth in this world might wipe out the use of the grapes in producing alcoholic liver injury, though I have little confidence that this will happen.   Nevertheless, a study of alcoholic liver injury may be a valuable tool in global sociology.

   In our Western countries, alcoholism is prominent in the economically less favored segment of an affluent society, with the possible exception of Portugal and Austria, where the poor wine producer has access to cheap but highly intoxicating byproducts.   To report a personal experience, between 1938 and 1946 I was the pathologist of Cook County Hospital in Chicago, a very large city hospital.   It has an extensive alcoholic clientele in which blacks were then barely represented.   One of my coworkers reviewed the extensive autopsy material of cirrhosis and emphasized in a Master's thesis the lack of black patients.   We assumed a genetic protection of the black population against alcoholism.   What we overlooked was that the protection was financial in that the blacks in the slums of Chicago were too poor to buy alcoholic beverages.   Recently, the increase of alcoholic liver injury in the United States was greater in blacks than in whites, and the highest increase was in black women, as reported in a study from Baltimore (4).   Thus, women were protected from alcoholic liver injury by a cultural barrier, rather than a genetic one; there is good statistical evidence that women are more susceptible to cirrhosis than men.   The data of Pequignot (5) indicate that the threshold of danger is low in female drinkers (20 grams ethanol per day, in contrast to 60 grams for males).   Our present social upheaval is reflected, at least in the United States, by a diminishing preponderance of alcoholic liver injury in the lower socio-economic groups.   Executives and their wives, and also Jews, are now more often victims of this disease than in the past. The previous belief that alcoholic liver injury is associated with social malfunction, exemplified by members of skid row, is rapidly fading.   We find it not necessarily associated with asocial behaviour, with absenteeism, or with a police record.   Particularly the gastroenterologist observes alcoholic hepatitis in socially well functioning persons of all strata of society, of both sexes, without evidence of nutritional disturbance.   The rapid change of the patterns of our social habits calls for a high index of suspicion of alcoholic liver injury, often confirmed only by liver biopsy, despite denial by the patient and even his family.

   A question not fully settled is genetic protection.   Epidemiologic statistical data accumulated by Lelbach (6) and Péquignot (5) as well as in Chile, show that anybody drinking a given amount of alcohol (between 60 and 80 grams per day) for a given period of time is at risk to develop cirrhosis and that this risk is considerably greater, almost a certainty, if the alcohol consumption exceeds 160 grams per day. However, the pattern and duration of alcohol intake vary. There are many definitions of a safe amount; I tell my students that the amount of alcohol which I drink is safe and it varies from day to day. But, to be serious, only 30 percent of proven alcoholics develop cirrhosis. I would be surprised if there were not genetic differences, since ethanol requires metabolic transformation to become injurious, and I do not know of any metabolic reaction which is not subject to genetic influences, hormonal or otherwise expressed. It is thus probably best to assume a genetic protection which is broken through in anyone if alcohol intake is excessively high.

What have we learned about the responsible agent in alcoholic liver injury? If we ignore congeners (7) as responsible for liver injury, the enemy can be of two types, a metabolic alteration or a topical toxin. Metabolically the main factor is the increased NADH and the limitation of its reoxidation. The augmented reduced state is incriminated in many effects, e.g. in the altered lactate/pyruvate ratio. Moreover, alcohol provides empty calories entailing wastage of energy. The topical effect may be exerted by ethanol or acetaldehyde or, probably less so, by acetate. This effect not only accounts for alterations of organelles like mitochondria, but acetaldehyde may also be involved in the immunologic injury.

What is the mechanism by which the enemy acts? Some effects are primary or direct, and others are secondary. Among the primary effects, one can list 1) respiratory inhibition with loss of ATP, 2) protein disaggregation within the hepatocytes, 3) the peroxidation by free radicals, the "lighting up" of the liver; this may be a link between ethanol and carcinogenesis, similar to the processes induced by many environmental factors, 4) the already mentioned wastage of energy; excess heat is produced both by nutritionally useless calories and by activity of the microsomal ethanol oxidizing system, both resulting in a faulty body economy, 5) the hypermetabolic state with relative oxygen deficiency on the periphery of the acinus (or center of the lobule) favoring necrotizing lesions in this location, 6) cell membrane alterations with effects on the receptors localized there, 7) alterations of the cytoskeleton consisting of contractile microfilaments of actin-myosin nature and rigid microtubules of tubulin character. The retention of proteins secreted by the hepatocyte, even in excess of triglycerides, as result of tubulin alterations and the recognition that alcoholic hyalin represents a lesion of the tubulin system are two important observations presented here. These changes may indeed not only explain the degenerative features of the cell, but may eventually be recognized as a main factor in cell necrosis. Dr. Farber is studying the latter, with emphasis on the disturbance of cellular calcium metabolism (8).

The most important secondary effects, often multifactorial, are as follows:

1) Steatosis is the hallmark of the initial alcoholic liver injury. Its pathogenesis has been appreciated for many years. Besides from increased

transport of triglycerides to the liver and their excess synthesis, it also results from a failure of fatty acid oxidation and secretion, and these last two phenomena reinforce each other in a vicious cycle.

2) Secondary metabolic alterations include hyperlipidemia reflecting increased lipoprotein secretion, ketoacidosis removing fat by ketone body formation, depressed gluconeogenesis and hyperuricemia.

3) The action of drugs is accentuated or inhibited, this depending upon either blockade or induction of the microsomal biotransformation system. This is not only important in drug therapy of alcoholics but may also influence the effect of illicit or addictive drugs; alcoholism is now widespread in the addict population of the United States. Moreover, the action of environmental chemical agents may be altered in alcoholics and toxicity of carbon tetrachloride is increased as we heard.

4) Nutritional disturbance results not only from faulty body economy but also from selectively impaired intestinal absorption. The malnutrition is more often reflected in obesity than in weight loss. Different responses to alcohol of starved and fed animals have been reported here.

5) The alteration of the immune status in alcoholics has several components. The hypergammaglobulinemia is caused, as in other chronic liver diseases, by a response of the lymphoid system to mainly intestinal antigens, bacterial in nature, or to endotoxins which are not taken up by the liver either because of reduced activity of the Kupffer cells or because of the bypass of blood from the parenchyma (9). Endotoxinemia is now invoked in the mechanisms of many systemic manifestations (10). Bacteremia and infection are common in alcoholics. In addition we become inceasingly convinced of the significance of hepatic immune injury in alcoholics from circulating antibodies or from lymphoid cells. Their action is directed against hepatocellular membrane antigens or against neoantigens, altered proteins, like the hyalin of Mallory. The roles of these immune reactions in diagnosis and in perpetuation of alcoholic liver injury are at present unfolding. They also cause some morphologic features with similarity to chronic viral hepatitis. This explains a frequent differential diagnostic problem, clinical and histologic. Lymphokinins secreted by specifically stimulated lymphocytes induce fibroblastic activity (11).

6) The just mentioned observation introduces the fibrogenic effect of alcohol. The fibrotic reaction of alcoholic liver disease and other chronic liver disorders and is now emerging as a main problem in these diseases. (12) To what degree the excess fibrogenesis is the result of a direct effect of alcohol or is stimulated by liver cell injury remains to be established. Again we encounter a vicious circle in that fibrosis favors liver cell injury, which in turn accentuates fibrosis.

7) Hormonal disturbances are also induced by alcohol.

Studies of tissue reactions in alcoholic liver injury by the use of light microscopy, electron microscopy, histology and biochemistry aid our understanding of pathogenesis and are also the basis of differential diagnosis by liver biopsy. Multiple sites are involved in view of the complex action of ethanol. Some of the changes are the effect of injury, but most may be adaptive. The cell membrane with the cytoskeleton, the Golgi apparatus and the cytosol are all altered, as is the rough endoplasmic reticulum accounting for disturbance of protein synthesis. However, much of the interest centers on mitochondrial injury, structural and functional, as a primary event. The great number of mitochondria creates difficulties in the histological evaluation since characteristic alteration of some does not exclude integrity of many others. But a particular argument involves the smooth endoplasmic reticulum, which appears increased in amount, though morphometric methods have rendered controversial results (13). It is the site of the microsomal biotransformation system and its quantity and morphologic appearance may be misleading since a hypertrophic one may be hypoactive in one or several aspects (14). Because of multiple heme proteins in this system, the rise of some, like cytochrome P-450, need not involve others, like cytochrome P-448. The activity of benzpyrene hydroxylase, related to the latter, was found not to be increased and these cytochromes are the ones engaged in the metabolism of carcinogens. The hepatic effect of ethanol is not restricted to the hepatocytes, but involves also fibroblasts and their precursors, lipocytes (15), as well as blood flow.

As to experimental models, we heard about work on isolated cells, on the perfused liver, and most important, on whole animals, particularly primates. Studies on experimental cirrhosis (16) indicated that in general the animal liver exhibits reactions less active than the human in two aspects. One is fibroplasia. The normal rodent liver, for instance, has only one-third of the collagen content, expressed as hydroxyproline per unit weight, of the adult human liver and a fully developed rat cirrhosis has as much collagen per gram as the normal human liver (17). The second concerns the inflammatory reaction, which is far more conspicuous in man than in experimental animals, including primates. This might explain why in all experimental models I know of, withdrawal of the toxic agent arrests the process and causes recovery, in contrast to human experiences. To what degree this applies to alcohol-induced injury in experimental models and particularly primates, remains to be established.

The hepatic diseases induced by ethanol - steatosis, hepatitis, cirrhosis - have been so well discussed that little can be added here. Carcinoma, however, was barely mentioned. In the Western world its incidence seems to be the same in the alcoholic as in hepatitis B-associated or cryptogenic cirrhosis, in contrast to Africa, where carcinoma is far more frequent in the hepatitis B-associated form (18). Morphologically, two precursor stages are known. One is foci of dysplastic cells (19) with significant cytologic aberrations from the norm. This is particularly characteristic of the hepatitis B-associated form and the dysplastic cells are rich in the "s component" of hepatitis B antigen (20). Such dysplastic foci may also be found in the cirrhosis of the alcoholic, but there cancer seems to arise more frequently in the center of regenerative nodules in which accentuated hyperplasia develops in nodular form. This architectural alteration, "nodule in nodule" (21), supports Farber's concept (22) of hepatocarcinogenesis by consecutive development of different cell populations with increasing loss of dependence on regulation following an initial event altering DNA. This raises the question whether ethanol is a carcinogen for which there is little evidence so far available, except that free radicals alter DNA. The other possibility is that cirrhotic transformation by itself favors carcinoma formation via abnormal regeneration, or because of the action of ubiquitous carcinogens on the more susceptible cirrhotic liver.

The diagnosis of alcoholic liver injury remains a difficult problem in view of the unreliability of the histories obtainable. This also concerns recognition of alcohol intake of a supposedly reformed alcoholic. Many clinical tests have been recommended for this purpose (23) and the ratio of alpha-aminobutyric acid/leucine was mentioned at this symposium. The pathologic diagnosis by liver biopsy is still an important tool although we have become aware of several conditions which produce in supposedly nonalcoholics the same picture as in very active alcoholic hepatitis, the changes including typical Mallory bodies. One is the lesion following intestinal bypass operation for obesity (24), and the second is the so-called fatty-liver hepatitis in obese women, often with diabetes. In both these instances, however, the question of unconfessed alcohol intake can never be fully excluded and this points to the importance of biochemical parameters of alcohol intake which have just been stressed.

The discussion of therapy was rewarding. It dealt with three problems. The first, the prevention and correction of alcoholism by pharmaco- and psychotherapy was well presented. The second, the therapy of the liver injury, dealt with the suppression of the hypermetabolic stage, with the use of antioxidants, with antiinflammatory therapy, possibly immunosuppressive, by steroids and otherwise, and with antifibroblastic therapy, which still remains more an experimental than a clinical procedure, although successful trials with colchicine (26) and penicillamine (27) have been reported. However, the latter may indeed be more antiinflammatory than antifibroblastic. Penicillamine side effects include aplastic anemia and nephrosis. We may more readily take the risk of penicillamine in Wilson's disease than in chronic hepatitis. The third aspect of therapy is symptomatic and has been so well discussed already that I cannot improve on it.

Much was said at this conference about alcoholic liver injury, but we hepatologists also learned about liver disease in general. The alcoholic injury can be compared to an experiment, undesirable as it is. Here, human beings do to themselves what we do to experimental animals and thus permit us to dissect biological processes induced by a toxic agent. I refer for instance to the effect of arginine on the urea cycle and to the complex reaction of the polyamines. The three metabolic pathways of ethanol in the hepatocytes can also be recognized with other substances, like vinyl chloride, an industrial hazard which produces hepatic fibrosis and angiosarcoma (28). Small amounts of this substance are metabolized by alcohol dehydrogenase in the cytosol, larger ones by catalase in the peroxisomes, and excessive doses in the microsomal biotransformation system of the endoplasmic reticulum (29).

Much as we have been enlightened about alcohol and the liver, there remain urgent problems for the future to be resolved, hopefully, at least in part, when the Canadian Hepatic Foundation will again convene a symposium on alcoholic liver injury. The first challenge today is to develop better psycho-social methods to prevent alcoholism and to wean alcoholics from their addiction. In this regard the pioneering work in Canada will doubtlessly continue. Secondly, we should establish the biochemical basis of the addiction or dependence. Some progress has been made. The combined study of alcohol and drug addiction may help us also. Indeed, it might be useful to look at alcohol as a drug even if no receptors or enkephalins (30) in the brain exist as is the case with other addictive drugs. A third question relates to the genetic differences in the tolerance to alcohol and the identification of persons at greatest risk. Fourthly, the diagnosis of past and continued alcohol abuse requires improvement, with good leads already being available. Less promising today is the fifth problem, the causal therapy of the sick liver cell and its protection. Even less hopeful is the problem of carcinogenesis. Finally, it is our obligation to continue the excellent epidemiologic work presented at the opening session, to identify the size of the problem and the cost of alcoholism to society (31) of which the liver injury represents a significant part.

At the end it is my privilege to thank the organizers for such an instructive meeting and for providing us also with a social environment of gratifying ambiance made even more pleasant by the excellent drinks. These "spiritual offerings" remind us that we need not necessarily preach abstinence, but should hope for tolerance and moderation. Some years ago I closed a similar conference (32) with a comment that I would like to repeat; namely, we do not want so much to add years to life, but rather life to years.

REFERENCES

1.   POPPER H: Entwicklung und Gegenwart der Hepatologie.   Leber Magen Darm 5: 175-179, 1975

2.   MARTINI GA: The role of alcohol in the etiology of cancer of the liver.   In Proceedings of the Third International Symposium on Detection and Prevention of Cancer New York, 1976, in press. New York, Marcel Dekker, Inc.

3.   LEE F: Cirrhosis and hepatoma in alcoholics. Gut 7: 77-85, 1966

4.   KRAMER K, KULLER L, FISHER R: The increasing mortality attributed to cirrhosis and fatty liver in Baltimore (1957-1966). Ann Intern Med 69: 273-282, 1968

5. PEQUIGNOT G, CHABERT C, EYDOUX H, COURCOL MA: Increased risk of liver cirrhosis with intake of alcohol. Rev Alcohol 20: 191-202, 1974

6. LELBACH WK: Epidemiology of alcoholic liver disease. In Progress in Liver Diseases, Volume V. H. Popper and F. Schaffner (eds.). New York, Grune & Stratton, 1976. pp. 494-515

7. SEIGERS CP, STRUBELT O, BREINING H: The acute hepatotoxic activity of alcoholic beverages and some of their congeners in guinea pigs. Pharmacology 12: 296-302, 1974

8. FARBER JL, EL-MOFTY SK: The biochemical pathology of liver cell necrosis. Am J Pathol 81: 237-250, 1975

9. PRYTZ H, BJORNEBOE M, JOHANSEN TS, ORSKOV F: The influence of portosystemic shunt operation on immunoglobulins and Escherichia coli antibodies in patients with cirrhosis of the liver. Acta Med Scand 196: 109-112, 1974

10. NOLAN JP: The role of endotoxin in liver injury. Gastroenterology 69: 1346-1356, 1975

11. CHEN T, ZETTERMAN R, LEEVY CM: Sensitized lymphocytes and hepatic fibrogenesis. Gastroenterology 65: 532-533, 1973

12. POPPER H, UDENFRIEND S: Hepatic fibrosis - correlation of biochemical and morphologic investigations. Am J Med 49: 707-721, 1970

13. OUDEA MC, COLLETTE M, DEDIEU P, OUDEA P: Morphometric study of the ultrastructure of human alcoholic fatty liver. Biomed Express 19: 1455-1459, 1973

14. HUTTERER F, KLION FM, WENGRAF A, SCHAFFNER F, POPPER H: Hepatocellular adaptation and injury. Structural and biochemical changes following dieldrin and methyl butter yellow. Lab Invest 20: 455-464, 1969

15. KENT G, GAY S, INOUYE T, BAHU R, MINICK OT, POPPER H: Vitamin A-containing lipocytes and formation of type III collagen in liver injury. Proc Nat Acad Sci, in press

16. POPPER H: Experimentelle Leberzirrhose. In Verhandlungen der Deutschen Gesellschaft fuer innere Medizin, 82. Band in press. Munich, Verlag J.F. Bergmann

17. KENT G, FELS IG, DUBIN A, POPPER H: Collagen content based on hydroxyproline determinations in human and rat livers. Its relation to morphologically demonstrable reticulum and collagen fibers. Lab Invest 8: 48-56, 1959

18. BLUMBERG BS, LAROUZE B, LONDON WT, WERNER B, HESSER IE,
     MILLMAN I, SAIMOT G, PAYET M: The relation of infection
     with the hepatitis B agent to primary hepatic carcinoma. Am J
     Pathol 81: 669-682, 1975

19. ANTHONY PP, VOGEL GL, BARKER LF: Liver cell dysplasia: a
     premalignant condition. J Clin Pathol 26: 217-223, 1973

20. POPPER H: Cancer of the liver; an overview. In Proceedings of the
     Third International Symposium on Detection and Prevention of
     Cancer, New York, 1976, in press. New York, Marcel Dekker,
     Inc.

21. POPPER H, STERNBERG SS, OSER BL, OSER M: The carcinogenic
     effect of Aramite in rats. A study of hepatic nodules. Cancer
     13: 1035-1046, 1960

22. FARBER E: Pathogenesis of liver cancer. Arch Pathol 98: 145-148,
     1974

23. HAMLYN AN, BROWN AJ, SHERLOCK S, BARON DN: Casual blood-
     ethanol estimations in patients with chronic liver disease.
     Lancet 2: 345-347, 1975

24. PETERS RL, GAY S, REYNOLDS TB: Postjejunoileal-bypass hepatic
     disease. Its similarity to alcoholic hepatic disease. Am J Clin
     Pathol 63: 318-331, 1975

25. THALER H: Die Fettleber und ihre pathogenetische Beziehung zur
     Leberzirrhose. Virchows Arch Pathol Anat 335: 180-210, 1962

26. KERSHENOBICH D, URIBE M, SUAREZ GH, ROJKIND M: Treatment
     of   cirrhosis   with   colchicine: a   randomized   trial.
     Gastroenterology 70: A128, 1976

27. RESNICK RH, BOITNOTT J, IBER FL, MAKIPOUR I, CERDA JJ:
     Penicillamine therapy in acute alcoholic liver disease.   In
     Collagen Metabolism in the Liver. H. Popper, K. Becker (eds.).
     New York, Stratton Intercontinental Book Corporation, 1975. pp.
     207-242

28. THOMAS LB, POPPER H, BERK PD, SELIKOFF I, FALK H: Vinyl-
     chloride induced liver disease. From idiopathic portal hyper-
     tension (Banti's syndrome) to angiosarcomas. N Engl J Med 292:
     17-22, 1975

29. WATANABE PG, McGOWAN GR, GEHRING PJ: Fate of ^{14}C vinyl
     chloride after single oral administration in rats. Toxicol Appl
     Pharmacol 26: 339-352, 1976

30. IVERSEN L, DINGLEDINE R: Enkephalin: the latest instalment.
         Nature 262: 738-739, 1976

31. BERRY RE, JR: Estimating the economic costs of alcohol abuse. N
         Engl J Med 295: 620-621, 1976

32. POPPER H: Zusammenfassung und Schlusswort des Praesidenten. In
         Alkohol und Leber. Internationales Symposium 2.-4. Oktober
         1970 in Freiburg i.Br. W. Gerok, K. Sickinger and H.H.
         Hennekeuser (eds.). Stuttgart, F.K. Schattauer Verglag, 1971.
         pp. 559-562

CONTRIBUTORS

N. R. Di Luzio, Ph.D.,
Department of Physiology,
Tulane University School of Medicine,
New Orleans, Louisiana.

W. L. Dunn, M.D.,
Department of Pathology,
University of British Columbia,
Vancouver, British Columbia.

Murray M. Fisher, M.D.,
Departments of Medicine and Pathology,
University of Toronto,
Toronto, Ontario.

Roy A. Fox, M.D.,
Department of Medicine,
Dalhousie University,
Halifax, Nova Scotia.

S. W. French, M.D.,
Department of Pathology,
Veterans Administration Hospital,
Martinez, California.

Ellen R. Gordon, Ph.D.,
McGill University Medical Clinic
Montreal General Hospital,
Montreal, Quebec.

Y. Israel, Ph.D.,
Department of Pharmacology,
University of Toronto,
Toronto, Ontario.

Kurt J. Isselbacher, M.D.,
            Department of Medicine,
            Massachusetts General Hospital,
            Boston, Massachusetts.

Jean-Gil Joly, M.D.,
            Clinical Research Center,
            Hôpital Saint-Luc,
            Montreal, Quebec.

Harold Kalant, M.D.,
            Department of Pharmacology,
            University of Toronto,
            Toronto, Ontario.

J.M. Khanna, Ph.D.,
            Department of Pharmacology,
            University of Toronto,
            Toronto, Ontario.

Charles S. Lieber, M.D.,
            Section of Liver Disease & Nutrition,
            Veterans Administration Hospital,
            Bronx, New York.

K. Lindros, Ph.D.,
            Research Laboratories of the
                State Alcohol Monopoly,
            Helsinki, Finland.

Frank Lundquist, M.D.,
            Department of Biochemistry A,
            University of Copenhagen,
            Copenhagen, Denmark.

Shohei Matsuzaki, M.D.,
            Section of Liver Disease & Nutrition,
            Veterans Administration Hospital,
            Bronx, New York.

M. James Phillips, M.D.,
            Department of Pathology,
            University of Toronto,
            Toronto, Ontario.

Hans Popper, M.D.,
            Mount Sinai School of Medicine of the
            City University of New York,
            New York, New York.

James G. Rankin, M.B.,
  Addiction Research Foundation,
  Toronto, Ontario.

Marcus A. Rothschild, M.D.,
  Radioisotope Service,
  New York Veterans Administration Hospital,
  New York, New York.

Emanuel Rubin, M.D.,
  Department of Pathology,
  Mount Sinai School of Medicine of the
  City University of New York,
  New York, New York.

W. Schmidt, Dr. Jur., M.S.W.,
  Addiction Research Foundation,
  Toronto, Ontario.

INDEX